Lifestyle Modifications in Pharmacotherapy

Lifestyle Modifications in Pharmacotherapy

THOMAS L. LENZ

Wolters Kluwer Health | Lippincott Williams & Wilkins

Philadelphia · Baltimore · New York · London
Buenos Aires · Hong Kong · Sydney · Tokyo

Acquisitions Editor: David B. Troy
Managing Editor: Karen M. Ruppert
Marketing Manager: Marisa A. O'Brien
Production Editor: Paula C. Williams
Designer: Doug Smock
Compositor: Circle Graphics
Printer: Data Reproductions Corp.

9 8 7 6 5 4 3 2 1

Library of Congress Cataloging-in-Publication Data

Lenz, Thomas L., 1969-
  Lifestyle modifications in pharmacotherapy / Thomas L. Lenz.
      p. ; cm.
  Includes bibliographical references and index.
  ISBN-13: 978-0-7817-7651-6 (alk. paper)
  ISBN-10: 0-7817-7651-1 (alk. paper)
  1. Chronic diseases—Prevention. 2. Lifestyles—Health aspects. 3. Health behavior. 4. Pharmacists. I. Title.
  [DNLM: 1. Health Behavior. 2. Chronic Disease—prevention & control.
3. Life Style. 4. Patient Education. 5. Pharmacists. W 85 L575L 2008]
  RC108.L47 2008
  616'.044—dc22

                                        2007012529

DISCLAIMER

Care has been taken to confirm the accuracy of the information present and to describe generally accepted practices. However, the authors, editors, and publisher are not responsible for errors or omissions or for any consequences from application of the information in this book and make no warranty, expressed or implied, with respect to the currency, completeness, or accuracy of the contents of the publication. Application of this information in a particular situation remains the professional responsibility of the practitioner; the clinical treatments described and recommended may not be considered absolute and universal recommendations.

The authors, editors, and publisher have exerted every effort to ensure that drug selection and dosage set forth in this text are in accordance with the current recommendations and practice at the time of publication. However, in view of ongoing research, changes in government regulations, and the constant flow of information relating to drug therapy and drug reactions, the reader is urged to check the package insert for each drug for any change in indications and dosage and for added warnings and precautions. This is particularly important when the recommended agent is a new or infrequently employed drug.

Some drugs and medical devices presented in this publication have Food and Drug Administration (FDA) clearance for limited use in restricted research settings. It is the responsibility of the health care provider to ascertain the FDA status of each drug or device planned for use in their clinical practice.

To purchase additional copies of this book, call our customer service department at **(800) 638-3030** or fax orders to **(301) 223-2320**. International customers should call **(301) 223-2300**.

Visit Lippincott Williams & Wilkins on the Internet: http://www.lww.com. Lippincott Williams & Wilkins customer service representatives are available from 8:30 am to 6:00 pm, EST.

This book is dedicated to my wife Nancy
and our three children Kaelie, Abbey, and Jack.

Preface

Disease prevention is an area of pharmacy practice that is rich with opportunity. Pharmacists have long been recognized as highly trusted and accessible healthcare providers and because of this have the opportunity to impact patients' lives by not only treating diseases but also preventing them. *Lifestyle Modifications in Pharmacotherapy* is a textbook that was written for both the student pharmacist and the practicing pharmacist as a tool to offer the skills necessary to counsel patients with chronic diseases on strategies to either reduce their risks for certain diseases or more effectively manage existing disease. The overarching goals for this book are to:

- Fill a current gap in the education of student pharmacists in the area of disease prevention by discussing the lifestyle modification strategies of proper nutrition, physical activity, weight control, tobacco cessation, and effective health behavior changes as they can be applied to pharmacy practice.
- Offer practical application of lifestyle modification strategies to patients who are at risk of developing certain diseases or patients who currently have certain diseases in which lifestyle modifications can be beneficial in preventing or controlling those diseases.
- Have the reader obtain the necessary information and skills to construct a wellness plan for a patient who has risk factors for certain chronic diseases or who may already have one or more chronic diseases.

ORGANIZATIONAL PHILOSOPHY

Lifestyle Modifications in Pharmacotherapy is organized into three major sections. Section I consists of five chapters that lay the foundation for the practical application sections of the book. It discusses in detail the lifestyle modification strategies of nutrition, physical activity, weight control, tobacco cessation, and health behavior change. The intent of these chapters is not to offer an exhaustive overview of each topic so as to create a nutritionist or exercise physiologist, but to provide student pharmacists and practicing pharmacists the necessary information they will need to effectively construct a wellness plan for a patient that complements their current treatment regimens.

Section II consists of 13 disease state chapters that take the information presented in Section I and practically apply that information to patients with specific conditions. These chapters begin by briefly explaining the epidemiology and pathophysiology of the disease state and are meant to complement information that the student pharmacist or practicing pharmacist has already obtained from other courses or experiences. Each of the chapters in Section II is similarly structured and contains five tables in consistently titled categories that are modified relative to the subject matter. This allows the reader to develop a consistent pattern of critical thinking when designing wellness programs for virtually any disease state.

Additionally, each chapter in Section II concludes with a case study that is germane to the information presented in that chapter. Approximately one half of the case studies in Section II are relevant to providing primary prevention lifestyle modification strategies to patients with certain risk factors, while the other half of the case studies are geared toward designing a wellness plan for the secondary prevention of disease for patients with existing chronic diseases. This allows the reader ample opportunities to practice both primary and secondary prevention strategy wellness plans. The answers to the case studies are provided in Appendix C. The approach of these chapters lends well toward an understanding and application of the material that builds skills rather than memorization.

Section III consists of three chapters that broadly discuss disease prevention in the specific population groups of children and youth, older adults, and women and minorities. The information provided in Section III can be used to supplement the disease states presented in Section II. For example, Chapter 8 discusses the prevention of coronary heart disease. The information in Section III can be used to apply the prevention of coronary heart disease to overweight children, older adults, women, or persons of certain ethnic origins.

To take full advantage of *Lifestyle Modifications in Pharmacotherapy* the reader should be at the academic level of a student pharmacist during any year of his or her academic pharmacy career or a practicing pharmacist. The disease states that are discussed are meant to supplement information about those diseases obtained from other courses. However, if the student has yet to be introduced to Non-Prescription Therapeutics or Pharmacotherapeutics, for example, the material is written in such a way that the novice pharmacy student should be able to understand the disease state adequately to be able to apply the lifestyle modification strategies. Additionally, the reader should first begin by reading the chapters in Section I. The reader can then go to any chapter in Section II to see how the information presented in Section I is applied to specific diseases. Section III can then be used to supplement information that may be necessary for writing a complete wellness plan for certain individuals. Once the reader has a good understanding of the basic concepts of Section I and has practiced implementing the concepts in patients with specific diseases in Section II, the book can then be used as a reference tool for years to come when designing pharmaceutical care plans for patients.

SPECIAL NOTE

As stated above, each chapter in Section II discusses a specific disease state. In particular, the specific practice guidelines that are recommended to manage each specific disease are presented, especially in the context of primary and secondary prevention of the disease. As of the time of publication of *Lifestyle Modifications in Pharmacotherapy*, the current practice guidelines are discussed. It is very likely, however, that new practice guidelines regarding the diseases discussed in Section II will be published before the second edition of this book is published. Therefore, it would behoove the reader to check whether a more current version of the practice guidelines for the diseases in which they are working with has been published. In an effort to assist with this, a URL link to the specific disease practice guidelines will be provided in the text whenever possible.

Reviewers

Monika Daftary, PharmD
Howard University
2300 4th Street, NW
Washington, DC 20059

Lesley-Ann Miller, PhD, MS, BA
West Virginia University
PO Box 9510
HSC North Room 1129A
Morgantown, WV 26506-9510

Sergey Semenov, PharmD
Medical Communications
220 E. 42nd Street
New York, NY 10017

Ralph Small, PharmD
Virginia Commonwealth University
1800 Locust Hill Road
Richmond, VA 23238

Acknowledgments

As with any large project, it takes a team effort to effectively create a quality product. *Lifestyle Modifications in Pharmacotherapy* is truly an example of teamwork. My colleagues at Creighton University have been instrumental in the design and creation of this project. I appreciate the leadership of the Dean of the School of Pharmacy and Health Professions, J. Chris Bradberry, Pharm.D., and I am indebted to the Chair of the Pharmacy Practice Department, Michael S. Monaghan, Pharm.D., for the tremendous latitude that he has provided me to pursue my career endeavors. Additionally, I would like to thank the President of Creighton University, Fr. John P. Schlegel, S. J., for his vision in applying Creighton's Jesuit Catholic mission to guide our students.

My students are a constant reminder of the excitement of gaining new knowledge. Their zeal for discovery and constant bombardment of difficult questions help to keep me up to date on current practice information and research. For this I am thankful as it creates a better teaching and learning environment and is the reason for a project such as this.

The staff at Lippincott Williams & Wilkins are unparalleled in their guidance, leadership, and expertise to create a product such as this. I would especially like to thank David Troy, Senior Acquisitions Editor, for sharing the same vision as I did at the beginning of this project, and Karen Ruppert and Meredith Brittain, Managing Editors, for their hard work and expertise to make this book a reality. Additionally, I would like to thank Paula Williams, Senior Production Editor, and Marisa O'Brien and Matt Hauber for their significant contributions to this project.

Most importantly, I could not have completed such a project if it were not for the continuous love and support of my family. My wife Nancy and our three children, Kaelie, Abbey, and Jack, are constant reminders of what is most important in life, and without their encouragement and support, this book would still be an idea rather than a reality. Thank you.

—Tom Lenz

Contents

Preface *vii*

SECTION I Disease Prevention Through Lifestyle Modification 1
   Introduction 1

CHAPTER 1 Nutrition 5

CHAPTER 2 Physical Activity 29

CHAPTER 3 Weight Control 57

CHAPTER 4 Tobacco Cessation 85

CHAPTER 5 Health Behavior Change 103

SECTION II Chronic Diseases 117
   Introduction 117

CHAPTER 6 Hypertension 119

CHAPTER 7 Dyslipidemia 133

CHAPTER 8 Coronary Heart Disease 145

CHAPTER 9 Stroke 159

CHAPTER 10 Peripheral Arterial Disease 173

CHAPTER 11 Heart Failure 185

CHAPTER 12 Diabetes Mellitus 197

CHAPTER 13 Obesity 215

CHAPTER 14 Metabolic Syndrome   227

CHAPTER 15 Cancer   239

CHAPTER 16 Osteoporosis   251

CHAPTER 17 Osteoarthritis   263

CHAPTER 18 Chronic Lung Disease   273

SECTION III Special Populations   285
            Introduction   285

CHAPTER 19 Children and Youth   287

CHAPTER 20 Older Adults   295

CHAPTER 21 Women and Minorities   301

SECTION IV Appendices   309
            A. Framingham 10-Year Coronary Heart Disease Risk Assessment 311
            B. Body Mass Index Table   315
            C. Case Study Answers   317

Glossary   359

Index   363

Disease Prevention Through Lifestyle Modification

INTRODUCTION

Knowledge and skills of disease prevention are becoming increasingly more important for healthcare professionals including pharmacists. Much evidence exists to show that the overall health of almost all populations is better if diseases are prevented rather than treated once they occur. Chronic diseases create a significant burden on the U.S. healthcare system at a societal and personal level as well as from a financial standpoint. The Centers for Disease Control and Prevention (CDC) reports that 70% of the deaths of all Americans and 75% of the U.S.'s annual healthcare costs are related to chronic diseases like those presented in Section II of this book. These data indicate that a focus on the prevention of these chronic diseases may produce better overall outcomes for patients and be cost effective for the U.S. healthcare system.

The figure in this introduction attempts to describe disease prevention as it affects the U.S. healthcare system with regard to the control and cost of diseases. The triangle on the far left of the figure shows the lack of focus on disease prevention in the way we in the United States currently practice pharmacy and medicine. This triangle represents an emphasis on treating patients once they become ill, with little emphasis on disease prevention. As a result, the triangle is tall and narrow to represent the high cost of healthcare and a shortened lifespan of years of quality life lived.

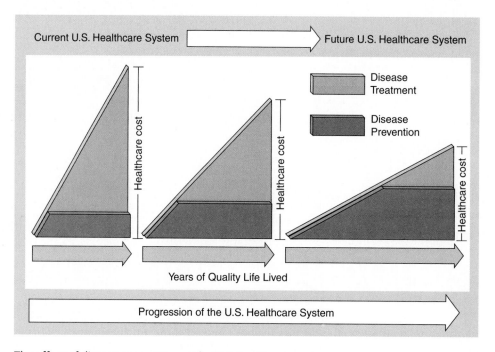

The effect of disease prevention on the U.S. healthcare system.

The triangle to the far right of the figure represents a healthcare system that places a great deal of emphasis on disease prevention. In this triangle disease prevention begins early in life to a significant extent, and is sustained throughout life. The triangle flattens out and becomes longer to represent the need for less disease treatment, lower healthcare costs, and a longer lifespan with a greater number of years of quality life lived when prevention is highly emphasized.

Looking at the figure in total, all three triangles represent the need for the U.S. healthcare system to progress from an emphasis on treating patients only when they are sick to a greater emphasis on the prevention of disease. The goal is to move from our current state of healthcare (left triangle) to a future state of healthcare that focuses more on disease prevention than on disease control (right triangle). The middle triangle represents the need for the progression of this process to occur over time. Approaching healthcare in this manner not only can increase the lifespan and years of quality life lived of an individual but also is more cost effective for the healthcare system as a whole.

Pharmacists have long been known to be highly accessible and trusted healthcare providers to the public. Many of the most commonly dispensed drugs in pharmacies are used to treat diseases in which lifestyle changes such as proper nutrition, physical activity, weight control, and tobacco abstinence are also recommended to prevent the disease. Therefore, pharmacists have frequent contact with patients who could potentially benefit from lifestyle modification information. Because of these factors, pharmacists are in an ideal position to offer patients information, guidance, and counseling regarding lifestyle changes that can help manage their medical conditions.

Section I consists of five chapters that lay the foundation for the practical application sections of this book. It discusses in detail the lifestyle modification strategies of nutrition, physical activity, weight control, tobacco cessation, and health behavior change. The intent of these chapters is to provide a background knowledge that will be needed in these lifestyle modification areas to effectively construct a wellness plan for a patient that complements their current treatment regimens. Information gained from these chapters can then be applied to the diseases that are presented in Section II.

CHAPTER 1

Nutrition

OBJECTIVES

At the end of this chapter the reader should be able to:

1. Recall the importance of proper nutrition for the treatment and prevention of chronic diseases.
2. Calculate the number of total daily calories appropriate for patients based on their individual information.
3. List the basic nutritional principles for carbohydrates, fats, proteins, vitamins, minerals, and water.
4. Highlight the important aspects of the 2005 Dietary Guidelines and how these guidelines can be applied with the U.S. Department of Agriculture's Food Guidance System for individual patients.
5. Discuss the role that alcohol may play on health outcomes.

Nutrition is a fundamental component necessary for growth, development, health, and well-being. Nutritional behaviors that promote health should begin at a very young age and continue throughout life with healthful eating habits.[1] Unhealthy eating can be a substantial contributor to many diseases that are considered preventable, such as heart disease, **cancer, obesity, diabetes mellitus, stroke,** and **osteoporosis.**[1,2] Each year, more than $33 billion in medical costs and $9 billion in lost productivity as a result of heart disease, cancer, stroke, and diabetes are attributed to a poor diet.[2]

NUTRITION AND CHRONIC DISEASES

Chronic disease can be caused by many factors that include both genetic and any number of lifestyle behaviors. As genetic factors are inherited at conception, the greatest opportunities for decreasing risks for the development of chronic diseases are to modify as many lifestyle behaviors as possible that contribute to specific diseases. For example, eating a healthful diet, along with **exercising,** moderating alcohol intake, and abstaining from smoking, decreases the risk for developing **cardiovascular disease,** stroke, cancer, diabetes, obesity, **metabolic syndrome, hypertension,** and hyperlipidemia.[1] More specifically, an eating plan that includes low amounts of sodium, saturated fat, and **cholesterol** and high amounts of fiber, potassium, calcium, and magnesium can help prevent and treat hypertension.[3] Likewise, an eating plan with adequate amounts of dietary calcium can decrease the incidence of osteoporosis.[4,5] Several other examples exist with other diseases and will be provided throughout the text as specific diseases are introduced. In addition, certain nutrients and other substances in foods may influence gene expression.[6] Some nutrients like vitamins and minerals can have a positive effect by helping prevent damage to DNA, whereas other substances like alcohol can have a negative effect by damaging DNA.[6]

The impact that a healthful eating plan can have on the prevention and treatment of chronic diseases cannot be understated. Knowing which foods place patients at greater risk for the development or further progression of specific diseases is essential information for pharmacists and all healthcare professionals. Providing patients with evidence-based information about the importance of healthy eating with regard to many chronic diseases is as important as providing good pharmaceutical care. The overarching goal when treating patients predisposed to chronic diseases such as cardiovascular disease, stroke, diabetes, cancer, and obesity is to decrease the overall risk for the development or progression of the disease. In most cases, a healthful eating plan is vitally important information and, therefore, pharmacists and other healthcare providers should be providing this information if proper patient counseling is being offered.

NUTRITION FOR HEALTHY LIVING

There are a total of six classes of nutrients that humans need to consume to maintain overall good health. These nutrients are carbohydrates, fats, proteins, vitamins, minerals, and water. A healthy eating plan comprises three basic principles that should be applied when consuming these nutrients.[4] These principles consist of (1) eating a balanced proportion of food from different food groups, (2) eating a wide variety of foods within each food group, and (3) eating in moderation.[4] Eating with these concepts in mind should allow for the consumption of all the necessary nutrients needed to provide **energy** to complete daily tasks, regulate metabolic processes, and allow for the growth and development of all tissues within the body while maintaining a healthy body weight.[6] Carbohydrates, fats, and proteins supply the body with calories or energy so that we can perform our activities of daily living. Vitamins, minerals, and water allow us to resist certain diseases and help our bodies perform adequate metabolic processes. In addition, abiding by the above-named principles will promote a healthy body weight and decrease risks for developing certain chronic diseases.[6]

FOOD AS ENERGY

The fundamental purpose of eating is to provide the body with adequate amounts of energy needed to perform many different metabolic and physiologic functions.[4] Many types of energy exist within the body. Examples include chemical, mechanical, electrical, and heat energy. More specifically, mechanical energy to move our bodies during exercise or during other daily activities is often thought of as the end result of eating because food gives us the "energy" to perform these tasks.[6] Proper nutrition also allows our bodies to perform many other important tasks that are not as outwardly obvious as exercise.

The energy that is gained from the food we eat is commonly expressed in terms of calories. A **calorie** is simply a measure of heat.[6] By definition, the energy it takes to raise the temperature of 1 g of water 1° Celsius is a calorie, sometimes called a gram calorie.[6] A gram calorie is very small and difficult to measure. Therefore, in human nutrition 1,000 calories (C) or 1 kilocalorie (**kcal**) is commonly used to express the energy obtained from the food we eat.[6] Throughout the text the abbreviations "C" and "kcal" may be used interchangeably.

Energy obtained from food for human use can be derived from three major sources: carbohydrate, fat, and protein. These three sources are collectively known as macronutrients. Calories can also be obtained from the consumption of alcohol. This source, however, contains little nutritional value outside of its contribution of calories to the diet. In general, a 1-g consumption of each of these sources results in the following number of calories in the human body:[6]

$$1 \text{ g carbohydrate} = 4 \text{ kcal}$$
$$1 \text{ g fat} = 9 \text{ kcal}$$
$$1 \text{ g protein} = 4 \text{ kcal}$$
$$1 \text{ g alcohol} = 7 \text{ kcal}$$

Alcohol consumption will be discussed later in this chapter; however, the remainder of the book will focus on carbohydrates, fats, and protein as the main sources of calorie consumption for its potential for use as energy.

The rate at which energy is used in the body is often referred to as metabolism or metabolic rate.[7] Metabolism or the sum total of all energy expended each day depends on three factors.[7] These factors include the **basal metabolic rate** (BMR), the thermic effect of food, and **physical activity.**[6] Basal metabolic rate is the energy that is required to complete cellular processes in the body necessary to sustain normal physiologic activities. The BMR accounts for the largest amount of daily energy expenditure. The thermic effect of food is the energy the body uses to absorb, transport, store, and metabolize food that has been consumed.[8] Energy use is greatest around 1 hour after ingestion and can last for up to 4 hours. Foods high in protein require the greatest thermic effect whereas high-fat foods require the lowest thermic effect.[8]

Physical activity is the least consistent factor that affects metabolism. Energy use for physical activity ranges from the energy required to get out of bed to that used for physical labor and exercise. Day-to-day variability in physical activity can be significant in many individuals.[6] For example, some days require us to be sedentary to study for an examination or complete a project at work, and other days, like weekends, allow us to be very active. Calculating the amount of energy or calorie consumption required to meet individual metabolism needs is an important component when counseling patients about a proper eating plan. For the purposes of this text, we will call this estimated energy requirements (EER).

Several equations are available that estimate the daily energy requirements or the EER. One widely accepted equation uses a formula with the variables of age, height, weight, and physical activity level.[9] Physical activity is represented in the formula as "PA," or physical activity coefficient, and can range from 1.0 for sedentary individuals to 1.45 and 1.48 for very active women and men, respectively. The physical activity coefficient chosen for the EER formula should represent the patient's physical activity level as closely as possible. This formula is provided in Table 1-1.

As stated above, physical activity can be the most variable component of the equation. It can also be the most difficult to estimate. The formula we will be using (listed in Table 1-1) to estimate EER allows for the choice of four different physical activity levels. A sedentary level should be used for individuals who perform mostly just activities of daily living, such as walking around the house, who mostly sit at work, and who engage in other forms of very light activity. A low activity level should be applied to individuals who are active 2 to 3 days per week doing light activity like walking, cycling, bowling, golf, and gardening. Active individuals are those who perform 30 to 60 minutes of physical activity at a moderate intensity on most days of the week. This can include a combination of household work and activities like walking, cycling, or other forms of exercise. Very active individuals are those who exercise at moderate to high levels on a daily basis for 60 minutes or longer.[4] These individuals probably also participate in sporting activities or have a job that requires physical activity in addition to their normal exercise routine.

As an example of estimating energy requirements, let's calculate the number of daily calories required for N.L., who is a 34-year-old female, is 5 foot 4 inches tall, weighs 140 pounds, and is considered active (45 minutes of moderate-intensity activity 5 to 6 days per week):

$$EER = 354 - 6.91 \times age + PA \times [9.36 \times weight + 726 \times height]$$

$$EER = 354 - 6.91 \times 34 + 1.27 \times [9.36 \times 63.6 + 726 \times 1.63]$$

$$EER = 2{,}378 \text{ kcal per day}$$

If N.L. wanted to maintain her current weight, she would need to eat approximately 2,378 calories daily. If she would like to lose weight, she would have to eat less than 2,378

TABLE 1–1   Calculating the Estimated Energy Requirements (EER)

Males aged ≥ 19 years:
$$EER = 662 - 9.53 \times age + PA \times [15.9 \times weight + 540 \times height]$$
Females aged ≥ 19 years:
$$EER = 354 - 6.91 \times age + PA \times [9.36 \times weight + 726 \times height]$$

Age = years
Weight = kilograms (kg; calculate by dividing weight in pounds by 2.2)
Height = meters (m; calculate by multiplying height in inches by 0.0254)
PA = physical activity coefficient (calculate using the following table)

	Sedentary	Low Active	Active	Very Active
Male	1.0	1.11	1.25	1.48
Female	1.0	1.12	1.27	1.45

Reprinted with permission from Dietary Reference Intakes for Energy, Carbohydrate, Fiber, Fat, Fatty Acids, Cholesterol, Protein, and Amino Acids (Macronutrients) by the National Academy of Sciences, Courtesy of the National Academies Press, Washington, D.C., 2005.

calories daily and, conversely, if she ate more than 2,378 calories per day she would gain weight. This concept will be discussed in greater detail in Chapter 3.

The U.S. Department of Agriculture (USDA) has established a table that estimates caloric intake on the basis of gender, age, and activity level.[10] This method of estimating a patient's caloric needs may be useful and practical as it does not require any calculations and is easy to interpret. This information can be found in Table 1-2.

Carbohydrates

As mentioned previously, there are six classes of nutrients that are needed to maintain overall good health. These six nutrients will be discussed in detail, starting with carbohydrates. Along with fats and proteins, carbohydrates are a major energy source for the human body. Each gram of carbohydrate yields approximately 4 kcal of energy. According to the Dietary Guidelines for Americans published by the U.S. Department of Health and Human Services (http://www.healthierus.gov/dietaryguidelines), carbohydrates should make up a majority of the calories (45 to 65%) we consume each day.[4] Therefore, carbohydrate consumption is an important component of our daily eating plan.

There are three major categories of carbohydrates: simple carbohydrates, complex carbohydrates, and dietary fiber.[6] Simple carbohydrates, often called sugars, can be

TABLE 1–2   Estimation of Daily Caloric Intake for Adults

Age (yr)	Males Activity Level[a] Sedentary	Moderately Active	Active	Females Activity Level[a] Sedentary	Moderately Active	Active
19–20	2,600	2,800	3,000	2,000	2,200	2,400
21–25	2,400	2,800	3,000	2,000	2,200	2,400
26–30	2,400	2,600	3,000	1,800	2,000	2,400
31–35	2,400	2,600	3,000	1,800	2,000	2,200
36–40	2,400	2,600	2,800	1,800	2,000	2,200
41–45	2,200	2,600	2,800	1,800	2,000	2,200
46–50	2,200	2,400	2,800	1,800	2,000	2,200
51–55	2,200	2,400	2,800	1,600	1,800	2,200
56–60	2,200	2,400	2,600	1,600	1,800	2,200
61–65	2,000	2,400	2,600	1,600	1,800	2,000
66–70	2,000	2,200	2,600	1,600	1,800	2,000
71–75	2,000	2,200	2,600	1,600	1,800	2,000
76+	2,000	2,000	2,400	1,600	1,800	2,000

Source: U.S. Department of Health and Human Services, U.S. Department of Agriculture. MyPyramid.gov. Available at: http://www.mypyramid.gov/professionals/pdf_calorie_levels.html. Accessed June 1, 2005.
[a] Calorie levels are based on the Estimated Energy Requirements (EER) and activity levels from the Institute of Medicine Dietary Reference Intakes Macro Nutrients Report, 2002.
Sedentary means less than 30 minutes a day of moderate physical activity in addition to daily activities.
Moderately active means at least 30 minutes up to 60 minutes a day of moderate physical activity in addition to daily activities.
Active means 60 or more minutes a day of moderate physical activity in addition to daily activities.

monosaccharides, disaccharides, trisaccharides, or higher saccharides. There are three monosaccharides: glucose, fructose, and galactose. The combination of two monosaccharides results in a disaccharide. Examples of disaccharides are sucrose (glucose + fructose), lactose (glucose + galactose), and maltose (glucose + glucose). Disaccharides and trisaccharides are often called refined sugars. Trisaccharides are commonly found in many foods as a sweetener. An example of a trisaccharide is high fructose corn syrup. Sugars can also be found naturally in foods like fruit (fructose) and milk (lactose).[6]

Complex carbohydrates, also called starches, are a combination of three or more glucose molecules called polysaccharides.[6] Most of the carbohydrates found in plants are polysaccharides. Unlike simple carbohydrates, starches are the storage form of carbohydrates. Stored carbohydrates are called glycogen. Sugars and starches supply energy to the body in the form of glucose. Added sugars, or caloric sweeteners, supply calories to the body but few or no nutrients. On the other hand, foods like fruits, vegetables, grains, and milk supply energy to the body as well as many needed nutrients such as vitamins, minerals, and dietary fiber. Therefore, choosing plenty of these foods, within the context of a calorie-controlled diet, can promote health and reduce chronic disease risk.[4]

Dietary fiber is non-starch carbohydrates and lignin that comes from plant foods and is not digested by enzymes in the small intestine.[4] Eating plants rich in dietary fiber has been shown to have several beneficial health effects including decreasing the risks for **coronary heart disease,** improving laxation, and possibly lowering the risk for type 2 diabetes.[4] The recommended daily intake of dietary fiber is 14 g/1,000 calories consumed.[4] Foods containing whole grains as well as fruits and vegetables contain high amounts of dietary fiber.

The mechanisms by which dietary fiber can prevent or improve diseases such as heart disease, certain forms of cancer, obesity, diabetes, and hypertension are currently unknown. Epidemiologic studies, however, have shown that an eating plan high in dietary fiber is associated with a lower risk for coronary heart disease. Given that coronary artery disease is the number one cause of death in the United States, it behooves all individuals, with disease and without, to consume the recommended amount of dietary fiber.[4] It should be noted, however, that a gradual increase in daily fiber is recommended for those currently consuming low amounts. A gradual increase in fiber will help curb gastrointestinal side effects associated with a sudden onset of a high-fiber intake.

Most Americans consume adequate amounts of grains each day. However, only a small percentage of these grains are whole grains.[4] Most of the grains consumed in the U.S. diet are refined grains that contain little dietary fiber. Diets rich in whole grains and fresh fruits and vegetables will supply the individual with an adequate intake of simple and complex carbohydrates as well as dietary fiber. A list of foods containing simple carbohydrates, complex carbohydrates, and dietary fiber is provided in Table 1-3.

Fats

Dietary fats and oils are an essential part of a healthful diet.[4] The type of fat and the total amount of fat consumed, however, do make a difference in potential health benefits. Dietary fat supplies essential **fatty acids** to our diet, serves as a carrier for the absorption of the fat-soluble vitamins A, D, E, and K and carotenoids, and is an important energy source.[4] Fats also serve as the building blocks of membranes and play key roles in regulating many biologic functions.[4] The recommended total fat intake is between 20 and 35% of the total daily calories recommended for adults. Eating plans that include a very

TABLE 1–3	Examples of Simple Carbohydrates (Sugars), Complex Carbohydrates (Starches), and Dietary Fiber
Sugars	Table sugar, brown sugar, confectioners sugar, raw sugar, dextrose, corn syrup, glucose syrup, fruits, vegetables, honey, sorbitol, mannitol, xylitol, milk, milk products, cereals and some baked goods
Starches	Flour, bread, rice, corn, oats, barley, potatoes, legumes, fruits, vegetables, pasta
Dietary fiber	Navy beans, kidney beans, lentils, oat bran, oats, legumes, citrus fruits, strawberries, apples with skin, rice bran, barley, whole-wheat breads and cereals, wheat bran, carrots, Brussels sprouts, turnips, cauliflower

Source: HHS Publication No. HHS-ODPHP-2005-01-DGA-A. Dietary Guidelines for Americans 2005, U.S. Department of Health and Human Services, U.S. Department of Agriculture. Available at: http://www.healthierus.gov/dietaryguidelines. Accessed June 1, 2005.

low intake of fat as well as those that contain a high amount of fat (>35% of total calories) have been shown to negatively impact health.[4] As stated earlier, 1 g of fat delivers 9 kcal of energy.

Fatty acids are the most common component in dietary fat that allows us to predict the degree of healthfulness of the fat we consume. Fatty acids can be saturated (**saturated fatty acids**) or unsaturated (**polyunsaturated fatty acids** [PUFAs] and **monounsaturated fatty acids** [MUFAs]). Most dietary fat calorie consumption should be obtained from unsaturated fatty acids.[4] Polyunsaturated fats and monounsaturated fats should represent approximately 10 and 20%, respectively, of the total daily caloric intake.[11,12] The remaining amount of fat intake (less than 10% in healthy individuals and less than 7% of total calories in those with elevated low-density lipoprotein, or LDL cholesterol) can come from saturated fats.

Saturated fats have been shown to be closely associated with increases in total and LDL cholesterol. The chemical makeup of saturated fatty acids shows that they contain all the hydrogen and carbon that the atoms can hold. At room temperature, they are usually in a solid state and do not combine readily with oxygen. The main sources of saturated fats in the typical American diet are from animals and some plants.[4,11,12]

To limit the intake of saturated fatty acids, the American Heart Association recommends substituting unsaturated fatty acids in their place. By definition, **unsaturated fatty acids** have at least one unsaturated hydrogen bond on the molecule.[4] Polyunsaturated oils are liquid at room temperature and when stored in the refrigerator. They have been shown to help reduce the amount of newly formed cholesterol and can help lower blood cholesterol levels when substituted for saturated fatty acids in the diet.[13]

Monounsaturated oils are liquid at room temperature but start to become solid when refrigerated. Monounsaturated fatty acids have also been shown to reduce blood cholesterol when consumed with a diet very low in saturated fats. Unsaturated fatty acids are most often found in the American diet in liquid vegetable oils.[12] Examples of saturated, polyunsaturated, and monounsaturated fatty acids are listed in Table 1-4.

Fatty acids contain a chemical makeup that consists of carbon atoms connected by double bonds.[12] Saturated fatty acids that occur in nature have hydrogen atoms attached to the same side of the double carbon bonds, in the *cis* position.[12] **Trans fatty acids** have

TABLE 1–4   Examples of Food High in Saturated and Unsaturated Fatty Acids and Dietary Cholesterol

Saturated fats	Beef, beef fat, veal, lamb, pork, lard, poultry fat, butter, cream, milk, cheeses and other dairy products made from whole milk, coconut oil, palm oil and palm kernel oil (often called tropical oils), cocoa butter
Polyunsaturated fats	Safflower, sesame, and sunflower seeds, corn and soybeans, many nuts and seeds, and their oils
Monounsaturated fats	Canola, olive, and peanut oils, avocados
Dietary cholesterol	Meat (especially organ meat), poultry, seafood (especially shrimp and crayfish), dairy products, egg yolks

Source: HHS Publication No. HHS-ODPHP-2005-01-DGA-A. Dietary Guidelines for Americans 2005, U.S. Department of Health and Human Services, U.S. Department of Agriculture. Available at: http://www.healthierus.gov/dietaryguidelines. Accessed June 1, 2005.

hydrogen atoms connected to the opposite side of the double carbon bonds, in the *trans* position.[12] *Trans* double bonds can occur in nature and can be found in meat and dairy products but can also be artificially created through the hydrogenation of vegetable and fish oils.[12] Trans fatty acids have been associated with a higher risk for coronary heart disease.[11,14–17] Therefore, it is recommended that trans fatty acid intake be reduced as much as possible to decrease the risks for certain chronic diseases such as cardiovascular disease.[4]

Butter vs. Margarine

As a result of a great amount of press in recent years, the question often arises, Which is healthier, butter or margarine? Butter contains high amounts of saturated fats whereas some margarines contain high amounts of trans fat. A great deal of data exists regarding the negative effects of too much saturated fat. A rise in LDL cholesterol levels has been associated with an increased dietary intake of trans fatty acids.[11,18–30] In addition, trans fatty acids have been associated with a higher risk for coronary heart disease.[11,14–17] Therefore, the debate is really about, "Which is worse, saturated fat or trans fat?"

The current Dietary Guidelines recommend that saturated fat intake should represent less than 10% of the total daily calories and even lower for those with heart disease.[4] It is recommended in the hypercholesterolemia guidelines (Adult Treatment Panel III) to keep the intake of trans fatty acids low and to try to use liquid vegetable oil, soft margarine, and trans fatty acid–free margarine in place of stick margarine, butter, and shortening.[11] Because there is currently no standard method to measure trans fatty acid content in food, it is difficult to estimate dietary intake.

With respect to the butter vs. margarine debate, the American Heart Association recommends using unhydrogenated vegetable oil such as canola or olive oil and to substitute soft margarines (liquid or tub) for butter or margarines that are harder or in stick form.[4] Choose margarines with liquid vegetable oil as the first ingredient and that contain no more than 2 g of saturated fat per tablespoon.

The best alternative is to choose a spread that contains plant sterols and stanols. These spreads are free of trans fat, taste like soft margarine, and have been shown to actually decrease blood cholesterol levels. Scientific studies show that 1.3 g per day of plant sterol esters or 3.4 g per day of plant stanol esters in the diet are needed to show a significant cholesterol lowering effect. To qualify for this health claim, a food must contain at least 0.65 g of plant sterol esters per serving or at least 1.7 g of plant stanol esters per serving.[31] The claim must specify that the daily dietary intake of plant sterol esters or plant stanol esters should be consumed in two servings eaten at different times of the day with other foods. The next best choice is soft margarine that is available in a tub, followed by butter, with the least desirable choice being margarine in the stick form.

Cholesterol is not a fat but is a fatlike substance found in animals. Cholesterol is not an essential nutrient that humans need to obtain from food because it is naturally produced in the liver.[6] The national average of dietary cholesterol intake in the United States is 256 mg/day.[11,32] Approximately one third of dietary cholesterol intake is obtained from the consumption of eggs.[11,33] It is recommended that Americans consume an average of 200 mg or less of dietary cholesterol daily.[11] High consumption of dietary cholesterol (10 mg/dL per 100 mg dietary cholesterol per 1,000 kcal) has been associated with an increased response in serum cholesterol.[11,34,35] In addition, higher intakes of dietary cholesterol have been associated with increases in LDL cholesterol, which then increases the risk for coronary heart disease (CHD).[11] Decreasing the intake of dietary cholesterol will decrease LDL cholesterol levels in most persons.[11] Examples of foods with high dietary cholesterol are listed in Table 1-4.

Protein

The third macronutrient is protein. Proteins consist of peptides, which are created when two or more amino acids are linked together.[6] The human body is able to manufacture some amino acids. These amino acids are commonly called non-essential amino acids because it is not essential that we supplement our diet with them. On the other hand, there are nine amino acids that the human body cannot manufacture. These are commonly referred to as essential amino acids because it is essential that we obtain these amino acids from the foods we eat to maintain good health. Foods that contain all nine essential amino acids are referred to as complete proteins. Foods that do not contain all nine essential amino acids are referred to as incomplete proteins.[6]

Proteins are important to consume in our diets for several reasons. Proteins help to regulate human metabolism by taking part in the formation of almost all enzymes and several hormones that control physiologic functions, such as regulation of the blood clotting system, acid-base balance, and the development of the human immune system.[6] Proteins play a key role in providing the structural basis and nutrients for most tissues in the body. This is especially important during times of growth, such as in childhood. As previously mentioned, protein also is a source of energy. Under normal conditions, protein is not a major energy source but can be converted to carbohydrate or fat during conditions of starvation or semistarvation. One gram of protein provides 4 kcal of energy.[6]

TABLE 1–5   Examples of Food High in Protein

Peanuts	Turkey
Soybeans	Salmon
Navy beans	Swordfish
Milk	Herring
Yogurt	Veal
Cheese	Lamb
Eggs	Pork
Beef	Wheat bread
Chicken	

Source: HHS Publication No. HHS-ODPHP-2005-01-DGA-A. Dietary Guidelines for Americans 2005, U.S. Department of Health and Human Services, U.S. Department of Agriculture. Available at: http://www.healthierus.gov/dietaryguidelines. Accessed June 1, 2005.

Because protein is not a major energy source, its percentage of the overall daily caloric intake is less, relative to carbohydrate and fat intake. It is recommended that proteins make up approximately 10 to 35% of the total daily calories.[6] Most Americans already consume enough protein in their daily diet. Sources for quality protein can be found in both plant and animal foods. Ironically, good food sources for protein are similar to foods that contain fiber, such as dry beans, lentils, and peas, as well as beef and chicken. A list of foods high in protein is provided in Table 1-5.

Vitamins

Vitamins are a complex group of organic substances needed to maintain normal and healthy physiologic processes.[6] Vitamins do not provide the body with energy and therefore do not possess a caloric value. They do, however, help regulate energy processes in the body. Some vitamins help activate enzymes that help muscles contract, transport gases such as carbon dioxide within the body, and aid in the release of energy stores. In addition, some vitamins such as vitamins E and C and β-carotene have been shown to help fight free radicals that have been shown to lead to certain forms of cancer and cardiovascular disease.[6] These vitamins are called antioxidants.

Vitamins can be divided into two groups: fat soluble and water soluble. The fat-soluble vitamins are A, D, E, and K. These vitamins are not soluble in water and can be stored in the body. There are nine water-soluble vitamins that include eight B-complex vitamins and vitamin C (ascorbic acid). The B-complex vitamins consist of thiamin, riboflavin, niacin, B_6, B_{12}, folate, biotin, and pantothenic acid. Water-soluble vitamins are not stored in the body like fat-soluble vitamins and, therefore, excess intake of water-soluble vitamins is usually excreted in the urine without harm in most cases. Key vitamins discussed throughout this text are listed in Table 1-6 and will again be addressed later in this chapter when reviewing the Dietary Guidelines for Americans 2005.

Minerals

Like vitamins, minerals provide no energy or calories for our bodies. They are inorganic elements that serve the body in two basic ways. Minerals are needed as a fundamental component to build many tissues within the body.[6] In addition, some minerals are also

TABLE 1–6   **Key Vitamins in Disease Prevention and Health Promotion**

Vitamin	Major Functions	Sources
A	Promotes bone development, maintains epithelial tissue in skin and mucous membranes	Whole and fortified milk, cheese, liver, carrots, green leafy vegetables
D	Increases intestinal absorption of calcium and promotes bone formation	Dairy products, fish oil, sunlight
E	Antioxidant to protect cell membranes	Whole-wheat products, vegetable oils, margarine, green leafy vegetables
B_{12}	Coenzyme for formation of DNA, red blood cell development, and maintenance of nerve tissue	Meat, fish, poultry, milk, eggs (animal sources only)
Folate	DNA formation and red blood cell development	Green leafy vegetables, legumes, nuts, fortified cereals, liver
C	Aids in absorption of iron, is an antioxidant, forms collagen for connective tissue	Citrus fruits, green leafy vegetables, strawberries, broccoli

Source: HHS Publication No. HHS-ODPHP-2005-01-DGA-A. Dietary Guidelines for Americans 2005, U.S. Department of Health and Human Services, U.S. Department of Agriculture. Available at: http://www.healthierus.gov/dietaryguidelines. Accessed June 1, 2005.

components of enzymes and hormones that are involved in the regulation of metabolism. Minerals are involved in normal heart rhythm, nerve impulse conduction, the immune system, acid-based balance, and many other important physiologic functions.[6] Key minerals discussed throughout the text are listed in Table 1-7 and will again be discussed later in the text as they relate to specific chronic diseases.

TABLE 1–7   **Key Minerals in Disease Prevention and Health Promotion**

Mineral	Major Functions	Sources
Potassium	Blunts the effect of salt on rising blood pressure, decreases risk for developing kidney stones, decreases bone loss	Baked white or sweet potatoes, bananas, oranges, orange juice, cooked dry beans, tomato products
Calcium	Bone formation, enzyme activation, muscle contraction, nerve impulse transmission	All dairy products such as milk, yogurt, egg yolk, dark green vegetables, peas
Magnesium	Protein synthesis, glucose metabolism, component of bone	Milk, yogurt, whole-grain products, fruits, vegetables
Iron	Hemoglobin and myoglobin formation	Organ meats, other meats, fish, nuts, whole-grain products, vegetables
Sodium	Increases blood pressure	Food processing for taste and as a preservative, table salt

Source: HHS Publication No. HHS-ODPHP-2005-01-DGA-A. Dietary Guidelines for Americans 2005, U.S. Department of Health and Human Services, U.S. Department of Agriculture. Available at: http://www.healthierus.gov/dietaryguidelines. Accessed June 1, 2005.

Water

Water, which provides no food energy, is considered the most essential nutrient for the human body. Most other nutrients needed by the body can only work if adequate amounts of water are present.[6] Water is essential for food digestion, normal metabolism, and the regulation of body temperature. In addition, water carries electrolytes that are essential to numerous physiologic processes. The recommended intake of water for adult males and females aged 19 and older is 3.7 and 2.7 L/day, respectively.[36] In conditions in which the environmental temperature is hotter than normal or during physical activity, water intake should be higher.

A balance of water intake and output should always be maintained so as not to dehydrate the body or alter the body's electrolyte balance. Water intake can come from the consumption of fluids and food as well as from the metabolism of foods to energy. About 20% of our daily total water intake comes from the food we eat.[6] A smaller but significant percentage of our water intake comes from the breakdown of fat, carbohydrate, and protein for energy. This process is known as metabolic water. Water loss can come from the combination of urine output, water in feces, loss through the lungs via exhaled air, and loss through the skin.

It has been shown that the combination of thirst and normal drinking behavior, especially the consumption of fluids with meals, is sufficient to maintain adequate amounts of fluid within the body.[4] Those individuals who are healthy and have sufficient access to fluid consume enough water to meet their needs. Extra water intake is warranted, however, for those exposed to heat stress, especially as a result of strenuous physical activity.[4] The American College of Sports Medicine (ACSM) recommends drinking 17 ounces of water approximately 2 hours before exercising to ensure adequate hydration during the exercise period.[36]

DIETARY GUIDELINES FOR AMERICANS 2005

First published in 1980 through a joint effort of the Department of Health and Human Services and the Department of Agriculture, the Dietary Guidelines for Americans (Dietary Guidelines) uses a scientific evidence-based approach to providing nutritional health information. The purpose of the Dietary Guidelines is to promote health and to reduce the risk of chronic diseases through diet and physical activity. As a result of its focus on health promotion and risk reduction, the Dietary Guidelines forms the basis of federal food, nutrition education, and information programs.[4] It should be noted that other nutritional guidelines and recommendations also exist from organizations such as the American Dietetic Association (ADA) and others. For the purposes of this book, the Dietary Guidelines will be used. The reader, however, can also reference the ADA dietary recommendations, which can be found at http://www.eatright.org/.

The Dietary Guidelines are important for our discussion because as stated earlier, major causes of morbidity and mortality in the United States are related to poor diet and sedentary lifestyle.[4] Specific diseases that have been linked to poor diet include cardiovascular disease, hypertension, **dyslipidemia,** type 2 diabetes, overweight and obesity, osteoporosis, constipation, diverticular disease, iron deficiency anemia, oral disease, malnutrition, and some cancers.[4] Combined with physical activity, which will be covered later, a healthful diet should enhance the health and well-being of most individuals. Therefore, healthcare providers who know the key recommendations in the Dietary Guidelines can effectively speak with their patients about individual changes they can make in their eating habits.[4]

The overarching themes of the Dietary Guidelines are to encourage most Americans to eat fewer calories, to be more physically active, and to make wiser food choices.[4] The basic premise is that nutrient needs should primarily be met through consuming foods. In some cases, fortified foods and dietary supplements may be useful if one or more nutrients that otherwise might be consumed in recommended amounts are consumed in less than recommended amounts. Dietary supplements, however, should not replace a healthful diet.[4] Two examples of healthful eating plans are the USDA Food Guide (http://www.mypyramid.gov), which is covered later in this chapter, and the Dietary Approaches to Stop Hypertension (DASH) eating plan, which is covered in Chapter 6.[37–39] It is important to note that these eating plans are not weight loss diets, but rather eating plans that promote overall good health. Eating plans for weight loss are covered in the Weight Control and Obesity chapters (Chapters 3 and 13, respectively).

The Dietary Guidelines provides examples of eating patterns consistent with a 2,000-calorie intake as a reference to maintain consistency. It should be noted that individual calorie intake will depend on variables such as age, sex, and activity level. At each calorie intake level, it is possible for individuals to eat nutrient-dense foods that allow them to meet their recommended nutrient intake without consuming the full calorie allotment.[4] The remaining calories are referred to as discretionary calories.[4] Discretionary calories allow individuals to consume foods and beverages that contain added fats, sugars, and alcohol.

The following is a listing of the key recommendations within selected chapters of the Dietary Guidelines for Americans 2005. It should be noted that several recommendations are made in the Dietary Guidelines. Individuals need not abide by all the recommendations to improve health; following just some of the recommendations can result in health benefits.[4] This concept is important for pharmacists and patients to understand because reasonable and adoptable recommendations provided to patients have a greater chance of being upheld rather than trying to institute all the recommendations for every patient.

Adequate Nutrients Within Calorie Needs

- Consume a variety of nutrient-dense foods and beverages within and among the basic food groups while choosing foods that limit the intake of saturated and trans fats, cholesterol, added sugars, salt, and alcohol.
- Meet recommended intakes within energy needs by adopting a balanced eating pattern, such as the USDA Food Guide or the DASH Eating Plan.
- People older than age 50 should consume vitamin B_{12} in its crystalline form (i.e., fortified foods or supplements).
- Women of childbearing age who may become pregnant should eat foods high in heme-iron or consume iron-rich plant foods with an enhancer of iron absorption, such as vitamin C–rich foods. This population should also consume adequate synthetic folic acid daily (from fortified foods or supplements) in addition to food forms of folate from a varied diet.
- Older adults, people with dark skin, and people exposed to insufficient ultraviolet band radiation (i.e., sunlight) should consume extra vitamin D from vitamin D–fortified foods or supplements.

Food Groups to Encourage

- Consume a sufficient amount of fruits and vegetables while staying within energy needs. Two cups of fruit and 2.5 cups of vegetables per day are recommended for a reference 2,000-calorie intake.

- Choose a variety of fruits and vegetables each day. In particular, select from all five vegetable subgroups (dark green, orange, legumes, starchy vegetables, and other vegetables) several times a week.
- Consume 3-ounce or more equivalents of whole grain products per day, with the rest of the recommended grains coming from enriched or whole grain products. In general, at least half of the grains should come from whole grains.
- Consume 3 cups per day of fat-free or low-fat milk or equivalent milk products.

Fats

- Consume less than 10% of calories from saturated fatty acids and less than 300 mg/day of cholesterol, and keep trans fatty acid consumption as low as possible.
- Keep total fat intake between 20 and 35% of calories, with most fats coming from sources of monounsaturated and polyunsaturated fatty acids, such as fish, nuts, and vegetable oils.
- When selecting and preparing meat, poultry, dry beans, and milk or milk products, make choices that are lean, low-fat, or fat-free.
- Limit intake of fats and oils high in saturated and trans fatty acids, and choose products low in such fats and oils.

Carbohydrates

- Choose fiber-rich fruits, vegetables, and whole grains often.
- Choose and prepare foods and beverages with little added sugars and caloric sweeteners, such as amounts suggested by the USDA Food Guide and the DASH Eating Plan.
- Reduce the incidence of dental caries by practicing good oral hygiene and consuming sugar- and starch-containing foods and beverages less frequently.

Sodium and Potassium

- Consume less than 2,300 mg (approximately 1 tsp of salt) of sodium per day.
- Choose and prepare foods with little salt. At the same time, consume potassium-rich foods such as fruits and vegetables.
- Individuals with hypertension, blacks, and middle-aged and older adults should aim to consume no more than 1,500 mg of sodium per day and meet the potassium recommendation (4,700 mg/day) with food.

Alcoholic Beverages

- Those who choose to drink alcoholic beverages should do so sensibly and in moderation, defined as the consumption of up to one drink per day for women and up to two drinks per day for men.

NUTRITIONAL APPLICATIONS

USDA Food Guide

In April 2005 the USDA released the newest food guidance plan called the MyPyramid Food Guidance System.[37] The MyPyramid plan is a fully interactive web-based system found at http://www.mypyramid.gov that is designed to make specific dietary recommendations based on individual characteristics. The system provides many options to help Americans make healthy food choices and to be active every day. The MyPyramid Food Guidance System is designed to implement the recommendations of the Dietary Guidelines for America 2005. It therefore makes the same key recommendations as those listed above in the discussion of the Dietary Guidelines. The advantage of the MyPyramid plan is that it is able to make specific dietary recommendations as to types and amounts of foods based on individual characteristics as well as suggest sample daily menus. The basic design of the MyPyramid plan is provided in Figure 1-1. A sample eating plan for a 2,000-calorie intake is provided in Table 1-8

Food Labeling and Consumer Nutrition

Most foods that we buy are required by law to have nutritional information printed on the package labeling. As a requirement, the nutritional information is to be printed in a specific and consistent manner so that two or more products can be compared with one another and an informed nutritional decision can be made as to the appropriateness of the food to a specific eating plan. Initial food labeling legislation was passed in 1973 but

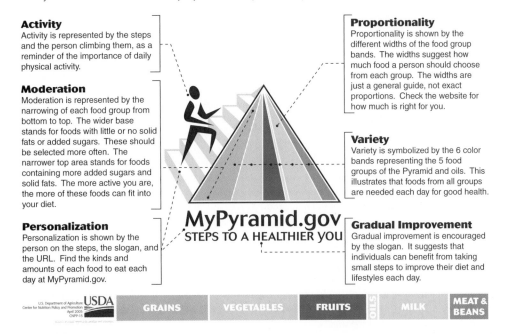

Anatomy of MyPyramid

One size doesn't fit all
USDA's new MyPyramid symbolizes a personalized approach to healthy eating and physical activity. The symbol has been designed to be simple. It has been developed to remind consumers to make healthy food choices and to be active every day. The different parts of the symbol are described below.

Activity
Activity is represented by the steps and the person climbing them, as a reminder of the importance of daily physical activity.

Moderation
Moderation is represented by the narrowing of each food group from bottom to top. The wider base stands for foods with little or no solid fats or added sugars. These should be selected more often. The narrower top area stands for foods containing more added sugars and solid fats. The more active you are, the more of these foods can fit into your diet.

Personalization
Personalization is shown by the person on the steps, the slogan, and the URL. Find the kinds and amounts of each food to eat each day at MyPyramid.gov.

Proportionality
Proportionality is shown by the different widths of the food group bands. The widths suggest how much food a person should choose from each group. The widths are just a general guide, not exact proportions. Check the website for how much is right for you.

Variety
Variety is symbolized by the 6 color bands representing the 5 food groups of the Pyramid and oils. This illustrates that foods from all groups are needed each day for good health.

Gradual Improvement
Gradual improvement is encouraged by the slogan. It suggests that individuals can benefit from taking small steps to improve their diet and lifestyles each day.

MyPyramid.gov
STEPS TO A HEALTHIER YOU

U.S. Department of Agriculture
Center for Nutrition Policy and Promotion
April 2005
CNPP-15
USDA

GRAINS   VEGETABLES   FRUITS   OILS   MILK   MEAT & BEANS

FIGURE 1–1   USDA MyPyramid Food Guidance System. (*Source:* U.S. Department of Agriculture. Center for Nutrition Policy and Nutrition. Anatomy of MyPyramid. April 2005. Available at: http://www.mypyramid.gov/downloads/MyPyramid_Anatomy.pdf. Accessed June 12, 2006.)

TABLE 1–8 USDA and DASH Eating Plan Recommendations

USDA Recommended Daily Amounts for a 2,000-Calorie per Day Intake		DASH Eating Plan Recommendations	
Food Group	Amount	Nutrient	Nutrient Target
Fruit[a]	2 cups	Fat (% of total kcal)	27%
		Saturated	6%
		Monounsaturated	13%
		Polyunsaturated	8%
Vegetables[b]	2.5 cups	Carbohydrates (% of total kcal)	55%
Grains[c]	6-oz equivalent	Protein (% of total kcal)	18%
Meat and beans[d]	5.5-oz equivalent	Cholesterol	150 mg/day
Milk[e]	3 cups	Fiber	31 g/day
Oils[f]	6 tsp	Potassium	4,700 mg/day
Discretionary calorie allowance[g]	267	Magnesium	500 mg/day
		Calcium	1,240 mg/day
		Sodium	1,500 mg/day

Sources: U.S. Department of Agriculture. MyPyramid.gov. Available at: http://www.mypyramid.gov. Accessed June 1, 2005. U.S. Department of Health and Human Services, National Institutes of Health. Facts about the DASH eating plan. Publication No. 03-4082. May 2003.

[a] Fruit group includes all fresh, frozen, canned, and dried fruits and fruit juices. In general, 1 cup of fruit or 100% fruit juice, or ½ cup of dried fruit can be considered as 1 cup from the fruit group.

[b] Vegetable group includes all fresh, frozen, canned, and dried vegetables and vegetable juices. In general, 1 cup of raw or cooked vegetables or vegetable juice, or 2 cups of raw leafy greens can be considered as 1 cup from the vegetable group.

[c] Grains group includes all foods made from wheat, rice, oats, cornmeal, and barley, such as bread, pasta, oatmeal, breakfast cereals, tortillas, and grits. In general, 1 slice of bread, 1 cup of ready-to-eat cereal, or ½ cup of cooked rice, pasta, or cooked cereal can be considered as 1-ounce equivalent from the grains group. At least half of all grains consumed should be whole grains.

[d] Meat and beans group. In general, 1 ounce of lean meat, poultry, or fish, 1 egg, 1 Tbsp. peanut butter, ¼ cup cooked dry beans, or ½ ounce of nuts or seeds can be considered as 1 ounce equivalent from the meat and beans group.

[e] Milk group includes all fluid milk products and foods made from milk that retain their calcium content, such as yogurt and cheese. Foods made from milk that have little to no calcium, such as cream cheese, cream, and butter, are not part of the group. Most milk group choices should be fat-free or low-fat. In general, 1 cup of milk or yogurt, 1½ ounces of natural cheese, or 2 ounces of processed cheese can be considered as 1 cup from the milk group.

[f] Oils include fats (from many different plants and from fish) that are liquid at room temperature, such as canola, corn, olive, soybean, and sunflower oil. Some foods are naturally high in oils, like nuts, olives, some fish, and avocados. Foods that are mainly oil include mayonnaise, certain salad dressings, and soft margarine.

[g] Discretionary calorie allowance is the remaining amount of calories in a food intake pattern after accounting for the calories needed for all food groups—using forms of foods that are fat-free or low-fat and with no added sugars.

then overhauled in 1990 with the passing of the Nutrition Labeling and Education Act.[6] The current food label, called "Nutrition Facts," is shown in Figure 1-2.

There are six basic sections to a "Nutrition Facts" label. Five of the six sections list specific information about the product, whereas the section at the bottom of the label does not change from food to food. Let's go through each section of the label and briefly explain the importance of each.[40]

Section 1: This section lists the serving size and the number of servings contained within the package and is the starting point when looking at a food label. Close attention should be made to the serving size because it affects the number of calories and all the nutrient amounts within the label. If a patient normally eats twice as much as the stated serving size, then the calories, nutrients, and percent daily value listed on the label need to be doubled.

Section 2: This section lists the total number of calories that are provided with each serving. In addition, it lists the number of calories that are supplied from fat. As we discussed earlier, it is recommended that 20 to 35% of total calories should come from fat. To calculate the number of fat calories in one serving, divide the calories for fat by the total calories and multiply by 100. For example if one serving contains 50 calories from

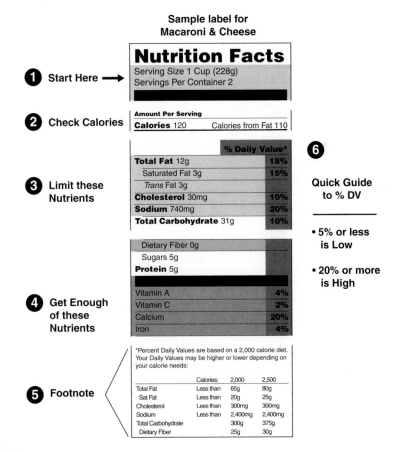

FIGURE 1–2   Food label: nutrition facts. *Source:* U.S. Department of Health and Human Services, U.S. Food and Drug Administration. Available at: http://www.cfsan.fda.gov/~dms/foodlab.html. Accessed July 27, 2006.

fat and the total number of calories is 160, the food consists of 31% fat calories (50/160 × 100 = 31.3%).

Sections 3 and 4: These sections combine to give the nutrient information about the product. Section 3 provides information about fats, cholesterol, and sodium. Americans generally consume enough or too much of these and they should therefore be limited in intake. Remember from earlier discussions that saturated fats should represent 10% or less of the total calories consumed. Even though the number of saturated fat calories is not provided, it can be easily calculated. Remember that 1 g of fat is equal to 9 calories of energy. To figure the number of calories that comes from saturated fat, simply multiply the grams of saturated fat by nine. Then use the same calculation as above to figure the percentage of saturated fat calories. The same can be done for monounsaturated and polyunsaturated fats. This same method can be used to figure the percentage of calories obtained from carbohydrates and proteins by multiplying the number of grams by four. As you may recall, 1 g each of carbohydrate and protein is equal to 4 calories.

To date there are no specific recommendations as to the amount of trans fatty acid one should consume. Therefore, the current recommendation is to limit the intake of trans fatty acid as much as possible.

Section 4 lists the nutrients that the typical American eating plan is deficient in or lacks in sufficient amounts. It is important to tell patients to pay close attention to this section as well to ensure that enough fiber, vitamins A and C, calcium, and iron are being consumed each day.

Sections 5 and 6: To the right of the label is listed the percent daily value (% Daily Value) of each of the nutrients. The percentages are based on a 2,000-calorie diet and, as stated above, will differ if more or less of the serving size is consumed. The % Daily Value helps to determine whether a serving of food is high or low in nutrient. In general, 5% Daily Value or less is considered low and 20% Daily Value or more is considered high. This generalization helps patients be good consumers so as to not get confused trying to remember specific amounts to eat or performing math calculations while comparing two products.

The bottom section of the label lists total amounts that should be consumed for a 2,000- or 2,500-calorie diet. This information does not change from label to label and for some packages that are small, it may not appear at all. Note, the daily value for some nutrients change as calories are increased, whereas others like cholesterol and sodium remain the same despite caloric intake. In addition, some nutrients like trans fat, sugars, and protein do not list a % Daily Value. These values are not listed for trans fat and sugar because no recommendations have been made for the total amount to eat each day. No value is provided for protein unless the food claims to be high in protein. Current scientific evidence suggests that protein is not a public health concern for adults and children older than 4 years of age.

More examples of food labels are provided in Figure 1-3 comparing two different types of milk. These two labels compare reduced-fat milk with non-fat milk. Note the amount of calories, total fat, and saturated fat listed on each label. Also note the amount of calcium listed on each label. Which type of milk provides adequate calcium intake but with fewer calories and less saturated fat?

Counting Calories

It is difficult for most individuals to count their daily calorie intake. Realistically, most people do not know how many calories they consume in the course of a day. It is dif-

REDUCED-FAT MILK
2% Milkfat

Nutrition Facts
Serving Size 1 Cup (236ml)
Servings Per Container 1

Amount Per Serving

Calories 120   Calories from Fat 45

% Daily Value*

Total Fat 5g	**8%**
Saturated Fat 3g	**15%**
Trans Fat 0g	
Cholesterol 20mg	**7%**
Sodium 120mg	**5%**
Total Carbohydrate 11g	**4%**
Dietary Fiber 0g	**0%**
Sugars 11g	
Protein 9g	**17%**

Vitamin A 10%   •   Vitamin C 4%
Calcium 30% • Iron 0% •Vitamin D 25%

*Percent Daily Values are based on a 2,000
calorie diet. Your daily values may be higher
or lower depending on your calorie needs:

NON-FAT MILK

Nutrition Facts
Serving Size 1 Cup (236ml)
Servings Per Container 1

Amount Per Serving

Calories 80   Calories from Fat 0

% Daily Value*

Total Fat 0g	**0%**
Saturated Fat 0g	**0%**
Trans Fat 0g	
Cholesterol Less than 5mg	**0%**
Sodium 120mg	**5%**
Total Carbohydrate 11g	**4%**
Dietary Fiber 0g	**0%**
Sugars 11g	
Protein 9g	**17%**

Vitamin A 10%   •   Vitamin C 4%
Calcium 30% • Iron 0% •Vitamin D 25%

*Percent Daily Values are based on a 2,000
calorie diet. Your daily values may be higher
or lower depending on your calorie needs:

FIGURE 1–3   Comparing milk labels. (*Source:* U.S. Department of Health and Human Services, U.S. Food and Drug Administration, Center for Food Safety and Applied Nutrition. How to understand and use the nutrition facts label. June 2000; updated July 2003 and November 2004. Available at: http://www.cfsan.fda.gov/~dms/foodlab.html. Accessed June 12, 2006.)

ficult, time consuming, and most likely not very accurate to try to add total calories, fat calories, grams of fiber, and so forth from labels of all that you consume each day. The main objective to counting calories is to capture a representative sample of all that is eaten during the course of several days. By doing this, eating patterns and trends can be discovered as well as knowing whether all the essential nutrients are consumed in adequate amounts. This process can also look at the intake of discretionary calories. Knowing this information can allow for specific recommendations to be made to patients based on their individual eating habits. Again, this is not realistic to do by hand, but fortunately there are several computer programs now available to assist in this process. Many of them can be purchased, but some are online and free of charge.

The USDA website www.mypyramidtracker.gov offers a free dietary tracking system called MyPyramid Tracker.[41] In addition to being an online dietary assessment tool, it also provides physical activity assessments, information on diet quality, physical activity status, related nutrition messages, and links to nutrient and physical activity information. The Food Calories/Energy Balance feature automatically calculates energy balance by subtracting the energy expended as a result of physical activity from food calories or energy intake. Use of this tool can help patients and healthcare professionals better understand energy balance status and enhance the link between good nutrition and regular physical activity. In addition, MyPyramid Tracker translates the principles of the Dietary Guidelines for Americans 2005 and other nutrition standards developed by the U.S. Departments of Agriculture and Health and Human Services.

Dark Chocolate and Disease Prevention

In recent years, foods that contain antioxidant vitamins and flavonoids have been linked with the prevention of cardiovascular disease. Flavonoids are polyphenolic compounds found abundantly in cocoa and to a slightly lesser extent in green tea, red wine, and apples. More particularly, the flavonoid found in dark chocolate has been linked to decreases in blood pressure, improvements in **endothelial dysfunction** that promote vascular homeostasis, improvements in antiplatelet activity, improvements in insulin sensitivity, increases in **high-density lipoprotein (HDL)** cholesterol concentrations, improvements in cognitive function, and antioxidant properties. Dark chocolate contains more flavonoids compared with milk chocolate and white chocolate because it contains more cocoa. The addition of milk to lighter colored chocolates inhibits flavonoid absorption, and a process called "dutching" to make chocolate less bitter destroys flavonoids.[42–44]

One study showed that 13 men and women between 55 and 64 years of age with mild isolated systolic hypertension who consumed 100 g of dark chocolate each day for 14 days experienced systolic and diastolic blood pressure decreases of 5.1 and 1.8 mm Hg, respectively, compared with those consuming 90 g of white chocolate daily for 14 days.[45] Additionally, another study using the same dark and white chocolate dosing as above for a period of 15 days in healthy volunteers showed that those ingesting the dark chocolate experienced significantly better insulin sensitivity ($P < 0.001$) and systolic blood pressure lowering ($P < 0.05$) compared with those ingesting white chocolate.[46] Other studies have shown that arterial stiffness and the force that the heart pushes against when ejecting blood are significantly improved after 1 day of eating 100 g of dark chocolate. This shows that there are improvements to the cardiovascular system after eating the flavonoids contained in dark chocolate.[43]

Although the future looks bright for the health benefits of eating dark chocolate, we should still caution our patients about its consumption. More studies need to be completed on large groups of people with and without heart disease to confirm preliminary published results. Other aspects to consider are that the ideal amount of flavonoids to elicit positive health responses has not been established, and the amount of flavonoid contained in each product is not currently being reported. In addition, we should still caution our patients that a significant amount of calories can be consumed by eating chocolate and this needs to be taken into consideration to maintain a healthy body weight. Lastly, dark chocolate may offer some very positive health benefits and be an excellent alternative for those with a sweet tooth who can afford the intake of discretionary calories.

ALCOHOL AND DISEASE PREVENTION

As previously stated, alcoholic beverages supply calories (7 kcal/g) but have few essential nutrients.[4] Therefore, consuming large quantities of alcohol can contribute to either excess weight gain, if food calorie intake remains the same, or malnutrition, if alcohol consumption is substituted for food consumption. The current recommendation for American adults on alcohol consumption is to do so in moderation.[4] Moderation is defined as the consumption of up to one drink per day for women and up to two drinks per day for men.[4] One drink is defined as 12 fluid ounces of regular beer, 5 fluid ounces of wine, or 1.5 fluid ounces of 80-proof distilled spirits. The definition of moderation is not intended as an average over several days, but rather the amount consumed on any single day.[4]

The effect of alcohol consumption varies depending on the amount consumed as well as on individual characteristics and circumstances.[4] Alcohol can be harmful if consumed in excess. Specifically, alcohol can alter judgment, lead to dependency or addiction, cause cirrhosis of the liver or inflammation of the pancreas, and damage the heart and brain. Consuming alcohol in amounts greater than moderate levels has been linked to increases in motor vehicle accidents and other injuries, violence, certain cancers (including breast cancer in women), stroke, and high blood pressure. The national treatment guidelines for high blood pressure (JNC 7) recommends that alcohol be consumed in moderation, as high blood pressure positively correlates with alcohol use.[3] A patient with high blood pressure who regularly consumes alcohol in amounts greater than moderation can decrease systolic blood pressure 2 to 4 mm Hg by limiting consumption to the recommended moderate levels.[4]

In addition, excessive alcohol consumption can lead to weight gain. The calorie intake for alcohol varies depending on the source. Twelve ounces of regular beer is equal to approximately 144 calories whereas light beer has about 108 calories for the same amount. Five ounces of white wine has approximately 100 calories and red wine has approximately 105 calories, whereas only 3 ounces of sweet dessert wine has 141 calories. Distilled spirits such as gin, rum, vodka, and whiskey at 80 proof have about 96 calories per 1.5 ounces.[4]

Moderate alcohol consumption has been linked to beneficial health effects in some individuals. Studies have shown that middle-aged and older adults who drink one to two alcoholic beverages per day or less have a lower relative risk for all-cause mortality compared with those of the same age who do not drink alcohol.[4,18,19] Light to moderate alcohol consumption has also been shown to decrease the risk for coronary heart disease and stroke, which are major contributors to all-cause mortality.[19] The mechanisms that explain these positive effects are not completely known, but several theories exist. The theories that have been presented to explain the positive effects of alcohol consumption include the following:[6,19]

- Decreases stress by having a relaxation effect
- Decreases the ability of platelets to stick together or clot by increasing the activity of the clot-dissolving enzyme in the blood
- Increases blood flow to the brain, which decreases certain brain diseases and stroke risk
- Improves insulin sensitivity
- Increases HDL cholesterol, or the good cholesterol, levels in the body
- Suppresses inflammatory markers
- Contains polyphenols and other phytochemicals (especially red wine), which can increase HDL cholesterol, have antioxidant activity, decrease platelet clotting, and promote vasodilation

The most widely reported theory regarding the benefits of alcohol consumption centers around its reported effect of increasing HDL cholesterol. The mechanism to explain this effect, however, has yet to be elucidated. In addition, red wine has received much attention regarding its proposed positive effects on health. Likewise, the mechanisms that explain these effects are yet to be discovered, but it is now thought that many of the cardiovascular benefits are primarily related to ethanol itself, regardless of the source.[19]

Some researchers in the health professions believe that alcohol consumption itself does not cause these positive health effects. Rather, it has been shown that adults who consume moderate amounts of alcohol are more likely to engage in lifestyle activities and have other social characteristics that promote positive health benefits compared with adults who do not drink.[20,21] For example, one study showed that adults who drink a moderate amount of alcohol are more likely to engage in leisure time physical activity.[20] Another study found that adults who abstain from drinking alcohol were more likely to be older, unemployed, have a lower income, lack health insurance, have diabetes, require medical equipment, and have a greater cardiovascular disease risk score compared with those who drink moderate amounts of alcohol.[21] All of these factors have independently been shown to be associated with poor health outcomes.[21] Therefore, it is unknown whether moderate alcohol consumption has a direct and positive effect on health or whether those who drink moderate levels of alcohol possess characteristics that promote health regardless of alcohol consumption.

Throughout this book we will talk about several strategies to promote health and reduce the risk of chronic diseases such as proper nutrition, as discussed in this chapter, physical activity, maintaining a healthy body weight, and smoking cessation. Current guidelines with regard to alcohol consumption state that it is not recommended that anyone begin drinking or drink more frequently on the basis of obtaining positive health benefits as discussed above.[4]

REFERENCES

1. Healthy People. Available at: http://www.healthypeople.gov/. Accessed June 1, 2005.
2. Centers for Disease and Prevention. Chronic disease prevention. Available at: http://www.cdc.gov/nccdphp/. Accessed June 1, 2005.
3. Chobanian AV, Bakris GL, Black HR, et al. Seventh report of the Joint National Committee on Prevention, Detection, Evaluation, and Treatment of High Blood Pressure. Hypertension 2003;42:1206–1252.
4. HHS Publication No. HHS-ODPHP-2005-01-DGA-A, Dietary Guidelines for Americans 2005, U.S. Department of Health and Human Services, U.S. Department of Agriculture. Available at: http://healthierus.gov/dietaryguidelines. Accessed February 6, 2007.
5. Hodgson SF, Watts NB, Bilezikian JP, et al. American Association of Clinical Endocrinologists medical guidelines for clinical practice for the prevention and treatment of postmenopausal osteoporosis: 2001 edition, with selected updates for 2003. Endocr Pract 2003;9:544–564.
6. Williams MH. Nutrition for Health, Nutrition and Sport, 7th ed. Boston: McGraw-Hill, 2005.
7. Hargreaves M. Skeletal muscle metabolism during exercise in humans. Clin Exp Pharmacol Psychol 2000; 27:225–228.
8. de Jonge L, Bray GA. The thermic effect of food and obesity. Obes Res 1997;5:622–631.
9. Brooks, GA, Butte NF, Rand WM, Flat JP, Caballero B. Chronicle of the Institute of Medicine physical activity recommendation: how a physical activity recommendation came to be among dietary recommendations. Am J Clin Nutr 2004;79:921S–930S.
10. U.S. Department of Health and Human Services, U.S. Department of Agriculture. My Pyramid. Available at: http://www.mypyramid.gov/professionals/pdf_calorie_levels.html. Accessed June 1, 2005.
11. National Institutes of Health, National Heart, Lung, and Blood Institute. Third report of the National Cholesterol Education Program (NCEP) Expert Panel on Detection, Evaluation, and Treatment of High Blood Cholesterol in Adults (Adult Treatment Panel III). NIH Publication No. 02-5215, September 2002.
12. American Heart Association. Available at: http://www.deliciousdecisions.org/. American Heart Association, 2002. Accessed June 1, 2005.
13. Mensink RP, Katan MB. Effects of dietary fatty acids on serum lipids and lipoproteins: a meta-analysis of 27 trails. Arterioscler Thromb 1992;12:911–919.
14. Willett WC, Stampfer MJ, Manson JE, et al. Intake of trans fatty acids and risk of coronary heart disease among women. Lancet 1993;341:581–585.
15. Pietinen P, Ascherio A, Korhonen P, et al. Intake of fatty acids and risk of coronary heart disease in a cohort of Finnish men: the Alpha-Tocopherol, Beta-Carotene Cancer Prevention Study. Am J Epidemiol 1997; 145:876–887.
16. Hu FB, Stampfer MJ, Manson JE, et al. Dietary saturated fats and their food sources in relation to the risk of coronary heart disease in women. Am J Clin Nutr 1999;70:1001–1008.

17. Kromhout D, Menotti A, Bloemberg B, et al. Dietary saturated and trans fatty acids and cholesterol and 25 year mortality from coronary heart disease: the Seven Countries Study. Prev Med 1995;24:308–315.
18. Holman CD, English DR, Milne E, Winter MG. Meta-analysis of alcohol and all-cause mortality. Med J Aust 1996;164:141–145.
19. Giles TD, Sander GE. Alcohol—a cardiovascular drug? Am J Geriatr Cardiol 2005;14:154–158.
20. Smothers B, Bertolucci D. Alcohol consumption and health-promoting behavior in a U.S. household sample: leisure time physical activity. J Stud Alcohol 2001;62:467–476.
21. Niami TS, Brown DW, Brewer RD, et al. Cardiovascular risk factors and confounders among nondrinking and moderate-drinking U.S. adults. Am J Prev Med 2005;28:369–373.
22. Lichtenstein AH, Ausman LM, Jalbert SM, Schaefer EJ. Effects of different forms of dietary hydrogenated fats on serum lipoprotein cholesterol levels. N Engl J Med 1999;340:1933–1940.
23. Judd JT, Clevidence BA, Muesing RA, Wittes J, Sunkin ME, Podczasy JJ. Dietary trans fatty acids: effects of plasma lipids and lipoproteins of healthy men and women. Am J Clin Nutr 1994;59:861–868.
24. Judd JT, Baer DJ, Clevidence BA, et al. Effects of margarine compared with those of butter on blood lipid profiles related to cardiovascular disease risk factors in normolipemic adults fed controlled diets. Am J Clin Nutr 1998;68:768–777.
25. Noakes M, Clifton PM. Oil blends containing partially hydrogenated or interesterified fats: differential effects on plasma lipids. Am J Clin Nutr 1998;68:242–247.
26. Aro A, Jauhiainen M, Partanen R, Salminen I, Mutanen M. Stearic acid, trans-fatty acids, and dairy fat: effects on serum and lipoprotein lipids, apolipoproteins, lipoprotein (a), and lipid transfer proteins in healthy subjects. Am J Clin Nutr 1997;65:1419–1426.
27. Almendingen K, Jordal O, Kierulf P, Sandstad B, Pedersen JI. Effects of partially hydrogenated fish oil, partially hydrogenated soybean oil, and butter on serum lipoproteins and Lp[a] in men. J Lipid Res 1995;36:1370–1384.
28. Wood R, Kubena K, O'Brien B, Tseng S, Martin G. Effect of butter, mono- and polyunsaturated fatty acid-enriched butter, trans-fatty acid margarine on serum lipids and lipoproteins in healthy men. J Lipid Res 1993;34:1–11.
29. Wood R, Kubena K, Tseng S, Martin G, Crook R. Effect of palm oil, margarine, butter, and sunflower oil on the serum lipids and lipoproteins of normocholesterolemic middle-aged men. J Nutr Biochem 1993;4:286–297.
30. Nestel PJ, Noakes M, Belling GB, McArthur R, Clifton PM, Abbey M. Plasma cholesterol lowering potential of edible-oil blends suitable for commercial use. Am J Clin Nutr 1992;55:46–50.
31. Zock PL, Katan MB. Hydrogenation alternatives: effects of trans fatty acids and stearic acid versus linoleic acid on serum lipids and lipoproteins in humans. J Lipid Res 1992;33:399–410.
32. Tippett KS, Cleveland LE. How current diets stack up: comparison of dietary guidelines. In: America's Eating Habits: Changes and Consequences. Washington, D.C.: U.S. Department of Agriculture, Economic Research Service, 1999:51–70.
33. Putnam J, Gerrior S. Trends in the U.S. food supply, 1970–1997. In: America's Eating Habits: Changes and Consequences. Washington, D.C.: U.S. Department of Agriculture, Economic Research Service, 1999:133–160.
34. Grundy SM, Barrett-Conner E, Rudel LL, Miettinen T, Spector AA. Workshop on the impact of dietary cholesterol on plasma lipoproteins and atherogenesis. Arteriosclerosis 1988;8:95–101.
35. National Research Council. Diet and Health: Implications for Reducing Chronic Disease Risk. Washington, D.C.: National Academy Press, 1989:171–201.
36. American College of Sports Medicine. Position stand on exercise and fluid replacement. Med Sci Sports Exerc 1996;28:i–vii.
37. U.S. Department of Agriculture. MyPyramid.gov. Available at: http://www.mypyramid.gov. Accessed June 1, 2005.
38. Sacks FM, Svetkey LP, Vollmer WM, et al. Effects on blood pressure of reduced dietary sodium and the dietary approaches to stop hypertension (DASH) diet. N Engl J Med 2001;344:3–10.
39. U.S. Department of Health and Human Services, National Institutes of Health. Facts about the DASH eating plan. Publication No. 03-4082, May 2003.
40. U.S. Food and Drug Administration, Center for Food Safety and Applied Nutrition. Available at: http://www.cfsan.fda.gov. Accessed June 1, 2005.
41. U.S. Department of Agriculture. MyPyramidTracker. Available at: http://mypyramidtracker.gov. Accessed June 1, 2005.
42. Katan MB, Zock, Mensink RP. Trans fatty acids and their effects on lipoproteins in humans. Ann Rev Nutr 1995;15:473–493.
43. Mensink RP, Katan MB. Effects of dietary trans fatty acids on high density and low density lipoprotein cholesterol levels in healthy subjects. N Engl J Med 1990;323:439–445.
44. Lichtenstein AH, Ausman LM, Carrasco W, Jenner JL, Ordovas JM, Schaefer EJ. Hydrogenation impairs the hypolipidemic effect of corn oil in humans: hydrogenation, trans fatty acids, and plasma lipids. Arterioscler Thromb 1993;13:154–161.

45. U.S. Food and Drug Administration. FDA Talk Paper. FDA authorizes new coronary heart disease health claim for plant sterol and plant stanol esters. September 5, 2000. Available at: http://www.fda.gov/bbs/topics/ANSWERS/ANS01033.html. Accessed February 6, 2007.

46. Steinberg FM, Bearden MM, Keen CL. Cocoa and chocolate flavonoids: implications for cardiovascular health. J Am Diet Assoc 2003;103:2215–2223.

47. Jeffery S. Chocolate, cocoa have positive acute effects on endothelial function. Available at: http://www.theheart.org/. May 21, 2004. Accessed May 16, 2005.

48. Rommelfanger J. Dark chocolate lowers blood pressure and reverses endothelial dysfunction. Available at: http://www.theheart.org/. August 27, 2003. Accessed May 16, 2005.

49. Taubert D, Berkels R, Roesen R, Klaus W. Chocolate and blood pressure in elderly individuals with isolated systolic hypertension. JAMA 2003;290:1029–1030.

50. Grassi D, Lippi C, Necozione S, Desideri G, Ferri C. Short-term administration of dark chocolate is followed by a significant increase in insulin sensitivity and a decrease in blood pressure in healthy persons. Am J Clin Nutr 2005;81:611–614.

CHAPTER 2

Physical Activity

OBJECTIVES

At the end of this chapter the reader should be able to:

1. Recall the importance of physical activity as it relates to health benefits and disease prevention.
2. Define the components of physical activity.
3. Explain the principles of an exercise prescription.
4. Develop an exercise prescription for a patient.
5. Calculate the energy expenditure of various types of physical activity.

The benefits of physical activity have been touted throughout history, but it was not until the 1950s that scientific evidence began to support these beliefs.[1] Early studies examined whether physical activity protected against **cardiovascular disease** for those people who performed intense physical activity in their jobs.[2] By the 1970s, enough information was available about the benefits of physical activity that the American College of Sports Medicine (ACSM, http://www.acsm.org), the American Heart Association (AHA, http://www.americanheart.org) and other national organizations began issuing physical activity recommendations to the public.[1]

Physical activity is defined as any bodily movement produced by skeletal muscles that results in the expenditure of energy.[1] Physical activity can be obtained in several ways, such as through one's job by hauling, lifting, pushing, and walking or through leisure-time activities such as sports, recreation, and hobbies. In addition, physical activity can be obtained from transportation activities such as walking, biking, or wheeling (for wheelchair users) to and from places such as work, school, place of worship, and stores.[1] It can also be obtained through household activities such as sweeping floors, washing windows, raking and mowing the lawn, and gardening.[1] **Physical inactivity** is defined as a lack of any regular pattern of physical activity beyond that required for daily functioning.[1]

Exercise is defined as physical activity that is planned or structured.[1] It involves repetitive bodily movements done to improve or maintain one or more of the components of **physical fitness:** cardiorespiratory endurance (aerobic fitness), muscular strength, muscular endurance, flexibility, and body composition.[1] **Cardiorespiratory endurance** (also called aerobic endurance or aerobic fitness) is the ability of the body's circulatory and respiratory systems to supply fuel and oxygen during sustained physical activity.[1] **Muscular strength** is the ability of the muscle to exert force during an activity. **Muscular endurance** is the ability of the muscle to continue to perform without fatigue. **Flexibility** is the range of motion around the joint. **Body composition** is the relative amount of muscle, fat, bone, and other vital parts of the body.[1] Body composition is important when considering overall health and managing body weight as it relates to overweight and obesity.

HEALTH BENEFITS OF REGULAR PHYSICAL ACTIVITY

Participating in regular physical activity can bring about many health benefits. Those who engage in a regular amount of moderate to vigorous intensity physical activity benefit by lowering their risk for developing coronary artery disease, **stroke, type 2 diabetes mellitus,** high blood pressure, colon cancer, and mental disorders such as anxiety and depression.[1,3] In addition, active individuals have lower premature death rates compared with those who are the least active. Engaging in physical activity, even when it begins later in life, can have a significant impact on lowering cardiovascular risks.[4] Therefore, enhancing the amount of physical activity can begin at any age. Table 2-1 lists several benefits of engaging in regular physical activity.

PHYSICAL ACTIVITY AND DISEASE PREVENTION

Regular physical activity has been shown to reduce the morbidity and mortality rates associated with many chronic diseases. Approximately 90 million Americans suffer from chronic illnesses.[5] Many of these illnesses such as **coronary heart disease, diabetes, obesity,** arthritis, **osteoporosis,** colon cancer, **hypertension,** and hyperlipidemia can be prevented or improved through regular physical activity.[5] Despite the benefits of regular physical activity, most adults and many children lead a relatively sedentary lifestyle and are not able to achieve these health benefits (Fig. 2-1).[5–11] As a result, individuals who are physically inactive are considered in many disease state treatment guidelines to have a risk factor for coronary heart disease. Therefore, increasing physical activity and physical fitness levels should be a priority for Americans of all ages.

A population who is physically inactive is not only at risk for several medical conditions, but is at a financial risk as well. For example, in 2000 the total cost associated with overweight and obesity was estimated to be $117 billion.[12] Other illnesses such as heart disease, cancer, diabetes, and arthritis cost an estimated $183, $157, $100, and $65 billion, respectively, in 2000.[12] One study found that obese individuals spend approximately 36% more than the general population on health services and 77% more on medications.[13] In addition, this same study found that the effects of obesity on spending were significantly larger than the effects of current or past smoking. Therefore, because regular physical activity helps prevent disease and promote health, it may actually decrease healthcare costs.

TABLE 2–1   **Health Benefits of Regular Physical Activity**

Reduces the risk of developing CHD	Reduces the risk of developing colon cancer and breast cancer
Reduces the risk of dying prematurely of CHD and other conditions	Helps people achieve and maintain a healthy body weight
Reduces the risk of stroke	Reduces the feelings of depression and anxiety
Reduces the risk of having a second heart attack in people who have already had one heart attack	Promotes psychological well-being and reduces feelings of stress
Lowers both total blood cholesterol and triglycerides and increases HDL	Helps build and maintain healthy bones, muscles, and joints
Lowers the risk of developing high blood pressure	Helps older adults become stronger and better able to move about without falling or becoming excessively fatigued
Helps reduce high blood pressure in people who already have hypertension	Improves health-related quality of life
Lowers the risk of developing type 2 diabetes mellitus	

Source: U.S. Department of Health and Human Services. Physical activity and health: a report of the Surgeon General. Atlanta: U.S. Department of Health and Human Services, Centers for Disease Control and Prevention, National Center for Chronic Disease Prevention and Health Promotion, 1996.

CHD, coronary heart disease; HDL, high-density lipoproteins.

Because physical inactivity is a risk factor for many diseases and conditions, making physical activity a priority in one's daily routine is critical. It is important to understand that physical activity need not be strenuous or be sustained for long periods to be beneficial. Moderate-intensity activity performed in short frequent bursts of 10 minutes or longer can yield health benefits. This concept will be covered in more detail later in this chapter. Promoting the benefits of physical activity to patients, including those who are physically challenged, should be an important part of patient care activities for all healthcare professionals, including pharmacists.

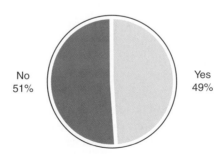

No
51%

Yes
49%

FIGURE 2–1   Percentage of U.S. adults participating in U.S. Surgeon General's recommended amounts of physical activity in 2005. (*Source:* Centers for Disease Control and Prevention, National Center for Chronic Disease Prevention and Health Promotion. Behavioral Risk Factor Surveillance System. Physical Activity—2005. Available at: http://apps.nccd.cdc.gov/brfss/list.asp?cat=PA&yr=2005&qkey=4418&state=All. Accessed June 14, 2006.)

BASIC EXERCISE PHYSIOLOGY

Exercise physiology is a subspecialty within the science of physiology that specifically looks at how organs, tissues, and cells in the body function as they relate to physical movement. In particular, exercise physiology focuses on energy transfer and the body's adaptation to training.[14] Understanding the physiology involved when patients perform physical activity and its impact on overall health is important for healthcare professionals as they talk with their patients about exercise.

Energy

Energy is defined as the ability to perform work and is revealed only when change takes place, like change in body position as a result of physical activity.[14] We receive energy to perform work through caloric intake from the food we eat. The energy in food is not transferred directly to the cells for biologic work. Rather, this "nutrient energy" is harvested and funneled through the energy-rich compound **adenosine triphosphate,** or ATP.[14] About 40% of the potential energy in food nutrients is transferred to the compound ATP.[14] When the terminal phosphate bond of the ATP is broken, the free energy that is liberated is harnessed and used to power all forms of biologic work. Therefore, ATP is considered the body's energy source.[14]

The major energy pathway for ATP used during physical activity differs depending on the intensity and duration of the activity. Those that are high in intensity and short in duration, such as sprinting and weight lifting, derive energy from the already present stores of intramuscular ATP and CP (creatine phosphate).[14] This energy source is often referred to as the immediate energy system. Activity that is high in intensity and long in duration, such as 1- to 2-minute activities like a 400-m or 800-m run or 100-m swim, generates energy from anaerobic reactions of glycolysis.[14] This energy source is referred to as the short-term energy system. Finally, activities that are low in intensity and long in duration such as walking, jogging, cycling, and mowing the yard generate energy from the aerobic system.[14] Oxygen consumption during activities such as these becomes an important factor in the process of ATP resynthesis. This system is called aerobic metabolism and is also referred to as the long-term energy system.[14] The aerobic system and its associated types of activities will be the focus of our discussions as it will be the energy system used by the majority of our patients.

Oxygen Consumption

Oxygen consumption is the process in which the body takes in oxygen and uses it to move the muscles during activity, especially aerobic activity.[14] As physical activity workload (measured as exercise intensity) increases, the body requires greater amounts of oxygen consumption to maintain that level of workload. At some point during a gradual increase in exercise intensity, an individual will reach a physiologic plateau of oxygen consumption. This oxygen consumption plateau is called **maximal oxygen consumption, maximal oxygen uptake, maximal aerobic power,** or simply **max $\dot{V}o_2$.**[14] Maximal oxygen consumption is assumed to be the individual's capacity for aerobic resynthesis of ATP. The measurement of an individual's max $\dot{V}o_2$ determines that person's ability to sustain a relatively high-intensity exercise.[14] Maximal oxygen consumption can be increased by participating in physical activity. This is what happens when we say we are "getting in shape."

It is not practical or even necessary to measure a patient's maximal oxygen consumption in the pharmacy setting. It is important, however, to understand the concept of oxygen consumption when placing individuals on an exercise program because it aids in the understanding and rationale behind "exercise intensity" and "exercise progression" as components of an exercise prescription. In most cases, we will not be counseling patients to improve their maximal oxygen consumption to the point of running a marathon. We can, however, apply this concept to sedentary individuals to improve physical functioning with daily activities. For example, modest improvements in oxygen consumption for a sedentary elderly individual may allow this person to effectively walk in a grocery store or take a walk in a park. Likewise, increasing the oxygen consumption of a sedentary parent with young children may allow that parent to actively play with his or her children outside in the yard. Specific activities designed to improve oxygen consumption will be provided later in this chapter.

COMPONENTS OF PHYSICAL ACTIVITY

Several components can be included in physical activity. These components include the following:[15]

- Warm-up
- Cool-down
- Aerobic conditioning
- Resistance training
- Stretching activities

It is important to understand that participation in all the components of physical activity is not necessary to gain health benefits. Likewise, an improvement in maximal oxygen consumption is also not necessary to gain health benefits and reduce the risks for disease.[15] The idea behind increasing physical activity is to "move more and sit less." In other words, any increases in physical movements that require energy expenditure are better than being sedentary. This concept applies to those individuals who are physically challenged as well. For example, individuals confined to a wheelchair can participate in aerobic conditioning, resistance training, and stretching activities that involve the upper body.

In addition to the activities listed above, it is also important to participate in recreational type activities such as tennis, basketball, and racquetball as well as leisure activities such as golf and bowling.[1,15] Household physical activities such as sweeping floors, scrubbing, washing windows, and raking and mowing the lawn are also activities that contribute to daily energy expenditures.[15] Also, incorporating ways to increase the number of steps taken each day in our daily activities is another good way to increase energy expenditure and has been shown to improve overall health. Examples of these types of activities are walking the dog, taking the stairs instead of the elevator, and parking the car farther away from one's destination and walking. These are all example of increasing the number of steps taken each day. Figure 2-2 is an exercise paradigm depicting components of physical activity and the relative amounts each individual should strive to obtain each week.[15,16]

Warm-up and Cool-Down

A warm-up before participating in physical activity is important to transition the body from rest to exercise, augment blood flow, increase metabolic rate, and stretch muscles.[15] It also decreases the susceptibility to injury and can enhance physical activity performance.[15] It is recommended that physical activity begin with 5 to 10 minutes of low-intensity stretching exercises of the major muscle groups followed by 5 to 10 minutes of progressive low-intensity aerobic activity sufficient to raise the heart rate above that of resting.[15] For example, individuals who choose brisk walking as their form of

Sparingly	2 – 3 Days/Wk	2 – 3 Days/Wk	3 – 5 Days/Wk	5+ Days/Wk	Every Day

Sedentary activities
- Sitting watching TV
- Playing video games
- Sitting at a computer

Leisure activities
- Golf
- Bowling
- Dance
- Ride bicycle
- Play frisbee
- Play catch/fetch with children/pets

Resistance Training/Stretching
- Lift weights at a health club
- Lift household items (e.g., soup cans, laundry detergent bottles)
- Use resistance bands
- Stretch all major muscle groups

Recreational Activities
- Play basketball, tennis, softball
- Ride bicycle
- Swim
- Canoe
- Ride horses

Aerobics Activities
- Walk
- Jog
- Ride bicycle
- Swim
- Exercise on stationary equipment

Daily Activities
- Walk, cycle, or jog to work, school, or the store
- Park farther away from your destination
- Take stairs instead of elevator
- Play with children and pets
- Household chores

FIGURE 2–2 Physical activity paradigm. (Adapted from ACSM Guidelines and Food Guide Pyramid. Available at: http://www.mypyramid.gov/.)

34

physical activity may begin with a warm-up period of slow walking. Likewise, brisk walking may serve as a good warm-up activity for jogging or running.

The cool-down period after physical activity provides a gradual return of the heart rate, blood pressure, blood circulation, and respiration to the preexercise state.[15] It reduces the potential for postexercise hypotension and dizziness, facilitates the dissipation of body heat, and reduces the risks of cardiovascular complications after exercise in those patients with heart disease.[15] Recommendations for the cool-down period are the same as those in the warm-up period but done so in the reverse order. That is, 5 to 10 minutes or longer of low-intensity physical activity followed by 5 to 10 minutes of stretching exercises of the major muscle groups.[15] Stretching exercises may be easier and more effective when done in the cool-down phase as compared with the warm-up phase.

Aerobic Conditioning

Current recommendations by the Centers for Disease Control and Prevention (CDC, http://www.cdc.gov) and the ACSM state that individuals who are currently not engaging in regular physical activity should begin by incorporating a few minutes of physical activity into each day, gradually building up to 30 minutes or more of accumulated moderate-intensity activities on most days of the week.[15,17] Individuals who are currently active but at less than recommended levels should adopt a more consistent activity pattern to include moderate-intensity physical activity for 30 minutes or more on 5 or more days of the week or vigorous-intensity physical activity for 20 minutes or more on 3 or more days of the week.[15,17] Those currently engaged in moderate-intensity activities for at least 30 minutes on 5 or more days of the week may achieve even greater health benefits by increasing the time spent or intensity of those activities.[15,17] Individuals who are currently engaging in vigorous-intensity activities for at least 20 minutes or more on 3 or more days per week are encouraged to continue this pattern of physical activity.[15,17] Explanations and examples of light-, moderate-, and vigorous-intensity physical activity will be provided later in this chapter.

Pedometers

Pedometers are becoming a popular device used to measure the accumulated step count of the wearer. They are worn on the hip and can measure the number of steps taken during a particular activity, or for a full day or full week. Most pedometers can also be set to measure distance as well as total calories expended by entering stride length and body weight, respectively.

An accumulated count of 10,000 steps per day has been widely publicized by the media as the goal step count for everyone. The 10,000 steps per day idea can be traced back to Japanese walking clubs and a business slogan used more than 30 years ago.[18] Initially, the idea of 10,000 steps per day had no scientific basis. Recently, however, studies have been published to look at the relationship between accumulating 10,000 steps per day and achieving the current recommendations for physical activity by the CDC, ACSM, and the Surgeon General of the United States.[19] One study suggests that individuals who accumulate 10,000 steps per day are more likely to meet the recommendations of accumulating at least 30 minutes of moderate-intensity physical activity on most days of the week.[19] It has previously been shown that exercise bout lengths should be at least 10 minutes long; however, this study showed that accumulating

10,000 steps per day does not guarantee meeting this current recommendation.[15,17] Additionally, another review of the literature showed that 10,000 steps per day may not be sustainable for some groups, including older adults and those with chronic diseases, and may not be enough for other groups like children.[18]

A more practical approach to using pedometers within an exercise prescription may be to have a patient wear the device before beginning an exercise program and record the number of steps accumulated after each day for 1 week. This will establish a baseline activity level for that patient. The exercise prescription can then recommend a step count for each day that is 5 to 25% above that of baseline. The lower percentages can be used for patients who are very sedentary or frail or with chronic diseases, whereas the higher percentages may be a more appropriate goal for younger patients who are without chronic diseases. Having a goal step count to achieve each day has been shown to be an effective motivator for physical activity and is a simple and relatively inexpensive technique to improve adherence.[20]

It should be noted that pedometers have been shown to be less accurate when walking at slower speeds.[21,22] Therefore, they may not pick up slow-moving activity that is performed around the house such as vacuuming and sweeping. In addition, they have been shown to be accurate in overweight and obese individuals when worn in the manufacturer's recommended position. Wearing a pedometer while riding in a car on smooth surfaces did not affect its ability to measure steps accurately.[21]

It should be noted that current recommendations state that the amount of physical activity completed each day does not have to be done all at the same time of day. Total amounts of physical activity may be accumulated throughout the day. For example, walking for 30 minutes each day can be broken up into three segments of 10 minutes each. Therefore, health benefits can be obtained from walking 10 minutes in the morning, 10 minutes at lunchtime, and 10 minutes in the evening.

Resistance Training

Resistance training allows the body to improve its muscular strength and muscular endurance.[15] Aerobic activities have been shown to have little effect on muscular strength and endurance, especially in the upper body, and therefore it is important to make a concerted effort to participate in resistance training exercises.[15] The maintenance and enhancement of muscular strength and endurance is important for individuals at any age as it allows for the completion of tasks of daily living as well as recreational and physical labor tasks such as mowing the grass, trimming the hedge, or moving heavy objects. Resistance training is especially beneficial for older individuals as it can improve and maintain balance, coordination, and mobility to maintain a high-standard quality of life and reduce the risk of falls.[15] In addition, research has shown that resistance training increases bone mass, which may be beneficial for middle-aged and older adults, in particular postmenopausal women who may experience a more rapid loss of bone mineral density.[15]

Current recommendations from the ACSM are to perform 8 to 10 separate exercises that train the major muscle groups that include the arms, shoulders, chest, abdomen, back, hips, and legs.[15] Individuals should perform a minimum of one set of 8 to 12 repetitions of each of the exercises to the point of muscle fatigue. Older adults and frail persons may want to perform 10 to 15 repetitions. Participation in these exercises should be done 2 to 3 days per week. It is further recommended that proper training on exercise technique should be taught by a trained professional before beginning a resistance training program to ensure safety and prevent injury.[15] In addition, it is recommended that participants not hold their breath while performing resistance training exercises as this can acutely increase blood pressure and, if possible, participants should exercise with a training partner who can provide feedback, assistance, and motivation.[15]

Stretching

Stretching is an important component of physical activity as it allows for increases in musculoskeletal function, balance, and agility; increases functional capabilities such as bending and twisting; and reduces injury potential by decreasing the risk for muscle strains, low back problems, and falls.[15] Stretching is particularly important for older adults to maintain mobility and functionality and prevent injury.

Stretching exercises should be performed on all major joints such as the hips, back, shoulders, knees, upper trunk, and neck region.[15] Exercises should incorporate slow movements that are sustained for 10 to 30 seconds.[15] The degree of stretch should not cause pain, but rather mild discomfort. At least four repetitions per muscle group should be performed at a minimum of 2 to 3 days per week and as an integral part of the warm-up and cool-down exercises. It is particularly important in older adults to precede stretching exercises with some type of warm-up activities to increase circulation and internal body temperature. It is also important to stretch smoothly and never bounce or stretch the joint beyond its pain-free range of motion.[15]

ESSENTIAL PRINCIPLES OF AN EXERCISE PRESCRIPTION

The purpose of an exercise prescription is to enhance physical fitness, reduce risk factors for chronic diseases, promote health, and ensure safety during exercise participation.[15] The essential components included in any exercise prescription are as follows:[15]

- Patient goals
- Type of physical activity (mode)
- Intensity
- Duration
- Frequency
- Rate of progression

These same six essential components of an exercise prescription can be applied to any individual regardless of age, fitness level, risk factors, and disease(s).[15] Exercise prescriptions should be developed with careful consideration of each patient's current health status, risk factors, personal goals, physical activity preferences, previous exercise experiences, and behavioral characteristics.

Patient Goals

Before an exercise program can be written, it is very important to consider the outcome or the end result and purpose of the individual patient participating in that program. Each patient should have an individual set of exercise goals and as a result an individually specific exercise prescription. No one exercise prescription is appropriate for all individuals. Some patients may have several goals whereas others may only have a few. The patient goals should be prioritized and addressed, with the most important goal(s) receiving the greatest amount of effort and attention. Some patients may need to increase cardiorespiratory endurance, whereas others may need upper body strength, and still others may need to decrease their risk for heart disease by lowering blood pressure or cholesterol levels. Whatever the goals may be, they should always be realistic and achievable, measurable, and mutually agreed on by the patient and the patient's physician and other healthcare providers involved, including the pharmacist.

Type of Physical Activity

The type of activity or exercise chosen, also called the mode of activity, is the first step in designing an exercise prescription. Several factors come into play when choosing the type of activity. The most important factor may be the personal preferences of the patient. Activities that are enjoyable to the patient are more likely to promote adherence to the activity. Exercise adherence may be the single most important factor leading to successful outcomes resulting from an exercise prescription.[15,23] Some patients will simply like to walk for their activity, whereas others would prefer to ride a bicycle or swim. Still others may prefer recreational activities such as basketball or racquetball. Other factors that may influence program adherence include convenience of the activity, schedule flexibility, or childcare concerns. These details should be addressed before making the decision as to which mode(s) of activity is best for the patient.

The type of activity must also match the physical abilities of the patient.[15,24] For example, recommending a jogging program to a patient with **osteoarthritis** of the knees would not be a wise choice for a mode of activity. It may be better to suggest that this patient participate in activities that are non-weightbearing. On the other hand, a patient who is at risk for the development of osteoporosis may benefit a great deal from participating in weightbearing activities, as they have been shown to build bone and increase bone strength. Likewise, patients who are elderly and frail should perform low-intensity resistance training activities instead of moderate- or high-intensity resistance training activities.

The greatest benefits in overall health and cardiovascular fitness come from the types of activities that involve the use of large muscle groups for prolonged periods and are rhythmic and aerobic in nature.[15] Examples include walking, hiking, running, machine-based aerobic equipment, swimming, cycling, rowing, dancing, cross-country skiing, rope skipping, or endurance games. In addition, moderate- to high-intensity recreational activities such as basketball, tennis, soccer, football, backpacking, and canoeing are excellent sources of activity that can improve overall health and cardiovascular fitness.[15]

Intensity

The intensity of physical activity refers to the workload of the particular activity. Physical activities can generally be placed into one of three intensity groups: light-intensity, moderate-intensity, or vigorous-intensity activities. Intensity and duration of the activity are inversely related. Higher-intensity activities require less time spent participating in that activity, whereas lower-intensity activities require more time spent participating in the activity to receive the same health benefits.

There are several ways to measure and monitor physical activity intensity. Below we will discuss four different ways that do not require prior fitness testing of the patient. In addition, this section will provide examples of activities that can be categorized into light-, moderate-, and vigorous-intensity activities.

Talk Test

The talk test method of measuring intensity is the simplest of all intensity measurements. You simply monitor the ability of the participant to carry on a conversation while exercising. A person participating in activity at a light-intensity level will be able to sing while doing the activity.[25] Someone active at a moderate-intensity level should be able to carry on a conversation comfortably while participating in the activity.[25] Lastly, a person participating in an activity that is considered vigorous will be too winded and out of breath to carry on a conversation.[25] This method is easy for patients to understand and measure themselves without a great deal of assistance from others.

Target Heart Rate

The second way to monitor physical activity intensity is to measure the patient's heart rate during the activity and determine whether it is within the predetermined heart rate parameters or the target heart rate zone.[15,26] Measuring heart rate while exercising is easy to do, but may take some practice for patients to measure on their own. It is recommended that they stop exercising briefly while measuring heart rate and feel for a pulse at the neck, the wrist, or chest. The preferred method is to find the radial pulse on the thumb side of the wrist by using the tips of the index and middle fingers. Pulses can be counted for a full 60 seconds or for 30 seconds, and that number is multiplied by two.

To calculate target heart rate, the patient's maximum heart rate (MHR) must first be estimated through a simple calculation,[26] which is to subtract the patient's age from 220. It is important to remember that this method is an estimation, with a possible error range of ±10 to 15 beats.[15,26]

For moderate-intensity physical activity, it is recommended that a person's target heart rate be 50 to 70% of his or her MHR.[26] For example, a 50-year-old male patient with an exercise prescription for a moderate-intensity walking program will have a target heart rate of 85 to 119 beats per minute (bpm). This was calculated as follows:

1. Calculate maximum heart rate (220–age):
   220–50 = 170 bpm
2. Calculate target heart rate (MHR × intensity percentage):
   50% level: 170 × 0.50 = 85 bpm
   70% level: 170 × 0.70 = 119 bpm

Therefore, while this patient is walking he should try to maintain a heart rate that is between 85 and 119 bpm.

For vigorous-intensity physical activity, it is recommended that the patient's target heart rate be 70 to 85% of the estimated maximum heart rate.[26] Therefore, if this 50-year-old patient had an exercise prescription for a vigorous-intensity jogging program, his target heart rate would be 119 to 145 bpm. This was calculated as follows:

1. Calculate maximum heart rate (220–age): (same as above)
   220–age (50) = 170 bpm
2. Calculate target heart rate (MHR × intensity percentage):
   70% level: 170 × 0.70 = 119 bpm
   85% level: 170 × 0.85 = 145 bpm

Therefore, while this patient is jogging he should try to maintain a heart rate that is between 119 and 145 bpm.

It should be noted that the target heart rate for light-intensity activities is usually not measured. If it were to be measured, however, it would be between the resting heart rate and 50% of the maximum heart rate. The same method as above is used to calculate the upper range of this target heart rate zone with a calculation of the lower level not needed.

Rate of Perceived Exertion

A third way to monitor physical activity intensity is simply to have the patient rate how he or she feels based on a scale that ranges from 6 to 20.[15,27,28] This rating scale is called the **Borg rating of perceived exertion** (RPE; Fig. 2-3).[15,27,28] It is generally agreed that an RPE of 12 to 14 or "somewhat hard" on the Borg scale correlates to physical activity being performed at a moderate level of intensity.[27,28] Through experience patients can monitor how their body feels while exercising and then adjust their intensity. This feeling should reflect how heavy and strenuous the exercise feels, combining all sensations and feelings of physical stress, effort, and fatigue (i.e., heart rate, respiratory rate, sweating, and muscle fatigue). If a patient describes the activity as "very light" (9 on the Borg scale) then he or she will want to increase the intensity. If the activity is

6	No exertion at all
7	
7.5	Extremely light
8	
9	Very light
10	
11	Light
12	
13	Somewhat hard
14	
15	Hard (heavy)
16	
17	Very hard
18	
19	Extremely hard
20	Maximal exertion

FIGURE 2–3   Borg scale rating of perceived exertion (RPE).

described as "extremely hard" (19 on the Borg scale), then he or she will want to decrease the intensity.[15,27,28]

It is also very important to note that the Borg RPE is the preferred method to assess physical activity intensity among patients who are taking medication that may affect their heart rate.[15,27,28] For example, a patient taking a β-blocker like metoprolol may have a difficult time using the "target heart rate" method to monitor intensity because the metoprolol may blunt the normal rise in heart rate response to exercise. Therefore, patients may "feel" as if they are exercising at a moderate- to vigorous-intensity level while their heart rate response may be only measuring a light- to moderate-intensity level. Therefore, teaching patients how to monitor intensity based on the Borg scale is practical and important for many patients with cardiovascular disease who are on certain heart rate–altering medications. The pharmacodynamics and pharmacokinetics of medications as they relate to physical activity will be covered in more detail later in this chapter.

Metabolic Equivalent Level

A fourth way of measuring physical activity intensity is by the **metabolic equivalent,** or MET level.[29] It becomes practical for certain patients to use the MET level of the activity to measure intensity because certain activities are commonly characterized as light, moderate, or vigorous, but many activities can be classified in any one or all three categories based on the level of effort of the participant. For example, riding a bicycle can range from an intensity of very light (riding flat surfaces at slow speeds) to moderate (riding a few hills at varying speeds) to vigorous (riding at greater than 10 mph on steep uphill terrain) depending on effort.[29]

The MET level provides a method to characterize physical activity at different levels of effort based on the amount of oxygen used by the body during that activity.[30,31] One MET is equal to the energy (oxygen) used by the body while sitting quietly doing little activity, such as reading a book. The harder the body works, the higher the MET level. Activities that burn 3 to 6 METs are considered moderate-intensity physical activity.[30,31] Those that burn greater than 6 METs are considered vigorous-intensity physical activity.[29–31] Table 2-2 presents various activities and their corresponding MET levels. Many more activities with associated MET levels can be found in Ainsworth et al.[31]

Duration

The duration portion of an exercise prescription is a measure of the length (usually measured in minutes) of the physical activity session. As mentioned earlier, the duration of an activity is inversely related to the intensity of the activity. Light-intensity activities can be sustained for a longer duration, and vigorous-intensity activities can only be sustained for short durations of time because of the greater oxygen requirements of the muscle.[32]

Current recommendations for physical activity duration vary slightly among several groups; however, they are all relatively similar. The CDC, National Institutes of Health Consensus Development Panel on Physical Activity and Cardiovascular Health, and the Surgeon General's report are all consistent in stating that the duration of aerobic endurance activity be at least 30 minutes.[1,17,33] The AHA recommends 30 to 60 minutes to promote health and prevent cardiovascular disease, and ACSM recommends 20 to 60 minutes of continuous or intermittent bouts (minimum of 10-minute bouts) of activity accumulated throughout the day.[15,34] A duration of

TABLE 2–2 Metabolic Equivalent Level of Various Activities

Activity	Moderate Activity 3.0–6.0 METs	Vigorous Activity >6.0 METs
Walking	Level surface inside or outside at 3.5 mph (3.8 METs) to 4 mph (5 METs) Hiking (6 METs)	Race walking (6.5 METs) Aerobic walking at 5 mph or greater (8 METs) Backpacking (7 METs) Mountain climbing, rock climbing (8 METs) Jogging in general (7 METs) Running at 10 min/mile pace (10 METs)
Bicycling	Level surface or few hills at 5–9 mph (4 METs) Stationary bike at light effort (5.5 METs)	More than 12–13.9 mph, leisure, moderate effort (8 METs) Stationary bike at vigorous effort (10.5 METs)
Dance	Water aerobics (4 METs) Ballroom, line, square, folk, modern, and disco (4.5 METs)	Aerobic dance (6.5 METs) High-impact aerobic dance (7 METs) Step aerobics (6- to 8-inch step; 8.5 METs) Water jogging (8 METs)
Leisure activities	Golf (wheeling or carrying clubs; 4.5 METs) Playing Frisbee (3 METs) Fishing while walking along river bank (4 METs) Fishing in stream wearing waders (6 METs)	
Recreational activities	Basketball (shooting baskets; 4.5 METs) Swimming (recreational; 6 METs) Canoeing or rowing a boat (light effort; 3 METs) Horseback riding (general; 4 METs) Baseball or softball (fast pitch or slow pitch; 5 METs)	Most competitive sports such as basketball (8 METs), football (8 METs), soccer (10 METs), rugby (10 METs), or racquetball (10 METs) Cross-country skiing (moderate effort; 8 METs) Canoeing or rowing (moderate effort; 7 METs) Running (5 mph or 12 min/mile; 8 METs)
Work in and around the house	Raking the lawn (4.3 METs) Digging, spading, filling garden, composting (5 METs) Weeding, cultivating garden (4.5 METs) Pushing power lawn mower (5.5 METs) Shoveling snow by hand (6 METs) Carpet sweeping, sweeping floors (3.3 METs) Washing windows, car (3 METs)	Moving household items upstairs (9 METs) Carrying groceries upstairs (7.5 METs) Carpentry, sawing hardwood (7.5 METs) Carrying heavy loads (8 METs) Shoveling, moderate (10–15 lb/min; 7 METs)

Source: Centers for Disease Control and Prevention. Available at: www.cdc.gov/nccdphp/dnpa/physical/measuring/met.htm. Accessed July 26, 2006.

30 minutes (either continuous or intermittent) is generally considered to be the goal for most individuals to attain.

Intermittent bouts of physical activity may be very useful and practical for certain individuals. Intermittent bouts of activity have been shown to improve exercise adherence in individuals who are not accustomed to physical activity and may be safer for patients who are severely deconditioned because it allows for more frequent rest and recovery until continuous exercise can be sustained.[35] In addition, some studies have shown that intermittent bouts of moderate- to high-intensity exercise of at least 10 minutes in duration can improve aerobic fitness.[36–38] Therefore, walking for 10 minutes in the morning, during a lunch break, and again in the evening can promote overall health, decrease the risks for cardiovascular disease, improve adherence, and may even increase aerobic fitness levels in almost all individuals.

Frequency

Frequency refers to the number of days per week the patient will partake in physical activity. This is a good time to again make the distinction between physical activity and exercise. As you may recall, physical activity is defined as any bodily movement produced by skeletal muscles that results in the expenditure of energy.[1] Exercise is defined as physical activity that is planned or structured and involves repetitive bodily movements done to improve or maintain one or more of the components of physical fitness.[1]

The U.S. Surgeon General (http://www.surgeongeneral.gov) recommends that physical activity be done on most days of the week.[1] ACSM recommends that 3 to 5 days of exercise be done each week.[15] Therefore, it is important to explain to our patients that being physically active in either recreational, leisure, resistance training, aerobic conditioning, or everyday activities counts toward the physical activity on most days of the week as the Surgeon General has recommended. Thus, a weekly activity log of a patient may include mowing the grass 1 day, golfing and gardening on 2 other days, and walking 3 days out of the week, showing the patient has participated in some form of physical activity 6 of 7 days of the week.

As just mentioned, the ACSM recommends 3 to 5 aerobic conditioning exercise sessions per week.[15] Activities included in this recommendation are walking, jogging, bicycling, stationary exercise equipment, swimming, and rowing. Patients exerting a higher exercise intensity can do so 3 days per week, whereas those exerting a lower intensity should do so more than 3 times per week to maintain or improve aerobic capacity ($\dot{V}o_2$).[15]

Rate of Progression

An exercise prescription should continually be evaluated for its effectiveness at achieving the individual goals of each patient. Therefore, when designing an exercise prescription the patient and healthcare provider should have a general plan for how the program progresses to meet the stated goals. This plan is called the rate of physical activity progression.

The rate of progression will depend on several factors, such as functional capacity, health status, age, individual goals, and the patient's tolerance for the physical activity program.[15] The current recommendations by the Surgeon General, CDC, and ACSM are that 30 minutes of moderate physical activity be done on most, if not all, days of the week.[1,15] It is important to understand that some patients will not be able to achieve this at the beginning of the program and that this may in fact be one of the primary goals of the program. Therefore, progressing to this level may be appropriate for some patients, whereas others may already be at this level and will want to progress to a greater intensity, frequency, or duration.

Physical activity progression is generally thought of in three separate stages: initial, improvement, and maintenance.[15] The initial stage is lower in intensity, duration, and frequency to decrease the risk of injury and muscle soreness. Adherence to the program is one of the primary goals of the phase. The intensity can start light and progress to moderate, and the duration can begin as low as 5 minutes but progress to 30 minutes by the end of 4 weeks. This phase usually lasts up to 4 weeks. Deconditioned individuals should be permitted more time to adapt to each stage within the program.[15]

The second stage is called the improvement stage.[15] The goal of this stage is to make gradual increases in duration, frequency, and intensity, with emphasis on duration and frequency to improve cardiorespiratory endurance. This stage will typically last 4 to 5 months.[15]

The third stage is the maintenance stage in which long-term maintenance and adherence to the physical activity program is the main goal.[15] During this stage, the major long-term goals of the physical activity program should be evaluated with the possibility of reassigning new goals to replace ones that have been accomplished.[15]

Energy Expenditure Goals

A goal in many exercise prescriptions is directed toward body weight, mostly weight loss. The amount of **total energy expenditure** (TEE) while performing an activity becomes important when designing a weight-loss program. The amount of energy or calories expended during physical activity can be calculated using a simple formula involving the MET level of the activity.[15] Therefore, this is a good time to discuss energy expenditure as it specifically relates to the exercise prescription.

The caloric expenditure of any physical activity can be estimated, but it is not an exact science. Several factors may influence energy expenditure of an activity, such as skill, coordination, and exercise efficiency as well as the variable intensities that may exist within an individual activity.[15] One method to approximate caloric expenditure of a specific activity uses the following formula:[15]

$$(\text{METs} \times 3.5 \times \text{body weight in kg})/200 = \text{kcal/min}$$

Thus, if the MET level of the activity is known and the weight of the patient is known, the number of calories expended performing that activity can be estimated.

Let's use an example: An exercise prescription you have designed for a 45-year-old male patient weighing 90 kg recommends that he walk at 3.5 mph for 30 minutes per day, 3 times per week. Waking at this intensity has a corresponding MET value of 3.8. Using the formula provided above we can figure the patient's caloric expenditure of his exercise prescription:

$$(3.8 \times 3.5 \times 90)/200 = 5.99 \ \text{kcal/min}$$

Therefore, our patient will burn almost 6 calories per minute or about 180 kcal per exercise session (5.99 kcal/min × 30 min = 179.7 kcal/day) while walking. In addition, he will burn approximately 539 kcal per week (179.1 kcal/day × 3 days/week) as a result of our exercise prescription.

PRESCRIBING PHYSICAL ACTIVITY

Increases in physical activity participation and cardiorespiratory fitness have been associated with a decreased risk for death from any cause and especially death associated with **coronary heart disease.**[15] The overall primary goals for becoming physically active are to decrease the risk for premature death, decrease the risk for developing chronic diseases, improve the management of existing chronic diseases, and improve overall quality of life. Individual patients, however, may have specific goals such as losing weight, increasing strength, or improving balance, but we should always try to keep in mind the major overarching ideals for participating in physical activity.

Legal Issues With Prescribing Exercise

Pharmacists are accustomed to recommending drug therapy and filling drug prescriptions. They are not accustomed to prescribing therapy. Therefore, the question frequently arises, "Is it legal for pharmacists to prescribe exercise?" The answer to this question is both simple and complex. The simple answer is that there are no laws that prohibit pharmacists or any other healthcare professionals from prescribing exercise. In fact, undergraduate students studying exercise sciences generally take a course in exercise prescription and are accustomed to writing exercise prescriptions for clients. The complex answer requires a bit more discussion.

As more and more adults with various disease states engage in exercise programs directed by pharmacists, the number of untoward events is likely to increase.[15] Negligence is the failure to conform one's conduct to a generally accepted standard of duty. This begs the question, "Is prescribing exercise an accepted standard of duty for a pharmacist?" The answer to this question lies in the disease state practice guidelines. For example, the practice guidelines for managing cholesterol (ATP III) state that exercise is an important and necessary component in the treatment of high cholesterol and the prevention of coronary heart disease.[39] Pharmacists are regularly involved in the treatment and disease state management of patients with high cholesterol. This involves counseling patients in the areas of medication therapy management, dietary counseling, and exercise programming. The same can be said for other diseases such as hypertension, diabetes, obesity, **metabolic syndrome,** and others. Therefore, reducing the risk for negligent behavior should be a priority for all pharmacists whether they are talking to patients about medication or exercise.[15]

Negligent risk can be prevented by obtaining as much education and knowledge about exercise as possible.[15] This may mean taking formal classes on exercise programming or informally educating oneself on the topic. In addition, following published guidelines for exercise recommendations, such as those from the ACSM or CDC as well as those in specific diseases, is important to decrease risk. Healthcare professionals are advised to keep up to date as information on new standards becomes available.[15] It is also important to understand that caring for patients is a team effort. Contacting the patient's physician and other healthcare professionals is important as they may offer valuable suggestions and be a source of motivation for the patient and a source for referring the patient when needed. Communication among all parties involved is always a good idea when caring for patients.

> Prescribing exercise to patients with chronic diseases does come with an increased liability risk. Anytime we as pharmacists care for a patient, we are accepting a certain amount of risk. As long as we are working within our duties as a pharmacist to care for patients, including disease state management, the added risk that we take is warranted. Patients can benefit greatly from pharmacists talking to them about exercise, and therefore it is a risk worth taking.

Becoming physically active, however, does come with a certain set of associated risks.[15] These risks should be evaluated and discussed with each patient and his or her physician before beginning an exercise program. The most common risks associated with physical activity are related to injury of the musculoskeletal system, which includes the bones, joints, tendons, and muscles.[40] Most of these types of injuries are not serious and can be minimized by taking sensible precautions and usually resolve with rest and over-the-counter (OTC) pain relievers.[40] Injuries such as these can be minimized through gradual increases in intensity, duration, and frequency, by performing proper warm-up and cool-down that includes stretching, and by avoiding excessive amounts of activity at one time.[40] Therefore, patients with little experience participating in physical activity should begin slowly by incorporating only a few minutes of physical activity into their day and gradually increasing the activity as their bodies adjust.[40,41]

Occasionally the press reports about an athlete who has died as a result of participating in a sport or physical activity. This may make some patients hesitant to take part in activities that are strenuous. It is important to tell worried patients that sudden death associated with physical activity is usually only associated with patients who have underlying cardiovascular disease and even in these patients it is very rare.[40,42] The CDC and ACSM recommend that patients with known cardiovascular disease or patients who have a prior history of a heart attack, stroke, or heart surgery have a physical evaluation by their physician before beginning a program of physical activity even at a moderate-intensity level.[15,40] It is also recommended that men older than age 40 and women older than age 50 who plan to participate in vigorous-intensity activity consult with their physician first.[40] In addition, it would be prudent for you as a pharmacist to contact an individual patient's physician to make him or her aware of your physical activity program. This keeps the physician informed of the patient's overall health and can be another source of encouragement and motivation for the patient to continue the program. Additionally, collaboration with the patient's physical therapist can be especially helpful when working with individuals with physical disabilities. Table 2-3 provides some tips for avoiding activity-induced injuries.

Sample Exercise Prescriptions

The current recommendation by the U.S. Surgeon General, the CDC, and the ACSM for physical activity is "every U.S. adult should accumulate 30 minutes or more of moderate-intensity physical activity on most, preferably all, days of the week."[1,15,17,41] Keeping this in mind, let's write an exercise prescription for a sample patient.

Sample Patient One

L.J. is a 47-year-old male with no prior cardiac history or history of chronic diseases. He does suffer from seasonal allergies for which he takes fexofenadine 180 mg once daily,

TABLE 2–3   Tips for Avoiding Activity-Induced Injuries

1. Listen to your body by monitoring fatigue, heart rate, and physical discomfort.
2. Be aware of signs of overexertion such as breathlessness and muscle soreness.
3. Be aware of warning signs of a heart attack such as chest pain that radiates to the arm or jaw, dizziness, and lightheadedness.
4. Begin activity with a proper warm-up and end with a proper cool-down that includes stretching of the major muscles in the body.
5. Start at an easy pace and increase the time or distance gradually.
6. Drink plenty of water before, during, and after the activity (drink a half cup of water for every 15 minutes of activity and consume even more in hot weather).
7. Exercise with a partner.
8. Modify recreational game rules and minimize competition.
9. Take precautions when exercising in the cold.

Centers for Disease Control and Prevention. Available at:
http://www.cdc.gov/nccdphp/dnpa/physical/life/risks.htm. Accessed July 26, 2006.

and he is slightly overweight. He takes no other medications. L.J. is sedentary and has been for approximately 15 years and has a family history of heart disease. He would like to begin an exercise program for the primary purpose of "getting back into shape." He states that he has access to a health club at work that offers aerobic and resistance training exercise equipment. L.J.'s exercise prescription is listed below.

Sample Patient One Exercise Prescription

GOALS
Short Term (4 weeks)
1. Increase overall activity by walking more at work and taking the stairs at least two to three floors at a time.
2. Do some form of physical activity for 30 minutes on most days of the week.
3. Have an overall adherence rating of 75% or greater.

Long Term (6 months)
1. Decrease risks for developing coronary heart disease as it runs in the family.
2. Have an overall adherence rating of 75% or greater.
3. Improve cardiorespiratory fitness level by assessing ease of household chores, yard work, and ability to exercise.
4. Achieve and maintain normal body weight.

TYPE OF ACTIVITY
Choose from walking, bicycling, and stationary aerobic equipment.
Choose from basketball, tennis, and racquetball for recreational activities and do usual yard work and household chores.

INTENSITY
Use target heart rate method at 50 to 70% of max heart rate
$220 - 47 = 173$ bpm (max heart rate)

Target heart rate = 87 to 121 bpm
50%: 173 × 0.50 = 86.5 bpm
70%: 173 × 0.70 = 121 bpm

DURATION

10 minutes once per day for week one
10 minutes twice per day for week two
10 minutes three times per day for weeks three and four
30 minutes per day beyond week four

FREQUENCY

2 times per week for week one
3 times per week for week two to four
3 to 5 times per week after week four

WARM-UP AND COOL-DOWN

Before the exercise period, perform 10 minutes of light-intensity activity as a warm-up. The same activity that is chosen for the exercise period can be used as the warm-up activity but at a lower intensity. Perform a 10-minute cool-down in the same fashion as the warm-up followed by 5 to 10 minutes of stretching activities.

ASSESSMENT PERIODS

After week two
After week four
At 3 months or as necessary
At 6 months or as necessary
Reassess goals after 6 months

Sample Patient Two

D.L. is a 58-year-old female with a history of hypertension, and she is slightly overweight. She leads a fairly active lifestyle but does not participate in structured aerobic exercise. She has come to your pharmacy to fill a prescription for metoprolol 25 mg twice daily. She is taking no other medication and has no family history for heart disease. She states that her physician told her she needs to get some exercise to help control her blood pressure. D.L.'s exercise prescription is provided below.

Sample Patient Two Exercise Prescription

GOALS

Short Term (4 weeks)

1. Do some form of structured aerobic exercise for 30 minutes on most days of the week.
2. Have an overall adherence rating of 75% or greater.

Long Term (6 months)

1. Manage blood pressure more effectively through exercise.
2. Decrease risks for developing coronary heart disease.
3. Achieve and maintain normal body weight.

Type of Activity

Choose from walking, bicycling, stationary aerobic equipment, swimming, or rowing for aerobic activity.

INTENSITY

Begin with light intensity and progress toward moderate intensity. D.L. is on the β-blocker metoprolol, so her exercising heart rate may be blunted by the drug. Thus, use the Borg scale to monitor physical activity intensity. Aim for an RPE of 12 to 14 or "somewhat hard" on the Borg scale as it correlates to physical activity being performed at a moderate level of intensity.

DURATION

10 to 20 minutes one to two times per day for week one and two
20 to 30 minutes per day for weeks three and four (may divide into intermittent sessions)
30 to 45 minutes per day after week four (may divide into intermittent sessions)

FREQUENCY

2 to 3 times per week for weeks one and two
3 to 5 times per week after week two

WARM-UP AND COOL-DOWN

Before the exercise period, perform 10 minutes of light-intensity activity as a warm-up. The same activity that is chosen for the exercise period can be used as the warm-up activity but at a lower intensity. Perform a 10-minute cool-down in the same fashion as the warm-up followed by 5 to 10 minutes of stretching activities.

ASSESSMENT PERIODS

After week two
After week four, monitor blood pressure for effectiveness
At 3 months or as necessary, monitor blood pressure for effectiveness
At 6 months or as necessary, monitor blood pressure for effectiveness
Reassess goals after 6 months

The exercise prescriptions for both L.J. and D.L. are similar in some ways; however, each has specific goals and progresses at a different pace based on individual circumstances. D.L. has hypertension and is taking a β-blocker and so the RPE method of monitoring intensity should be used as her heart rate may be affected by the medication. L.J. is younger but more sedentary and therefore his exercise prescription progresses more slowly.

OVERCOMING BARRIERS TO PHYSICAL ACTIVITY

With so much positive information written about the effects of regular participation in physical activity, it is sometimes difficult to understand why a majority of the population in the United States is still not active at the recommended levels. There are many barriers that exist that can keep people from becoming physically active. Understanding common barriers to physical activity and addressing potential barriers that may influence an individual patient's compliance are important to discuss at the time of the initial exercise prescription.

Barriers to physical activity can come from both environmental and personal sources.[43,44] Environmental barriers can include the accessibility and location of parks, trails, sidewalks, and recreation centers.[43,44] They can also include factors such as street design, density of housing, availability of public transportation, water and air pollution, crime, and dangerous automobile traffic.[43,44] It is important to address the individual circumstances of each patient and devise creative solutions to overcome environmental barriers that may inhibit program adherence. Many personal variables also exist such as physiologic, behavioral, and psychological factors that may affect the adherence to a well laid out exercise prescription.[43,44] The 10 most common reasons for adults failing to adopt a physically active lifestyle are listed in Table 2-4, along with suggestions for overcoming these barriers.

PHARMACOKINETICS AND PHARMACODYNAMICS AND PHYSICAL ACTIVITY

In the practice of pharmacy we are accustomed to screening drug therapy for interactions with other drugs, herbals, and foods. It has been shown that certain medications may also interact with physical activity. This drug–exercise interaction can be looked at from both a pharmacodynamic and a pharmacokinetic perspective. From a pharmacodynamic perspective, some medications may inhibit or enhance the ability to perform physical activity. On the other hand, participating in physical activity may change the pharmacokinetic parameters of some medications, which can affect their ability to work as they were intended.

Pharmacodynamics

Pharmacodynamics is the study of biochemical and physiologic effects of drugs and their mechanism of action. Of particular importance with regard to physical activity are the effects that some medications can have on exercising heart rate and blood pressure and the resulting effects on exercise capacity or $\dot{V}O_2$.[15] A drug that decreases a patient's heart rate during exercise will have a direct effect on **cardiac output.** As you may recall, cardiac output is heart rate multiplied by stroke volume or the volume of blood ejected from the left ventricle of the heart after each heart beat. Therefore, cardiac output during exercise will be affected if the heart rate does not increase to normal exercising levels. This will then decrease the amount of blood and, as a result, oxygen, to the working muscles during exercise. A decrease in the oxygen delivery to working muscle will then lead to a decrease in physical activity performance and make exercise feel as if it were more strenuous and intense.

It is very important to consult patients who are taking medication that may alter exercise heart rate and exercise capacity to provide realistic expectations from physical activity. In addition, it is also important to note that even though exercise heart rate and exercise capacity may not reach the patient's expectations, all the benefits of participating in physical activity previously mentioned in this chapter can still be achieved. Therefore, these patients should be continually encouraged to participate in regular physical activity.

An example of this type of drug–exercise interaction is with β-blockers. Drugs in this class have been shown to decrease heart rate at rest and during exercise. Newly diagnosed patients with hypertension are often prescribed a β-blocker to control their blood

| TABLE 2–4 | Suggestions for Overcoming Physical Activity Barriers |

Barrier	Suggestion
Lack of time	Schedule physical activity into your daily routine as if you were scheduling an appointment and do so several days in advance rather than during the same day
	Make time for physical activity during lunch hour, or instead of a coffee break, take a fitness break
	Choose activities that require minimal preparation time such as walking or stair climbing
Social influence	Explain your goals to your family and friends and ask them to support you and even join your efforts
	Plan social activities that involve physical activity such as walking or biking to a restaurant
	Join a group that is physically active such as a hiking, biking, or walking club that meets regularly
Lack of energy	Educate patients that doing physical activity will increase energy levels
	Choose a time of day to exercise when energy levels are high
Lack of motivation	Plan ahead and make physical activity part of the daily schedule and even mark it on the calendar
	Make an activity log and record when you have exercised
	Exercise with a friend so you can motivate each other
	Join an exercise group or class
	Use a pedometer to monitor daily steps
	Inform the patient's physician of physical activity plans to gain his or her support and aid in motivating the patient
Fear of injury	Educate patients regarding proper warm-up, cool-down, and stretching activities as well proper exercise techniques
	Wear a good pair of shoes if walking or jogging is the activity of choice
	Choose activities with minimal risk
	Recommend a physical examination for patients with significant cardiac history and for those with significant injury concerns
Lack of skill	Choose activities that require little skill such as walking or climbing stairs
	Exercise with a friend who has the same skill level
	Take a class to learn the skill or proper techniques
Lack of resources	Choose activities that require minimal equipment such as walking or jumping rope
	Identify inexpensive and convenient resources within the community such as worksite, community, and park and recreation programs
	Use soup cans or laundry detergent bottles filled with water or sand to provide resistance to strengthen the upper body instead of buying weight equipment
Weather conditions	Develop a plan for exercising during inclement weather such as walking at an indoor mall, climbing stairs, or indoor cycling
	Participate in cold-weather activities such as cross-country skiing or warm-weather activities such as outdoor swimming

(continued)

TABLE 2–4	Suggestions for Overcoming Physical Activity Barriers *(Continued)*
Barrier	**Suggestion**
Travel	Stay in places with exercise facilities or a pool
	Pack a jump rope in your suitcase
	Find a local shopping mall or large department store and walk
Family obligations	Exercise with the family by playing in the yard, take a family walk, or walk or ride bikes to a restaurant
	Hire a babysitter and look at the cost as a worthwhile investment in your physical and mental health
	Exercise at home by jumping rope or riding a stationary bike while the kids are sleeping or playing
	Join a health club that offers childcare services
	Trade babysitting time with a friend, neighbor, or family member who also has small children
Retirement years	View retirement as a time to become more active instead of less
	Spend time gardening, walking the dog, and playing with grandchildren. Children with short legs and grandparents with slower gaits can be great walking partners
	Participate in activities that you previously did not have time for such as ballroom dancing, square dancing, or swimming
	Ride a stationary bike while reading your favorite book

Source: Centers for Disease Control and Prevention. Available at:
http://www.cdc.gov/nccdphp/dnpa/physical/life/overcome.htm. Accessed July 26, 2006.

pressure and advised to participate in physical activity. It would be prudent to talk with patients such as these regarding the effect of their new medication on their ability to perform exercise and at the same time stress the importance of physical activity in controlling blood pressure and decreasing the risks of cardiovascular disease. Table 2-5 lists medications and their corresponding effect on exercising heart rate, blood pressure, and exercise capacity.

Pharmacokinetics

Pharmacokinetics is a discipline within pharmacology that studies a drug's absorption, distribution, metabolism, and excretion to predict how the drug will perform once it is administered.[45] Physiologic changes that result from physical activity such as blood flow redistributions, respiratory changes, skin temperature and hydration changes, metabolic rate, gastrointestinal transit time, and plasma protein changes attributable to water loss can all affect how a particular drug will perform.[45]

Most pharmacokinetic changes are a result of alterations in blood flow during exercise. At rest, the liver receives the greatest percentage of blood flow (27%), followed by the kidneys (22%) and the muscles (20%).[45] During exercise at moderate intensity, blood flow dramatically shifts in these areas so that the greatest amount goes to the muscles (71%), with the liver and kidneys only getting 3% each of the total blood volume. Some drugs are highly dependent on blood flow to the liver and kidneys for metabolism and excretion.[45] Therefore, the pharmacokinetic parameters of some drugs may be altered as a result of exercise. Blood flow to the skin at rest is approximately 6% of the total blood

TABLE 2–5 **Pharmacokinetic and Pharmacodynamic Changes Resulting From Exercise**

Drug or Drug Classification	Pharmacokinetic Changes as a Result of Exercise	Pharmacodynamic Changes During Exercise		Effect on Exercise Capacity
		Heart Rate	**Blood Pressure**	
β-blockers		↓	↓	↑ in pts with angina ↓ or ↔ in pts without angina
Atenolol Propranolol	↓ renal clearance$_{ss}$ ↑ plasma concentration$_{ss}$ ↓ half-life$_{ss}$ ↓ AUC$_{ss}$ ↓ clearance$_{ss}$			
Propranolol	↔ maximal concentration$_{ct}$, time to maximal concentration$_{ct}$, half-life$_{ct}$, AUC$_{ct}$, protein binding$_{ct}$, clearance$_{ct}$, bioavailability$_{ct}$, volume of distribution$_{ct}$			
Carvedilol	↔ plasma concentration$_{ss}$			
Calcium-channel blockers				↑ in pts with angina
Verapamil	↔ clearance$_{ss}$ ↔ volume of distribution$_{ss}$ ↔ half-life$_{ss}$	↓	↓	↔ in pts without angina
ACE inhibitors	ND	↔	↓	↑ or ↔ in pts with CHF ↔ in non-CHF
Digoxin	↓ plasma concentration$_{ss}$ ↑ skeletal muscle concentration$_{ss}$ ↔ time of onset$_{ct}$, time to maximal drug concentration$_{ct}$, half-life$_{ct}$	↓ in pts with AF and possibly CHF	↔	↑ in pts with AF and CHF

(*continued*)

TABLE 2-5   Pharmacokinetic and Pharmacodynamic Changes Resulting From Exercise (*Continued*)

Drug or Drug Classification	Pharmacokinetic Changes as a Result of Exercise	Pharmacodynamic Changes During Exercise		Effect on Exercise Capacity
		Heart Rate	Blood Pressure	
Amiodarone	ND	↓	↔	↔
Nitrates	ND	↑ or ↔	↓ or ↔	↑ in pts with angina ↔ in pts without angina ↑ or ↔ in pts with CHF
Sympathomimetic agents	ND	↑ or ↔	↑, ↓ or ↔	↔
Bronchodilators	ND	↔	↔	↑ in pts limited by bronchospasm
Theophylline	↑ half-life$_{ss}$ ↓ clearance$_{ss}$	↔	↔	ND
Insulin	↑ absorption$_{ss}$ ↓ plasma glucose$_{ss}$	↔	↔	↔
Aspirin	↑ intestinal permeability$_{ss}$ ↓ gastroduodenal permeability$_{ss}$ ↔ plasma concentration$_{ss}$, half-life$_{ss}$, clearance$_{ss}$	↔	↔	↔
Warfarin[a]	ND	ND	ND	ND

Sources: Adapted with permission from American College of Sports Medicine. ACSM's Guidelines for Exercise Testing and Prescription, 7th ed. Baltimore: Lippincott Williams & Wilkins, 2006:261–266; and Lenz TL, Lenz NJ, Faulkner MA. Potential interactions between exercise and drug therapy. Sports Med 2004;34:293–306.
[a]No pharmacokinetic or pharmacodynamic data; however, increases in physical activity have been shown to significantly decrease the international normalized ratio (INR), making the warfarin less effective.
↓, decrease; ↑, increase; ↔, no change; pts, patients; ss, single-session exercise regimen; AUC, area under the curve; ct, continuous training exercise regimen; AF, atrial fibrillation; CHF, congestive heart failure; ND, no data.

volume, whereas it is doubled to 12% during moderate-intensity exercise.[45] This change in blood flow as well as the skin temperature and hydration changes during exercise can affect the pharmacokinetics of medications delivered via a transdermal patch.

Physical activity can have a profound effect on blood glucose levels if insulin is administered around the same time as physical activity is performed. Insulin absorption has been shown to significantly increase when injected into the leg just before performing leg exercises because of blood flow increases in the leg muscles.[45] As a result, plasma glucose decreases from the rapid absorption of the insulin. Insulin absorption has shown no change if administered in a non-working muscle just before exercise, such as the arm before performing leg exercises. Therefore, it would be a good idea to counsel diabetic patients taking insulin to choose injection sites wisely when exercising. Using an injection site that is not in a muscle that is about to be involved in physical activity or performing physical activity at times other than those close to the injection times are good suggestions. In addition, patients with diabetes should consider other preventive hypoglycemic techniques such as increasing carbohydrate intake or reducing the total insulin dose.

It is important to note that even though exercise may alter certain pharmacokinetic parameters, it may not clinically affect the patient.[45] In most cases, the clinical effect of pharmacokinetic changes resulting from physical activity is unclear. Most studies that have been published have involved young, healthy volunteers and not patients with preexisting diseases. In addition, most studies have been conducted with single bouts of exercise and not with a continuous training program, so it is relatively unknown whether the pharmacokinetics of most drugs are different in trained versus untrained individuals.[45] Therefore, given the lack of knowledge in this area and the potential for therapeutic consequences, it would be prudent for the pharmacist and other healthcare providers to be aware that there is a potential for drug–exercise interactions and to investigate the possibility of exercise causing pharmacokinetic changes when drug therapy problems arise. Table 2-5 provides examples of pharmacokinetic changes of some drugs resulting from exercise.

REFERENCES

1. U.S. Department of Health and Human Services. Physical activity and health: a report of the Surgeon General. Atlanta: U.S. Department of Health and Human Services, Centers for Disease Control and Prevention, National Center for Chronic Disease Prevention and Health Promotion, 1996.

2. Yu S, Yarnell J. Exercise for the prevention of cardiovascular disease: how vigorous and how often? Cardiovasc Rev Rep 2004;25:274–276.

3. Centers for Disease Control and Prevention. Available at: www.cdc.gov/nccdphp/dnpa/physical/importance/why/htm. Accessed July 26, 2005.

4. Petrella RJ. Can adoption of regular exercise later in life prevent metabolic risk for cardiovascular disease? Diabetes Care 2005;28:694–701.

5. U.S. Department of Health and Human Services. Physical activity fundamental to preventing disease. U.S. Department of Health and Human Services, Office of the Assistant Secretary for Planning and Evaluation, June 20, 2002.

6. Paffenbarger RS, Hyde RT, Wing AL, et al. The association of changes in physical-activity level and other lifestyle characteristics with mortality among men. N Engl J Med 1993;328:538–545.

7. Sherman SE, D'Agostino RB, Cobb JL, et al. Physical activity and mortality in women in the Framingham Heart Study. Am Heart J 1994;128:879–884.

8. Kaplan GAA, Strawbridge WJ, Cohen RD, et al. Natural history of leisure-time physical activity and its correlates: association with mortality from all causes and cardiovascular diseases over 28 years. Am J Epidemiol 1996;144:793–797.

9. Kushi LH, Fee RM, Folsom AR, et al. Physical activity and mortality in postmenopausal women. JAMA 1997;277:1287–1292.

10. Lee CD, Blair SN, Jackson AS. Cardiorespiratory fitness, body composition, and all-cause and cardiovascular disease mortality in men. Am J Clin Nutr 1999;69:373–380.

11. Wei M, Kampert JB, Barlow CE, et al. Relationship between low cardiorespiratory fitness and mortality in normal-weight, overweight, and obese men. JAMA 1999;282:1547–1553.

12. U.S. Department of Health and Human Services. The Surgeon General's call to action to prevent and decrease overweight and obesity. Rockville, MD: U.S. Department of Health and Human Services, Public Health Service, Office of the Surgeon General, 2001.

13. Strum R. The effects of obesity, smoking and problem drinking on chronic medical problems and health care costs. Health Affairs 2002;21:245–253.

14. McArdle WD, Katch FI, Katch VL. Exercise Physiology: Energy, Nutrition, and Human Performance, 5th ed. Philadelphia: Lippincott Williams & Wilkins, 2004.

15. American College of Sports Medicine. Guidelines for Exercise Testing and Prescription, 6th ed. Philadelphia: Lippincott Williams & Wilkins, 2000.

16. U.S. Department of Agriculture. Available at: http://www.mypyramid.gov. Accessed July 26, 2005.

17. Centers for Disease Control and Prevention. Available at: www.cdc.gov/nccdphp/dnpa/physical/recommendations/adults.htm. Accessed July 26, 2005.

18. Tudor-Locke C, Bassett DR. How many steps/day is enough? Preliminary pedometer indices for public health. Sports Med 2004;34:1–8.

19. Le-Masurier GC, Sidman CL, Corbin CB. Accumulating 10,000 steps: does this meet current physical activity guidelines? Res Q Exerc Sport 2003;74:389–394.

20. Rooney B, Smalley K, Larson J, Havens S. Is knowing enough? Increasing physical activity by wearing a pedometer. WMJ 2003;102(4):31–36.

21. Le-Masurier GC, Tudor-Locke C. Comparison of pedometer and accelerometer accuracy under controlled conditions. Med Sci Sports Exerc 2003;35:867–871.

22. Swartz AM, Bassett DR, Moore JB, Thompson DL, Strath SJ. Effects of body mass index on the accuracy of an electronic pedometer. Int J Sports Med 2003;24:588–592.

23. Ryan RM, Fredrick CM, Lepes D, Rubio N, Sheldon KM. Intrinsic motivation and exercise adherence. Int J Sports Psychol 1997;28:335–354.

24. Hagerman PS. Aerobic endurance training program design. In: Earle RW, Baechle TR, eds. NSCA's Essentials of Personal Training. Champaign, IL: Human Kinetics, 2004:399–424.

25. Centers for Disease Control and Prevention. Available at: www.cdc.gov/nccdphp/dnpa/physical/measuring/talk_test.htm. Accessed July 26, 2005.

26. Centers for Disease Control and Prevention. Available at: http://www.cdc.gov/nccdphp/dnpa/physical/measuring/target_heart_rate.htm. Accessed July 26, 2005.

27. Borg G. Perceived Exertion and Pain Scales. Champaign, IL: Human Kinetics, 1998.

28. Centers for Disease Control and Prevention. Available at: www.cdc.gov/nccdphp/dnpa/physical/measuring/perceived_exertion.htm. Accessed July 26, 2005.

29. Centers for Disease Control and Prevention. Available at: www.cdc.gov/nccdphp/dnpa/physical/measuring/met.htm. Accessed July 26, 2005.

30. Ainsworth BE, Haskell WL, Leon AS, et al. Compendium of physical activities: classification of energy costs of human physical activities. Med Sci Sports Exerc 1993;25:70–80.

31. Ainsworth BE, Haskell MC, Whitt ML, et al. Compendium of physical activities: an update of activity codes and MET intensities. Med Sci Sports Exerc 2000;32(Suppl):S498–S516.

32. Sharkey BJ. Intensity and duration of training and development of cardiorespiratory fitness. Med Sci Sports 1970;2:197–202.

33. National Institutes of Health: Consensus Development Panel on Physical Activity and Cardiovascular Health. Physical activity and cardiovascular health. JAMA 1996;276:214–246.

34. Fletcher GF, Balady SN, Blair SN, et al. Benefits and recommendations for physical activity programs for all Americans. A statement for health professionals by the Committee on Exercise and Cardiac Rehabilitation of the Council of Clinical Cardiology, American Heart Association. Circulation 1996;94:857–862.

35. Jakicic JM, Wing RR, Butler BA, Robertson RJ. Prescribing exercise in multiple short bouts versus one continuous bout: effects on adherence, cardiorespiratory fitness, and weight loss in overweight women. Int J Obes 1995;19:893–901.

36. Ebisu T. Splitting the distance of endurance running: on cardiorespiratory endurance and blood lipids. Jpn J Phys Educ 1985;30:37–43.

37. Hardman AE. Issues of fractionization of exercise (short vs long bouts). Med Sci Sports Exerc 2001; 33(6 Suppl):S421–S427.

38. Murphy MH, Hardman AE. Training effects of short and long bouts of brisk walking in sedentary women. Med Sci Sports Exerc 1998;30:152–157.

39. National Institutes of Health, National Heart, Lung, and Blood Institute. Third report of the National Cholesterol Education Program (NCEP) Expert Panel on Detection, Evaluation, and Treatment of High Blood Cholesterol in Adults (Adult Treatment Panel III). NIH Publication No. 02-5215, September 2002.

40. Centers for Disease Control and Prevention. Available at: http://www.cdc.gov/nccdphp/dnpa/physical/life/risks.htm. Accessed July 26, 2005.

41. Pate RR, Pratt M, Blair SN, et al. Physical activity and public health: a recommendation from the Centers for Disease Control and Prevention and the American College of Sports Medicine. JAMA 1995;273:402–407.

42. Pratt M. Exercise and sudden death: implications for health policy. Sports Sci Rev J 1995;4:106–122.

43. Centers for Disease Control and Prevention. Available at: http://www.cdc.gov/nccdphp/dnpa/physical/life/overcome.htm. Accessed July 26, 2005.

44. U.S. Department of Health and Human Services, Public Health Services, Centers for Disease Control and Prevention, National Center for Chronic Disease Prevention and Health Promotion, Division of Nutrition and Physical Activity. Promoting physical activity: a guide for community action. Champaign, IL: Human Kinetics, 1999.

45. Lenz TL, Lenz NJ, Faulkner MA. Potential interactions between exercise and drug therapy. Sports Med 2004;34:293–306.

3

Weight Control

At the end of this chapter the reader should be able to:

1. Discuss the prevalence of obesity and its impact on public health.
2. Compare and contrast body weight versus body composition.
3. Explain the three phases of a weight-control program.
4. Summarize the recommended strategies for weight control.
5. Develop a weight-loss program for a patient using the five-step weight-loss program.

IMPACT OF OVERWEIGHT AND OBESITY

In the past several years the issue of weight control, particularly weight loss, has become a regular part of our national rhetoric. Today, more than ever in our history, many Americans are advised to lose weight for medical reasons. It is estimated that approximately 64.5% of U.S. adults are either overweight or obese, with 30.5% of U.S. adults being obese or extremely obese (Fig. 3-1).[1] **Obesity** is a chronic disease with complex political, social, psychological, environmental, economic, and metabolic causes and consequences.[2]

Because of its prevalence, obesity has become a significant public health problem in the United States. It increases the risks of chronic diseases and health conditions such as heart disease, **stroke, type 2 diabetes, cancer** (specifically endometrial, breast, prostate, and colon), hyperlipidemia, **hypertension,** hyperinsulinemia, **osteoarthritis, chronic obstructive pulmonary disease,** gallbladder disease, and all-cause mortality.[3,4] In addition, obesity is associated with social stigma, poor self-esteem, and economic disadvantage.[4]

An estimated $100 billion is spent annually in the United States to treat obesity-related conditions. Direct costs associated with obesity account for 5 to 10% of the

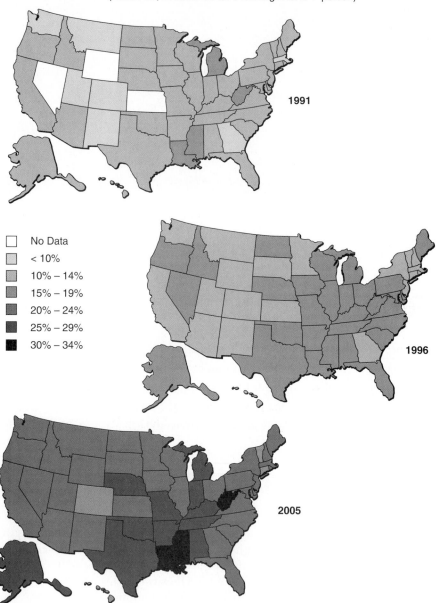

Obesity Trends Among U.S. Adults
BRFSS, 1991, 1996, 2005

(BMI ≥ 30, or about 30 lbs overweight for 5'4" person)

No Data
< 10%
10% – 14%
15% – 19%
20% – 24%
25% – 29%
30% – 34%

1991

1996

2005

FIGURE 3–1   Obesity trends among U.S. adults. (*Source:* U.S. Department of Health and Human Services, Centers for Disease Control and Prevention. CDC's Behavioral Risk Factor Surveillance System [BRFSS]. Overweight and Obesity: Obesity Trends: U.S. Obesity Trends 1985–2005. Accessed July 28, 2006, at http://www.cdc.gov/nccdphp/dnpa/obesity/trend/maps/index.htm.)

healthcare dollars spent annually.[5] In addition, approximately 71% of women and 62% of men in America are attempting to lose weight at any given time.[6] Overweight and obesity have been designated as the second leading cause of preventable death in the United States.[7,8]

The standard method used to define obesity is called **body mass index** (BMI).[2] BMI can be calculated by using one of the following two formulas:[2]

$$[\text{weight (pounds)}/\text{height (inches}^2)] \times 703$$

OR

$$[\text{weight (kg)}/\text{height (m}^2)]$$

In addition, BMI can be estimated through the use of tables such as the one in Appendix B by simply knowing the patient's height and weight. The clinical guidelines on the identification, evaluation, and treatment of overweight and obesity in adults (Obesity Guidelines, http://www.cdc.gov/nccdphp/dnpa/obesity/recommendations. htm) defines a normal BMI as 18.5 to 24.9 kg/m².[2] Overweight is defined as having a BMI of 25.0 to 29.9 kg/m², and obesity and extreme obesity are defined by a BMI of 30.0 to 39.9 kg/m² and ≥ 40 kg/m², respectively.[2] The classifications for overweight and obesity according to BMI are listed in Table 3-1.

BODY WEIGHT AND BODY COMPOSITION

As stated above, BMI is considered the current standard for assessing a patient's size as it relates to his or her health risks.[2] It does, however, have some limitations. Only two variables, height and weight, are used when measuring BMI. This method does not account for the amount of lean tissue or fat tissue that a patient possesses. Therefore, two individuals may have the exact same height and weight, and as a result the same BMI, but have very different body compositions and therefore different health risks.

Take for example patient number one: a 30-year-old sedentary male who is 6-foot tall (72 inches), weighs 222 pounds, and has 25% body fat. The BMI for this individual is 30 kg/m², which puts him in the obese category. On the other hand, patient number two is a 30-year-old highly active male who is a former college athlete and remains active through regular exercise and weight lifting. Patient number two is also 6-foot tall and

TABLE 3–1   Classification of Overweight and Obesity According to BMI

BMI kg/m²	Classification
<18.5	Underweight
18.5–24.9	Normal
25–29.9	Overweight
30–34.9	Obesity class I
35–39.9	Obesity class II
≥40	Extreme obesity or obesity class III

Source: Clinical Guidelines on the Identification, Evaluation, and Treatment of Overweight and Obesity in Adults. Bethesda, MD: National Institutes of Health, U.S. Department of Health and Human Services, 1998. NIH Publication No. 98-4083.

weighs 222 pounds but only has 15% body fat but also has a BMI of 30 kg/m². This patient is clearly healthier than patient number one because of the lower percentage of body fat and participation in regular exercise. However, patient number two also has a BMI that is considered to be obese.

For most average Americans, BMI works well to give healthcare practitioners an idea of a patient's health risks as they relate to body size. However, it may behoove practitioners to also consider physical activity level and body composition when assessing certain patients.

Body composition can be defined as the substances that make up the different components of the body grouped together as like tissues or materials. Four major body components are included in body composition: fat-free mass, total body fat, body water, and bone density.[9] The two components that are the most commonly assessed are fat-free mass and total body fat. **Fat-free mass,** also called lean body mass, primarily consists of protein and water. The major component of fat-free mass is muscle tissue, but also includes internal organs. **Total body fat** consists of both essential fat and storage fat.[9]

Body Fat

Essential body fat is a minimum amount of fat needed in the brain, heart, cell membranes, nerve tissue, and bone marrow for the body to function normally.[9] In adult males, essential fat represents approximately 3% of the total body weight. Adult females are required to have an additional 9 to 12% of their total body weight be essential body fat for reproductive processes. Therefore, adult women are required to have 12 to 15% of their total body weight be essential body fat.[9]

An acceptable level of total body fat for adult males is 15 to 20% or less and for adult females is 24 to 30% or less.[9] A body fat percentage in the overweight range is 21 to 24% for males and 31 to 36% for females. Anything over 25% and 37%, respectively, for men and women is considered obese with respect to percentage of body fat.[9]

Storage fat is nothing more than excess deposits of fat. Approximately 50% of excess body fat is stored just under the skin and is called subcutaneous fat.[9] Other amounts of excess fat are stored more deeply in the body and are known as visceral fat. Men and women distribute excess fat differently. Male-type obesity, also called android-type obesity, accumulates in the abdominal region and especially in the deep visceral tissue.[9] It is sometimes referred to as apple-shaped obesity because excess fat is stored centrally in the upper body and lower trunk region. Although it is not fully understood, it is believed that fat is deposited in the abdominal region of men because of an overproduction of the hormone cortisol.[9] Female-type obesity, also called gynoid-type obesity, tends to accumulate in the hips, buttocks, and thighs of women.[9] This type of obesity is sometimes referred to as pear-shaped obesity because excess fat is stored in the lower body.

Much has been reported about the risks that are associated with where excess body fat is stored. Fat cells that are stored in the deep, visceral tissues, such as in males, appear to be biochemically different from those stored in the lower body, such as in females. Deep visceral fat cells are highly metabolically active and can be easily mobilized.[9] As a result, android-type obesity has been associated with increased risk for heart disease and diabetes compared with gynoid-type obesity by being associated with metabolic disorders such as hypertriglyceridemia, increasing the atherogenic small, dense low-density lipoprotein (LDL) cholesterol (bad cholesterol), decreasing high-density lipoprotein (HDL) cholesterol (good cholesterol), and increasing hypertension as well as increasing insulin resistance, hyperinsulinemia, and impaired glucose tolerance.[9]

WEIGHT CONTROL

The concept of weight control can include three separate phases: cessation of weight gain, weight loss, and weight maintenance.[2] It is common for many to think only of weight loss and not the other two phases of weight control, especially weight maintenance, as it is so important. Focusing only on weight loss rather than on weight loss followed by weight maintenance assumes that this concept is a short-term fix to a problem rather than a long-term plan to fight a chronic disease.

Obesity is considered a chronic disease that incorporates long-term treatment strategies similar to those used for treating other chronic diseases such as hypertension or hyperlipidemia.[2] Therefore, weight maintenance is probably the most important component of a weight-control program because, in the overall picture, it continues for many years, whereas cessation of weight gain and weight loss are relatively short periods comparatively. Strategies for each of the components of a weight-control program are similar and will be discussed in detail below.

Cessation of Weight Gain

The guidelines for treating overweight and obesity state that the first goal in weight control is to prevent further weight gain.[2] This may sound obvious, but can be an important first step when counseling patients about weight control. Some patients tend to gain weight more rapidly than others. Stopping this from occurring and maintaining a consistent body weight for a period of time (even if it is too much weight) can be a victory. Focusing on this aspect of weight control may be more applicable for those patients who are extremely obese (BMI > 40 kg/m^2) rather than those who are overweight or mildly obese.

Weight Loss

The Obesity Guidelines recommend an initial reduction of body weight by approximately 10% from baseline.[2] Even a modest reduction of 10% body weight has been shown to significantly decrease the severity of obesity-related risk factors.[2] The Obesity Guidelines state that it is reasonable to achieve a 10% weight loss in approximately 6 months.[2] Once this initial goal is achieved, reevaluation of the patient's weight-control status is recommended. If further weight loss is warranted, a new weight-loss goal should be set and again reevaluated once this new goal is achieved.[2]

As stated above, reaching the initial weight-loss goal can realistically take approximately 6 months. In doing so, gradual weight loss occurs at a rate of approximately 0.5 to 2 pounds/week. Patients with a BMI in the typical range of 27 to 35 kg/m^2 can reach a 10% weight loss in 6 months by losing 0.5 to 1 pound/week with a caloric deficit of 300 to 500 kcal/day.[2] Patients with a BMI of greater than 35 kg/m^2 will need to be treated more aggressively to achieve a 10% weight loss in 6 months by creating a caloric deficit of 500 to 1,000 kcal/day, which should yield a weight loss rate of approximately 1 to 2 pounds/week.[2]

Weight loss ideally should be a slow, gradual, and steady process. Rapid weight loss (rates greater than 2 pounds/week) is not desirable because it often leads to a rapid regain of the lost body weight. In addition, rapid weight loss can lead to increases in gallstones and electrolyte abnormalities and is counterproductive to the patient's self-esteem when the weight is regained.[2] The media tends to influence some patients' expectations into thinking that rapid weight loss is easy and healthy. Therefore, stressing the point that gradual weight loss leads to greater long-term weight-control success is important.

It is realistically difficult for many patients to continue to lose weight at a rate of 1 to 2 pounds/week after approximately 6 months on a weight-loss program.[2] This is mostly because of changes in the resting metabolic rate and difficulties adhering to the treatment strategies. Some patients can be successful beyond 6 months, but for those who are not, it is critical to stress the importance of a weight-maintenance program.[2]

Weight Maintenance

Weight maintenance is perhaps the most important aspect of a weight-control program. As stated above, significant health benefits can be achieved through a 10% decrease in body weight, and this weight loss can be achieved in approximately 6 months. The Obesity Guidelines recommend that the weight-maintenance treatment period continue indefinitely.[2] Therefore, weight maintenance becomes the most important aspect of weight control because of its duration of the treatment period. The key to achieving the health-related benefits of weight loss is to prevent the weight from being regained.

A successful weight-maintenance program is defined in the Obesity Guidelines as a weight regain of less than 3 kg (6.6 lbs) in 2 years and a sustained reduction in waist circumference of at least 4 cm.[2] The key to a successful weight-maintenance program is continual observation, monitoring, and encouragement by one or more healthcare providers of patients who have successfully lost weight.[2] Long-term monitoring and encouragement from pharmacists can be accomplished in several ways. Contact with patients can be made in the pharmacy every time the patient comes to pick up a prescription or through regularly scheduled appointments. In addition, pharmacists can offer group meetings, or contact patients via telephone or email. Pharmacists are logistically in an excellent position to assist patients in maintaining weight that has been lost. Pharmacists can also use the weight-maintenance strategies of emphasizing a healthy eating plan, regular exercise, and behavior modification that are continued indefinitely for patients of normal weight to prevent future weight gain.

STRATEGIES FOR WEIGHT CONTROL

An effective weight-control program incorporates a combination of several treatment strategies.[2] Available strategies include dietary therapy, physical activity, behavior therapy, pharmacotherapy, and surgery.[2] These strategies, in particular dietary therapy, physical activity, and behavior therapy, can and should be used in combination in any of the three phases of weight control. The Obesity Guidelines recommend that everyone participate in the lifestyle-modification components of dietary therapy and physical activity unless they are contraindicated.[2] Incorporating these treatment strategies is important because they have not only been shown to improve the success of a weight-loss and weight-maintenance program but have also been shown to decrease some of the comorbidities associated with obesity. These topics are also covered in Chapter 13.

The fundamental principle of a weight-control program involves caloric balance. The caloric balance equation consists of (1) calorie intake from food and (2) energy expenditure from physical activity in relation to the amount of calories an individual patient requires throughout a day.[2] The number of calories needed by an individual patient during a day can be calculated by using the equation provided in Table 1-1 in

Chapter 1. Total daily net calories are the number of calories consumed in a day minus the number of calories expended through physical activity and metabolic activity. The number of calories expended through physical activity can be calculated through the use of the TEE equation provided in Chapter 2.

During the weight-loss phase, the goal is to create a **caloric deficit.** A caloric deficit means that a patient's net calories at the end of the day were fewer than that required to maintain the current body weight. A caloric deficit can be created by eating fewer calories than required each day or by expending calories through physical activity or a combination of both. It is important to understand that even if a patient consumes a perfectly balanced eating plan according to the Nutritional Guidelines, body weight can still increase if too many calories of this perfectly balanced eating plan are consumed.[10] Although it is important to eat the right kinds of foods, it may be more important in the weight-loss phase to eat foods in moderation to create a caloric deficit to achieve the weight-loss goal.

During the weight-maintenance phase, the goal is to have the daily net calories and the required daily calories equivalent. This is primarily achieved through a consistent eating pattern along with daily physical activity through a structured exercise program. It is recommended that patients in the weight-maintenance phase participate in at least 30 to 60 minutes of a daily exercise regimen.[3] As a result, it is thought that the most important component of a weight-maintenance program is a consistent, structured exercise program.[3]

A **positive caloric balance** is what occurs when a patient gains or regains weight. During this process, the **net daily calories** are greater than what is required each day. To prevent this from occurring, a consistent eating plan and physical activity plan are required.

Dietary Therapy

The dietary therapy component of weight loss focuses on teaching patients how to modify their individual diet to decrease calorie intake. It appears that the success of the weight-loss phase of a weight-control program is more dependent on the dietary therapy component compared with the other weight-loss strategies.[2] It is very important that calorie-reduction recommendations are not too aggressive and are made with the goal of slow and progressive weight loss through moderate calorie reduction. In addition, the composition of the diet should be balanced and structured in a way that decreases other possible cardiovascular risk factors such as hypertension, **dyslipidemia,** and **diabetes mellitus.**[2]

The focus of weight loss through dietary therapy is to create a caloric deficit by decreasing the caloric intake. To achieve this caloric deficit, a low-calorie diet is recommended that consists of at least 1,000 to 1,200 kcal/day for most women and 1,200 to 1,600 kcal/day for most men.[11] The specific caloric intake for each patient should be individualized and chosen with the patient's baseline caloric intake and body weight in mind. Healthcare practitioners should emphasize to patients that moderate dietary changes should be incorporated, not drastic ones. This will help maintain patient compliance to the weight-loss regimen and produce slow and progressive weight loss. A diet that is individually designed to create a deficit of 500 to 1,000 kcal/day should be adequate to produce a 1- to 2-pound weight loss per week.[11] A diet that consists of very low calorie intake, often called very low–calorie diets or VLCD (<800 kcal/day), will require extra dietary supplementation and are only recommended in specific patients for short periods.[2] The amount of weight loss is similar with low-calorie diets and VLCD; however, the incidence of weight regain is greater with VLCD.[2,11] Only specialized practitioners with experience in the use of VLCD should recommend this type of therapy.[2]

Resistance Training and a VLCD

It is recommended that the proper strategies for losing weight incorporate calorie reduction, physical activity, and behavior therapy.[3] Severely restricting calorie intake to lose weight, or VLCD, has been shown to result in a dramatic and sustained decrease in resting metabolic rate (RMR).[12–14] In addition, VLCD has been shown to produce a weight loss that consists largely of lean tissue (muscle tissue).[12,15] One study reported that 40% of the weight that was lost in those who decreased body weight via calorie restriction alone was in lean tissue.[16] Therefore, patients who attempt to lose weight through VLCD are actually creating more harm than good. One of the main goals in a weight-loss program is to increase resting metabolism so that a greater amount of calories can be expended throughout the day, even at rest. Another main goal is to maintain lean tissue. A greater amount of lean tissue not only leads to a more favorable body composition, but it also helps to improve muscular fitness and maintain an adequate resting metabolism.

One particular study set out to assess the effects of a resistance-training program on a VLCD with respect to the loss of lean body weight and on the decrease in RMR.[12] Twenty participants (17 women, 3 men) were randomized to one of two treatment groups for 12 weeks. The participants had a mean age of 36 years and a baseline BMI of 35 kg/m^2. The first group followed a standard treatment protocol that consisted of aerobic exercise four times per week that gradually increased in duration from 20 minutes per session to 60 minutes per session. In addition, this group consumed a VLCD consisting of a liquid formula ingested five times per day that had a total daily caloric value of 800 kcal. The second group participated in resistance exercises that consisted of 10 exercise stations at which four sets of 8 to 12 repetitions were performed three times per week. This group also followed the same diet regimen as in the control group.[12]

The results showed that both groups lost a significant amount of body weight compared with baseline, but the control group lost significantly more body weight compared with the resistance-training group (−18.1 kg vs. −14.4 kg, respectively, $P < 0.05$).[12] The control group, however, lost a significant amount of lean body weight compared with baseline (−4.1 kg, $P < 0.05$), whereas the resistance-training group did not lose lean body weight. In addition, the resistance-training group increased its RMR by 63.3 kcal/day, which compares with the control group that actually decreased its RMR by 210.7 kcal/day.[12] Therefore, those patients who lifted weights during the weight-loss process actually burn more overall calories throughout the day, which can result in indirect weight loss.

This study shows that by incorporating resistance training into a VLCD, patients can maintain lean body tissue and RMR.[12] Although a VLCD is not recommended for the average patient wishing to lose weight, many individuals attempt this form of weight loss. Therefore, it would behoove the healthcare professional counseling patients who are using VLCD methods about the adverse consequences associated with such a strategy. In addition, it is also important for the patient to understand that many of those who use the VLCD strategy tend to regain the weight that was lost. This weight that is regained does not recoup the lean tissue that was lost during the weight-loss phase, and therefore the patient's overall body fat percentage will increase even if the body weight returns to baseline. This can be especially damaging to the body composition for those who frequently lose and regain weight via the VLCD method. The net result is that these individuals become "fatter" over time by the gradual increase in body fat percentage even if the baseline body weight remains relatively the same.

In the weight-loss phase, success is dependent on modifying the patient's diet to create a caloric deficit while providing for all the necessary dietary allowances and also maintaining food preferences of the patient. The keys to success in the weight-loss phase for dietary therapy are to (1) educate the patients regarding the calorie value of foods they are choosing as well as the composition (carbohydrate, fats, and protein) by reading the nutrition label, (2) avoid overconsumption of high-calorie foods, (3) reduce portion size, and (4) maintain adequate water intake.

In the weight-maintenance phase, success is dependent on the ability to modify the patient's eating plan in a way that creates permanent and maintainable changes. Maintaining a relatively consistent calorie intake, along with a structured exercise program, will allow the patient the greatest ability to maintain the weight that had been lost. Keys to success in the weight-maintenance phase of a weight-control program are (1) making realistic changes to the eating plan that the patient can adhere to, (2) maintaining a relatively consistent caloric intake on a daily basis, and (3) incorporating a structured exercise regimen, as this has been shown to help maintain changes to the eating plan.

Specific information regarding balanced eating plans for patients can be found in Chapter 1. Patients in a weight-control program should incorporate these same strategies to consume the appropriate types of food; however, they will need to eat less to create a caloric deficit. Please refer to Chapter 1 for more information about proper nutrition.

Physical Activity

It has been shown that greater amounts of weight loss can occur by decreasing calorie intake alone versus expending calories through exercise alone.[2] However, the combination of the two strategies has shown to yield the greatest success in a weight-control program.[2] Even though reducing caloric intake will have the greatest effect in the weight-loss phase, exercise is important because it decreases the loss of fat-free mass–associated weight loss and improves cardiovascular and metabolic health independent of weight loss.[3,11] In addition, as stated earlier, **physical activity** may be one of the most important components involved in the maintenance of weight loss. Maintaining body weight can occur directly by increasing caloric expenditure through physical activity. It can also occur indirectly by promoting a positive behavior change wherein the patient decreases food consumption. The influence of physical activity on food intake is not well known, but it is thought to have a possible impact on calorie intake in some individuals.[17]

Participation is aerobic exercise is very beneficial for weight loss as well as weight maintenance because it directly decreases daily net calories to help create a negative or neutral caloric balance. In addition, it can independently improve the cardiovascular and metabolic risk by improving cardiovascular fitness levels with or without weight loss.[2,18–29] Improving cardiovascular fitness has also been shown to improve quality of life in overweight patients by improving mood, self-esteem, and physical function in daily activities.[2,30] Participation in regular physical activity has been shown to decrease the risk for **cardiovascular disease** and diabetes by helping to lower blood pressure and **triglycerides,** increasing HDL cholesterol, and improving glucose tolerance independent of weight loss.[2,30] Recall that the current guidelines on physical activity recommend that every American participate in at least 30 minutes of accumulated physical activity on most days of the week.[31,32] This guideline is important because adopting this recommendation can help reduce the risks for certain diseases and help to maintain current body weight. It may not, however, have a significant impact on weight loss. Patients who are recommended to lose weight will most likely need to participate in a more intensive exercise regimen (upward of 60 minutes of aerobic activity) to be successful at achieving their weight-loss goals.[3] Likewise, those patients trying to prevent weight regain may also have to participate in a more intensive exercise regimen to be successful at maintaining their newly lost weight.[3]

Participation in resistance-training physical activity is important in a weight-control program because it helps to decrease the loss of fat-free tissue (i.e., muscle) during the weight-loss phase.[2,3] Resistance-training activities can be done through the use of weight equipment at the local fitness center and in home gyms or by simply lifting household items such as soup cans or laundry detergent bottles filled with water or sand. Please refer to Chapter 2 for more information regarding resistance training.

Depending on the prior experiences and the length of time the patient has been sedentary, the physical-activity program should begin very slowly and proceed gradually. For some patients, an initial program may begin with increasing the activities of daily living. Examples of this could include work around the house such as vacuuming, ironing, cooking, gardening, or painting a room.[11] Other patients may begin at a level that includes a slow 10-minute walk around the neighborhood, riding a stationary bicycle, or swimming at a slow pace. Still others may be able to work at a greater intensity by walking more briskly, rowing or cycling at a greater intensity, or using other non-impact aerobic machines. Recreational sports such as tennis, racquetball, and basketball are also good activities that will increase caloric expenditure and improve the patient's cardiovascular profile.

It is important to remember that overweight and obese patients are at increased risk for orthopedic injuries if they participate in high-impact activities such as running. These types of activities should be avoided until the patient has lost a sufficient amount of weight and has improved aerobic capacity with other activities.

The activities that are appropriate for each patient should be individualized. Decisions on the type and amount of activity will depend on the patient's comorbidities, prior experiences, and specific preferences.[3] Many patients should begin with non–weight-bearing activities or very low–intensity weight-bearing activities and progress to greater-intensity activities. Many of the activities that are chosen, such as walking or cycling, can be performed for short amounts of time (i.e., 5 to 10 minutes) several times per day. It is important to begin a program with short-duration activities that are preferable to the patients. This will be more encouraging and enjoyable and lead to better compliance. The progression of the activities should begin with 2 to 3 days/week and progress to most days of the week. It is important also to emphasize an increase in duration over intensity for the initial several weeks of the program. This will decrease the risks for injury and improve compliance. The American College of Sports Medicine (ACSM, http://www.acsm.org) recommends that overweight and obese adults progress to a minimum of 150 minutes of moderate-intensity exercise per week and, when possible, progress to greater than 200 minutes of moderate-intensity exercise per week.[3] Greater and more effective results will be experienced with a longer duration of activity. Therefore, patients who have weight loss as their goal should attempt to increase physical activity duration up to 60 minutes per day.[3]

Sedentary Patients With Normal BMI vs. Active Patients With Obese BMI

It is well documented and proven that individuals with a body mass index (BMI) greater than 30 kg/m^2 are at increased risk for several obesity-related diseases. It is also well known and documented that individuals who are sedentary are at increased risk for disease, especially cardiovascular disease. Many patients who are obese may be successful on a weight-loss program at decreasing their body weight with proper eating habits and exercise, but may still not reach a BMI that is below 30 kg/m^2 (the defining BMI for obesity). Therefore, the question often arises from patients, "Do I need to obtain a BMI of less than 30 mg/m^2 to gain health benefits?" In addition, many individuals who are not obese feel that they do not need to exercise as they perceive their health risks to be low as long as they are not overweight or obese. Therefore, the question often arises, "Which is a more significant predictor of morbidity and mortality, overweight and obesity or physical inactivity?" Also, "Do individuals who are obese but remain active have a lower morbidity and mortality risk compared with patients who are of normal weight but are sedentary?"

A study published in 1999 by Blair and Brodney set out to answer these questions.[12] The authors reviewed the available literature related to disease risk outcomes associated with BMI, body composition, and physical-activity habits. A total of 24 studies were found to meet the criteria appropriate to answer the objectives of the study. Specific data were available to study the outcomes of all-cause mortality, cardiovascular disease mortality, **coronary heart disease,** hypertension, type 2 diabetes, and cancer as they relate to BMI and physical activity.[12] It was discovered that all outcome measures except one showed that individuals who are active appeared to be protected against the health risks associated with overweight and obesity.[12] In addition, the review showed that physical activity not only decreases health risks associated with overweight and obesity, but that active obese individuals have a lower morbidity and mortality than normal-weight individuals who are sedentary.[12] Lastly, the review showed that physical inactivity and low cardiorespiratory fitness levels are as important as overweight and obesity as predictors for mortality.[12] The outcome measure that did not protect against health risks was cancer owing to an inadequate amount of data to analyze.[12]

Therefore, it is important to remind our patients that what they see on the outside of the body should not lead to conclusions as to what is happening on the inside of the body. Patients who are participating in regular physical activity are obtaining lots of health benefit even if they are not successful at decreasing body weight. The primary goal of a weight-control program should be to decrease overall morbidity and mortality risks. This goal can be achieved as a result of increased physical activity even if the patient does not lose a single pound of body weight. Our society often judges individuals based on outward appearance. Healthcare professionals should counsel patients who are having difficulties in a weight-control program to decrease discouraging feelings because many "good things" are happening in their bodies to improve their health even if their outward appearance does not change. Likewise, healthcare professionals should counsel sedentary, normal-weight patients of the risks associated with a sedentary lifestyle and that a normal body weight may not equal a healthy body.

Many overweight and obese patients have been sedentary for years. As a result, these patients may lack the confidence, motivation, and skills needed to participate in physical activities. Therefore, some patients may need supervision when first beginning a physical-activity program. Safety should always be the highest priority for patients beginning a physical-activity program, especially if they have little experience being physically active.[2] Physical injury may be one of the primary reasons for discontinuation of physical activity in obese patients.[17] A patient who becomes injured while exercising will be increasingly difficult to motivate to continue the program after the injury heals.[11] Overweight and obese patients must always obtain clearance from their physician before beginning an exercise program.[3] Some patients may require testing for cardiopulmonary disease before beginning depending on their symptoms and comorbidities.[11]

Behavior Therapy

Behavior therapy is a critical aspect of a weight-control program because it incorporates techniques that can be used to overcome barriers that exist within the dietary therapy and physical-activity programs.[11] Most patients have a difficult time adhering to a weight-loss program for longer than 6 months in part because of the lifestyle changes that have occurred.[2] Therefore, behavior therapy is important in both the weight-loss and weight-maintenance phases of weight control and should be continued indefinitely.

As with other aspects of a weight-loss program, behavior therapy needs to be individualized. Before attempting to motivate the patient for change, the practitioner must first evaluate the patient's readiness for change and self-motivation level. The behavior therapy plan should include important themes such as setting appropriate and achievable goals and focusing on the main outcomes of the program. The most important outcome of a weight-loss program should be to improve the patient's health.[11] Monitoring progress is a continuous and ongoing process and is the responsibility of both the patient and the healthcare practitioner. Behavior therapy is recommended along with dietary therapy and physical activity for all patients with a BMI of 25 kg/m² or greater.[11] Behavior therapy is covered in more complete detail in Chapter 5.

Pharmacotherapy

The use of medication to treat obesity is appropriate if the patient has a BMI of 27 to 29.9 kg/m² with the existence of comorbidities.[11] Obesity medications are appropriate to use in patients with a BMI of 30 kg/m² or greater regardless of the presence of comorbidities.[11] There are currently six commonly used drugs that have U.S. Food and Drug Administration (FDA) approval to be used for weight loss.[34] Since 1973 only two of these six drugs have been approved, and these same two drugs are the only ones approved for long-term use. The two drugs are orlistat and sibutramine.

It is important to note that sibutramine has been shown to produce significant increases in both **systolic** and **diastolic blood pressure** as well as heart rate.[11] Therefore, sibutramine should not be used in patients with a history of coronary artery disease, stroke, **heart failure,** or arrhythmias and should be used with caution in patients with pulmonary hypertension.[35] Measuring blood pressure at baseline and throughout treatment is recommended regardless of whether comorbidities exist. Medications with FDA approval for weight loss are listed in Table 3-2.

TABLE 3–2   Medications Approved for Weight Loss

Drug Class	Individual Agent
Lipase inhibitor	Orlistat
Noradrenergic/serotonergic agent	Sibutramine
Noradrenergic agent	Phentermine
	Diethylpropion
	Phendimetrazine
	Benzphetamine

Combination Therapy

Several clinical trials have demonstrated that combining the weight-control strategies of behavior therapy, reduced-calorie eating plans, and increased physical activity provides better outcomes for long-term weight reduction compared with implementing only one or two of these strategies.[2] The guidelines state that the implementation of combination therapy provides the best opportunity for weight loss and long-term weight control. Therefore, the guidelines specifically state, "Weight loss and weight maintenance therapy should employ the combination of low calorie diet (LCD), increased physical activity and behavior therapy."[2]

WEIGHT-LOSS GOALS

Three primary goals are associated with a weight-control program. At minimum, prevention of further weight gain is the first goal. Second, a reduction in body weight should be the focus, and third, maintaining the lower body weight for the long term is the final and lasting weight-control goal.

Some patients may not be successful in a weight-loss program. For these patients, prevention of further weight gain can be considered a partial therapeutic success.[2] If this weight-gain prevention can be maintained, this should be viewed as an important first step in a weight-control program. Healthcare practitioners should recognize the importance of this goal for patients who are not able to immediately lose weight.[2] Cessation of weight gain may warrant the need for some patients to maintain this goal for an extended period through the use of weight-maintenance strategies.[2]

The initial goal of weight-loss therapy should be to reduce body weight by approximately 10% from baseline. A 10% weight loss has been shown to significantly reduce the risk factors associated with obesity.[2] Further weight loss should be attempted if the patient was successful with the initial 10% loss and if further assessments indicate such an outcome.[2] Weight loss at a rate of 1 to 2 pounds/week commonly occurs for up to 6 months. A caloric deficit of 500 to 1,000 calories/day is often sufficient to yield a 1- to 2-pound/week loss. After 6 months, weight loss may plateau unless a more restrictive weight-loss regimen is implemented.[2]

Maintaining weight that has been lost is the most challenging phase of weight control for most patients. The Obesity Guidelines recommend long-term observing, monitoring, and encouraging of patients who have lost weight.[2] Successful weight maintenance is defined as a weight regain of less than 3 kg in 2 years and a sustained reduction in weight circumference of at least 4 cm.[2] This phase of weight control should be continued indefinitely.

WEIGHT CONTROL IN PHARMACY PRACTICE

Pharmacists are well positioned within the community to treat and manage weight-control issues for patients. The community pharmacy practice setting offers easy access and follow-up, whereas those who practice in a clinical setting can offer ideal weight-control therapy as they can easily collaborate with other healthcare professionals within the same clinical setting.

The following practice case scenario will present a patient who follows a five-step process designed to assess and create a personalized weight-control program. Figure 3-2 is a weight-loss program worksheet that can be used with this process.

Weight-Loss Program Worksheet

Name: _____

Date of initial consultation: _____

Gender: Male / Female

Age: _____ yr

Height: _____ inches

Height: _____ meters (calculate by multiplying height in inches by 0.0254)

Weight: _____ lb

Weight: _____ kg (calculate by dividing weight in pounds by 2.2)

PA = physical activity coefficient (calculate using the following table)

	Sedentary	Low active	Active	Very active
Male	1.0	1.11	1.25	1.48
Female	1.0	1.12	1.27	1.45

STEP 1: Calculate Body Mass Index (BMI) and Classify

BMI = [weight (kg) / height (m^2)]

BMI = [_____ kg / (_____ m)^2]

BMI = _____ kg/m^2

Classification of overweight and obesity according to BMI (circle)

<18.5 kg/m^2	Underweight
18.5–24.9 kg/m^2	Normal
25–29.9 kg/m^2	Overweight
30–34.9 kg/m^2	Obesity class I
35–39.9 kg/m^2	Obesity class II
≥40 kg/m^2	Obesity class III or extreme obesity

STEP 2: Calculate the Estimated Energy Requirement (EER)

Males aged > 19 years:

EER = 662 − 9.53 × age (yr) + PA × [15.9 × weight (kg) + 540 × height (m)]

EER = 662 − 9.53 × _____ yr + _____ × [15.9 × _____ kg + 540 × _____ m]

EER = _____ kcal

Females aged > 19 years:

EER = 354 − 6.91 × age (yr) + PA x [9.36 × weight (kg) + 726 × height (m)]

EER = 354 − 6.91 × _____ yr + _____ × [9.36 × _____ kg + 726 × _____ m]

EER = _____ kcal

 FIGURE 3–2 Weight-loss program worksheet. MET, metabolic equivalent; RPE, rating of perceived exertion.

STEP 3: Calculate Current Caloric Intake and Eating Patterns

Day 1 total calories: _____ kcal

Day 2 total calories: _____ kcal

Day 3 total calories: _____ kcal

Day 4 total calories: _____ kcal

Average total daily calories: _____ kcal

Suggested caloric deficit from food consumption per day: _____ kcal (multiply by 7 to get weekly caloric deficit = _____ kcal)

STEP 4: Design Exercise Prescription and Calculate Energy Expenditure

Examples of physical activity the patient prefers:

_____

_____

Weight-loss goals:

1._____

2._____

3._____

Exercise Prescription:

        Mode: _____

              Associated MET level: _____

        Intensity: _____ (% max heart rate or RPE)

        Duration: _____ minutes

        Frequency: _____ times per week

        Rate of Progression:

        _____

        _____

Energy expenditure:

(METs × 3.5 × body weight in kg)/200 = kcal/min

(_____ × 3.5 × _____ kg)/200 = _____ kcal/min (calories expended per minute of activity)

Multiply answer by the duration = calories expended per exercise session (kcal/session)

_____ kcal/min × _____ minutes = _____ kcal/session

Multiply answer by frequency = calories expended per week (kcal/week)

_____ kcal/session × _____ times per week = _____ kcal/week

FIGURE 3–2 *(Continued)*

STEP 5: Design a Weight-Loss Program

A. Current body weight: _____ lb

B. Weight-loss goal: _____%

C. Weight-loss goal in pounds: _____ lb (Step A × Step B)

D. Goal body weight: _____ lb (Step A – Step C)

E. Goal BMI classification: _____ (obtain from chart in Step 1)

F. Weekly calories decreased from food consumption: _____ kcal (obtain from Step 3)

G. Caloric expenditure per week from physical activity: _____ kcal (obtain from Step 4)

H. Total weekly caloric deficit: _____ kcal (Step F + Step G)

I. Amount of body weight lost per week: _____ lb (Step H/3,500 kcal)

J. Approximate time to achieve the goal weight: _____ weeks (Step C/Step I)

FIGURE 3–2   (*Continued*)

Sample Patient

C.J. is a 45-year-old male accountant who comes to your pharmacy to participate in the weight-control program. C.J. is 5′11″ tall and weighs 245 pounds. He states that he has been sedentary for several years, and has no current medical conditions and no family history of heart disease, stroke, diabetes, or cancer. C.J. would like to lose weight because he has been recommended to do so by his physician and because he desires to "become more healthy."

Step 1: Calculate Body Mass Index and Classify

BMI can be calculated by using one of the following two formulas: [weight (pounds)/height (inches^2)] × 703, or [weight (kg)/height (m^2)]; or by estimating through the use of tables such as the one in Appendix B.[2] Using the first formula listed as well as C.J.'s height (5′11″ or 71″) and weight (245 lbs) stated above, his calculated BMI is **34 kg/m^2.** According to Table 3-1, C.J. is categorized as class I obesity.

Step 2: Calculate the Estimated Energy Requirements

Recall from Chapter 1 that we can calculate the amount of energy or calorie consumption required to meet our individual metabolism needs, or the **estimated energy requirements (EER)**.[9] This can be done through the use of a formula such as the one in Table 3-3. The variables that we need for this calculation are gender (male), age (45 years), physical-activity level (sedentary), height (1.8 m), and weight (111.4 kg). Notice from Table 3-3 that C.J. receives a physical-activity (PA) coefficient of 1.0 as a result of being sedentary. Therefore, using the formula for males older than 19 years, EER = 662–9.53 × age + PA × [15.9 × weight + 540 × height], C.J. requires approximately **2,976 kcal** to maintain his current weight of 245 pounds. Other formulas also exist to calculate EER, and the values from the various calculations may differ slightly from one another.

TABLE 3–3   Calculating Estimated Energy Requirement (EER)

Males aged ≥ 19 years:

EER = 662–9.53 × age + PA × [15.9 × weight + 540 × height]

Females aged ≥ 19 years:

EER = 354–6.91 × age + PA × [9.36 × weight + 726 × height]

Age = years

Weight = kilograms (kg; calculate by dividing weight in pounds by 2.2)

Height = meters (m; calculate by multiplying height in inches by 0.0254)

PA = physical activity coefficient (calculate using the following table)

	Sedentary	Low active	Active	Very active
Male	1.0	1.11	1.25	1.48
Female	1.0	1.12	1.27	1.45

Reprinted with permission from Dietary Reference Intakes for Energy, Carbohydrate, Fiber, Fat, Fatty Acids, Cholesterol, Protein, and Amino Acids (Macronutrients) by the National Academy of Sciences, Courtesy of the National Academies Press, Washington, DC, 2005.

Step 3: Calculate Current Calorie Intake and Eating Patterns

It is important to assess baseline calorie consumption and eating patterns to offer specific eating plan recommendations for individual patients. To do this, patients should complete a 3- to 4-day food diary and return it within 1 week of the initial visit. Patients should be instructed to record all food and drink that is consumed in a 24-hour period for 3 to 4 consecutive days as well as the time of day at which it is consumed. It is beneficial to have one of the days be a weekend day to compensate for the possibility that some individuals may have slightly different eating habits on weekends or days that do not constitute normal daily routines.

Once the patient has completed and returned the food diary, calorie consumption can be calculated by entering the information into the U.S. Department of Agriculture (USDA) dietary tracking system called MyPyramid Tracker.[36] This can be found on the USDA website at www.mypyramidtracker.gov. MyPyramid Tracker is a free dietary analysis program that can be accessed from any computer with Internet capabilities. Individual users can log into their personal accounts with a username and password and track their dietary intake over time. Other dietary analysis software is commercially available. The advantages of MyPyramid Tracker are that it is a free service from the USDA and patients can be taught how to use the system themselves to keep track of their own dietary intake over a long period on their own computers.[36]

C.J. completed the food diary and returned it to the pharmacy for analysis. Figure 3-3 shows the entries in C.J.'s food diary. After calculation it was discovered that C.J. had a caloric intake as follows: Day 1 = 4,021 kcal; Day 2 = 3,482 kcal; Day 3 = 3,266 kcal; Day 4 = 2,918 kcal (weekend). The average caloric intake from the 4 days was 3,422 kcal. Figure 3-4 shows the results received from MyPyramid Tracker for C.J. Therefore, our baseline assessment of C.J.'s caloric intake is that he consumes approximately **3,422 kcal/day.** This can then be compared with the EER calculated in Step 2 above. Please note that

Name: C.J.	Date: Wednesday, October 12, 2005		Day # 1
Food or Drink		**Amount**	**Time of Day**
Coffee, black, decaf		2 cups	6:15 am
McDonald's sausage biscuit with egg		1 sandwich	7:00 am
Orange juice		2 cups	7:00 am
Snickers candy bar		1 candy bar	10:15 am
Pepsi		1 can	10:30 am
Turkey sandwich with butter		1 sandwich	12:00 noon
Potato chips, baked		2 cups	12:00 noon
Pepsi		1 can	12:00 noon
Chocolate chip cookie		1 cookie	12:00 noon
Pepsi		1 can	3:00 pm
Chicken and rice dinner		2.5 cups	6:30 pm
Bread, homemade, French, whole wheat		1 slice	6:30 pm
Butter		1 pat	6:30 pm
Red wine		2 glasses	6:30 pm
Popcorn, buttered, microwave		1 bag	9:00 pm

FIGURE 3–3   Food diary for sample patient.

Name: C.J.	Date: Thursday, October 13, 2005		Day # 2
Food or Drink		**Amount**	**Time of Day**
Coffee, black, decaf		2 cups	6:20 am
Doughnuts, glazed		3	7:00 am
Snickers candy bar		1 candy bar	9:30 am
Taco Bell, beef tacos		3 tacos	12:15 pm
Pepsi		2 cans	12:15 pm
Potato chips, baked		About 10 chips	2:45 pm
Soup, beef and noodle		3 cups	6:00 pm
Bread, homemade, French, whole wheat		1 slice	6:00 pm
Butter		1 pat	6:00 pm
Red wine		2 glasses	6:00 pm
Cheesecake		1 slice	6:00 pm
Popcorn, buttered, microwave		½ bag	9:00 pm

FIGURE 3–3   (*Continued*)

Name: *C.J.*	Date: Friday, October 14, 2005		Day # 3
Food or Drink		**Amount**	**Time of Day**
Coffee, black, decaf		2 cups	6:00 am
McDonald's, ¼ pounder with cheese		1	11:30 am
Lettuce salad		1	11:30 am
Coke		2 cans	11:30 am
Spaghetti with meat sauce		4 cups	5:30 pm
Italian bread		3 slices	5:30 pm
Red wine		1 glass	5:30 pm
Movie theater popcorn		5 cups	7:30 pm
Coke		2 cans	7:30 pm

FIGURE 3–3   (*Continued*)

Name: C.J.	Date: Saturday, October 15, 2005		Day # 4
Food or Drink	**Amount**		**Time of Day**
Coffee, black, decaf	2 cups		7:30 am
Doughnuts, glazed	3		7:30 am
Pepsi	1 can		10:00 am
Peanut butter and jelly sandwich	1.5 sandwiches		12:30 pm
Potato chips, Pringles	About 20 chips		12:30 pm
Pepsi	1 can		12:30 pm
Steak, without bone	8 oz		5:45 pm
Baked potato, with butter and sour cream	1 large		5:45 pm
Mixed vegetables	1 cup		5:45 pm
Beer, lite	2 bottles		5:45 pm

FIGURE 3–3   (*Continued*)

MyPyramid Tracker can calculate the EER, and the value may be slightly different from the one we calculated in Step 2.

After reviewing C.J.'s eating habits and daily caloric intake, a suggestion should be made as to the number of calories that C.J. could decrease from his total daily caloric intake. The Obesity Guidelines recommend a caloric deficit of 500 to 1,000 kcal/day if weight loss is attempted via calorie restriction alone. If exercise is incorporated, a lesser caloric deficit can be attempted, which may improve adherence to a new eating plan. Because C.J. will be participating in an exercise program, it would be reasonable to suggest a **500-kcal decrease in caloric consumption per day.** This value can then be multiplied by 7 to obtain the weekly caloric deficit from decreased food consumption (**500 × 7 = 3,500 kcal**).

Healthy Eating History

Food Energy Intake History for CJ_Sample_Pt

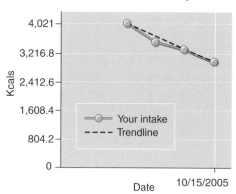

Average kcals: 3,421.8
Average Percent Estimated
Energy Requirement: 111.5%

View History for: 1 day I 1 week I 1 month I
3 months I 6 months I 1 year

Date	Kcals	Estimated energy requirement (%)
10/12/2005	4,021	144%
10/13/2005	3,482	109%
10/14/2005	3,266	102%
10/15/2005	2,918	91%

FIGURE 3–4   Caloric intake history for sample patient. (*Source:* U.S. Department of Agriculture, Center for Nutrition Policy and Promotion, MyPyramid.gov. MyPyramid Tracker. Accessed July 28, 2006, at http://www.mypyramidtracker.gov/.)

Step 4: Design Exercise Prescription and Calculate Energy Expenditure

Chapter 2 discusses the designing of exercise prescriptions to meet the individual needs and outcomes of patients. An exercise prescription designed for overweight and obese patients must emphasize three important points. First, the type(s) of exercise that the patient chooses to do should be safe. Given the extra load in excess body fat that the patient carries, weight-bearing activities should be performed with caution to prevent joint injuries, especially in patients with osteoarthritis in the lower extremities. Second, it should be stressed to patients that extending the duration of the exercise session over the intensity will result in more effective weight loss and is safer as it may result in less risk for injury. Lastly, compliance is likely the most important aspect of the exercise prescription that will lead the patient to successful weight loss. Therefore, choosing activities that reduce the risk for injury and that the patient enjoys doing will offer the greatest chances of achieving the weight-loss goals.

After interviewing C.J., he states that he currently does not have a preference of exercising outdoors or indoors and states that there is a fitness center for which he has access to in the building where he works. In addition he used to enjoy riding his bike several years ago but would also like to do some walking. Therefore, based on this information a sample exercise prescription for C.J. could be as follows:

  Goals: (1) lose 10% body weight within 6 months; (2) decrease the risks for obesity-related diseases
  Type of exercise (mode): stationary bicycling
  Intensity: 40 to 50% maximum heart rate (MHR), progressing to 50 to 70% MHR
  Duration: 30 minutes per exercise session initially
  Frequency: 4 times per week for first 2 weeks
  Rate of progression: As C.J. becomes more comfortable exercising and has some success losing weight, his exercise prescription can be altered by incorporating

longer exercise durations and greater frequencies as well as the possibility of walking. His exercise prescription should be reevaluated at 2 weeks and then every 4 weeks until the first weight-loss goal is attained.

Based on this exercise prescription, the amount of calories that C.J. expends from exercise can be calculated. Recall from Chapter 2 that this can be calculated by knowing C.J.'s weight (111.4 kg) and the MET (**metabolic equivalent**) level of the activity he will participate in while exercising. MET levels of common activities can be obtained from Table 2-2 as well as from two references authored by Ainsworth et al.[37,38] The formula to calculate energy expenditure is as follows:

$$METs \times 3.5 \times body\ weight\ in\ kg/200 = kcal/min$$

Using C.J.'s body weight (111.4 kg) and an MET level of 5.5 for stationary bicycling (obtained from Table 2-2), C.J. will expend approximately **321 kcal per exercise session** or approximately **1,284 kcal/week** if he exercises four times per week. Note that he can expend more calories by increasing the duration and frequency of exercise.

Step 5: Design a Weight-Loss Program

Based on the assessment information gathered in Steps 2 through 4, we can now put together an individual weight-loss program with specific goals and timelines. Recall from Chapter 1 that a caloric deficit of 3,500 kcal is equal to losing 1 pound of body fat. Therefore, if we combine calorie restriction and physical activity to create a daily caloric deficit, we can calculate the approximate amount of time it will take to lose the desired weight. Figure 3-5 shows a completed weight-loss program worksheet for our sample patient.

C.J. currently weighs 245 pounds and our initial weight loss goal is 10% within 6 months. Therefore, the initial goal for C.J. would be to lose 24.5 pounds, yielding a body weight of 220.5 pounds. This would put C.J.'s BMI at 30.8 kg/m². This BMI would still be classified as class I obesity, but his BMI would be significantly lower from his baseline of 34.2 kg/m².

Using the estimation that 3,500 kcal is equal to 1 pound of body fat, a total weight loss of 24.5 pounds would mean that C.J. would need a total caloric deficit (decreased calories plus physical activity) of 85,750 kcal. In Step 4 we figured that if C.J. followed the current exercise prescription of riding the stationary bicycle four times per week for 30 minutes per session, he would expend 321 kcal per exercise session or 1,284 kcal per week. In addition, we established in Step 3 that C.J.'s current caloric intake was 3,422 kcal per day. If he decreases 500 kcal per day from his total daily food consumption, this would create a weekly caloric deficit of 3,500 kcal (500 kcal × 7 days). The combination of caloric restriction and physical activity would yield a weekly caloric deficit of 4,784 kcal (1,284 kcal + 3,500 kcal). This program would allow C.J. to lose approximately 1.4 pounds of weight per week (4,784 kcal/3,500 kcal per lb of fat), which is within the recommended range of weight loss according to the Obesity Guidelines.[2] Therefore, to achieve a goal weight of 220 pounds it would take C.J. approximately 17.5 weeks or about 5 months. This estimation assumes that C.J. will adhere to the program as well as continuing to exercise with this current exercise prescription. If C.J. increases his exercise duration or frequency, the initial goal weight will be achieved more quickly.

Reassessment

Once C.J. has been successful at reaching his initial goal weight of 220 pounds, he may want to try to lose even more weight. Whether he decides to continue on a weight-loss

Weight-Loss Program Worksheet

Name: _C.J._

Date of initial consultation: _January 23, 2006_

Gender: (Male) Female

Age: _45_ yr

Height: _71_ inches

Height: _1.8_ meters (calculate by multiplying height in inches by 0.0254)

Weight: _245_ lb

Weight: _111.4_ kg (calculate by dividing weight in pounds by 2.2)

PA = physical activity coefficient (calculate using the following table)

	Sedentary	Low active	Active	Very active
Male	(1.0)	1.11	1.25	1.48
Female	1.0	1.12	1.27	1.45

STEP 1: Calculate Body Mass Index (BMI) and Classify

BMI = [weight (kg) / height (m^2)]

BMI = [_111.4_ kg / (_1.8_ m)^2]

BMI = _34_ kg/m^2

Classification of overweight and obesity according to BMI (circle)

<18.5 kg/m^2	Underweight
18.5–24.9 kg/m^2	Normal
25–29.9 kg/m^2	Overweight
(30–34.9 kg/m^2)	(Obesity class I)
35–39.9 kg/m^2	Obesity class II
≥40 kg/m^2	Obesity class III or extreme obesity

STEP 2: Calculate the Estimated Energy Requirement (EER)

Males aged > 19 years:

EER = 662 − 9.53 × age (yr) + PA × [15.9 × weight (kg) + 540 × height (m)]

EER = 662 − 9.53 × _45_ yr + _1.0_ × [15.9 × _111.4_ kg + 540 × _1.8_ m]

EER = _2,976_ kcal

Females aged > 19 years:

EER = 354 − 6.91 × age (yr) + PA x [9.36 × weight (kg) + 726 × height (m)]

EER = 354 − 6.91 × _____ yr + _____ × [9.36 × _____ kg + 726 × _____ m]

EER = _____ kcal

FIGURE 3–5 Weight-loss program worksheet for sample patient. MET, metabolic equivalent; RPE, rating of perceived exertion.

STEP 3: Calculate Current Caloric Intake and Eating Patterns

Day 1 total calories: __4,021__ kcal

Day 2 total calories: __3,482__ kcal

Day 3 total calories: __3,266__ kcal

Day 4 total calories: __2,918__ kcal

Average total daily calories: __3,422__ kcal

Suggested caloric deficit from food consumption per day: 500_____ kcal (multiply by 7 to get weekly caloric deficit = __3,500__ kcal)

STEP 4: Design Exercise Prescription and Calculate Energy Expenditure

Examples of physical activity the patient prefers:

__bicycling, walking indoors or outdoors, has access to a fitness center at work__

_____

Weight-loss goals:

1. _Lose 10% body weight within 6 months_____

2. _Decrease risk for obesity-related diseases_____

3._____

Exercise Prescription:

Mode: _stationary bicycling_____

Associated MET level: __5.5__

Intensity: _40-50% MHR__ (% max heart rate or RPE)

Duration: __30___ minutes

Frequency: ___4____ times per week

Rate of Progression:

___Focus should be on increasing duration (30–60 min) and frequency___

___(5-6 times/week) over intensity (50-70% MHR)___

Energy expenditure:

(METs × 3.5 × body weight in kg)/200 = kcal/min

(__5.5___ × 3.5 × __111.4__ kg)/200 = __10.7__ kcal/min (calories expended per minute of activity)

Multiply answer by the duration = calories expended per exercise session (kcal/session)

__10.7__ kcal/min × ___30___ minutes = __321___ kcal/session

Multiply answer by frequency = calories expended per week (kcal/week)

__321___ kcal/session × ___4____ times per week = _1,284__ kcal/week

FIGURE 3–5 *(Continued)*

STEP 5: Design a Weight-Loss Program

A. Current body weight: __245__ lb

B. Weight loss goal: __10__ %

C. Weight loss goal in pounds: __24.5__ lb (Step A × Step B)

D. Goal body weight: __220.5__ lb (Step A − Step C)

E. Goal BMI classification: __obesity class I__ (obtain from chart in Step 1)

F. Weekly calories decreased from food consumption: __3,500__ kcal (obtain from Step 3)

G. Caloric expenditure per week from physical activity: __1,284__ kcal (obtain from Step 4)

H. Total weekly caloric deficit: __4,784__ kcal (Step F + Step G)

I. Amount of body weight lost per week: __1.4__ lb (Step H/3,500 kcal)

J. Approximate time to achieve the goal weight: __17.5__ weeks (Step C/Step I)

FIGURE 3–5   (*Continued*)

program or switch to a weight-maintenance program, reassessment of certain variables is warranted. A follow-up nutritional analysis (Step 3) may be a good idea at this time with the focus on creating a balanced eating plan that is more in line with the 2005 Dietary Guidelines.[10] In addition, C.J. may want to try other forms of exercise such as weight-bearing activities, in which case a new exercise prescription can be written to include these activities and the caloric expenditures that they will create (Step 4). Assessing compliance issues with C.J. should be an ongoing process throughout the initial weight-loss period but should be reassessed at this time.

REFERENCES

1. Flagel KM, Carroll MD, Ogden CL, Johnson CL. Prevalence and trends in obesity among US adults, 1990–2000. JAMA 2002;288:1723–1727.
2. Clinical Guidelines on the Identification, Evaluation, and Treatment of Overweight and Obesity in Adults. Bethesda, MD: National Institutes of Health, U.S. Department of Health and Human Services; 1998. NIH Publication No. 98-4083.
3. ACSM Position Stand on the Appropriate Intervention Strategies for Weight Loss and Prevention of Weight Regain for Adults. Med Sci Sports Exer 2001;33:2145–2156.
4. Nawaz H, Katz DL. American College of Preventive Medicine Practice Policy. Weight management counseling for overweight adults. Am J Prev Med 2001;21:73–78.
5. Centers for Disease Control and Prevention. State-specific prevalence of obesity among adults with disabilities—eight states and the District of Colombia, 1998–1999. MMWR Morb Mortal Wkly Rep 2002;51:805.
6. Levy A, Heaton A. Weight control practices of U.S. adults trying to lose weight. Ann Intern Med 1993; 119:661–666.
7. National Institutes of Health, National Heart, Lung, and Blood Institute. Clinical Guidelines of the Identification, Evaluation, and Treatment of Overweight and Obesity in Adults—Executive Summary. NIH Publication No. 98-4083, 1998.
8. National Institutes of Health, National Heart, Lung, and Blood Institute. The Practical Guide: Identification, Evaluation, and Treatment of Overweight and Obesity in Adults. NIH Publication No. 00-4084, 2000.
9. Williams MH. Nutrition for Health, Nutrition and Sport, 7th ed. Boston: McGraw-Hill, 2005. Chapter 10: 377–409.
10. HHS Publication number: HHS-ODPHP-2005-01-DGA-A, Dietary Guidelines for Americans 2005, U.S. Department of Health and Human Services, U.S. Department of Agriculture. Available at: http://healthierus.gov/dietaryguidelines. Accessed February 6, 2007.

11. The Practical Guide. Identification, Evaluation, and Treatment of Overweight and Obesity in Adults. Bethesda, MD: National Institutes of Health, U.S. Department of Health and Human Services; 2000. NIH Publication No. 00-4084.

12. Blair SN, Brodney S. Effects of physical activity and obesity on morbidity and mortality: current evidence and research issues. Med Sci Sports Exerc 1999;31(Suppl):S646–S662.

13. Bryner RW, Ullrich IH, Sauers J, et al. Effects of resistance vs. aerobic training combined with an 800 calorie liquid diet on lean body mass and resting metabolic rate. J Am Coll Nutr 1999;18:115–121.

14. Elliot DL, Goldberg L Kuehl KS, Bennett WM. Sustained depression of the resting metabolic rate after massive weight loss. Am J Clin Nutr 1989;49:93–96.

15. Leibel RL. Changes in energy expenditure resulting from altered body weight. N Engl J Med 1995;332:621–628.

16. Krotkiewsk M, Grimby G, Holm G, Szczepanik J. Increased muscle dynamic endurance associated with reduction on a very-low calorie diet. Am J Clin Nutr 1990;51:321–330.

17. Wallace JP. Obesity. In: Durstine JL, Moore GE, eds. ACSM's Exercise Management for Persons With Chronic Diseases and Disabilities. Champaign, IL: Human Kinetics, 2003:149–156.

18. Anderson S, Holme I, Urdal P, Hjermann I. Diet and exercise intervention have favorable effects in blood pressure in mild hypertension: the Oslo Diet and Exercise Study (ODES). Blood Press 1995;4:343–349.

19. Fortmann SP, Haskell WL, Wood PD. Effects of weight loss on clinic and ambulatory blood pressure in normotensive men. Am J Cardiol 1998;62:89–93.

20. Katzel LI, Bleeker ER, Colman EG, Rogus EM, Sorkin JD, Goldberg AP. Effects of weight loss vs aerobic exercise training on risk factors for coronary disease in healthy, obese, middle-aged and older men. A randomized and controlled study. JAMA 1995;274:1915–1921.

21. Stefanick ML, Mackey S, Sheehan M, Ellsworth N, Haskell WL, Wood PD. Effects of the NCEP Step 2 diet and exercise on lipoprotein in postmenopausal women and men with low HDL-cholesterol and high LDL-cholesterol. N Engl J Med 1998;339:12–20.

22. King AC, Haskell WL, Taylor CB, Kreamer HC, DeBusk RF. Group- vs home-based exercise training in healthy older men and women. A community-based clinical trial. JAMA 1991;266:1535–1542.

23. Ronnemaa T, Marniemi J, Puukka P, Kuusi T. Effects of long term physical exercise on serum lipids, lipoproteins and lipid metabolizing enzymes in type 2 (non-insulin dependent) diabetic patients. Diabetes Res 1988;7:79–84.

24. Wood PD, Stefanick ML, Dreon DM, et al. Changes in plasma lipids and lipoproteins in overweight men during weight loss through dieting as compared to exercise. N Engl J Med 1988;319:1173–1179.

25. Frey-Hewitt B, Vranizan KM, Dreon DM, Wood PD. The effect of weight loss by dieting or exercise on resting metabolic rate in overweight men. Int J Obes 1990;14:327–334.

26. Hammer RL, Barrier CA, Roundy ES, Bradford JM, Fisher AG. Calorie-restricted low-fat diet and exercise in obese women. Am J Clin Nutr 1989;49:77–85.

27. Bertram SR, Venter I, Stewart RI. Weight loss in obese women—exercise vs. dietary education. S Afr Med J 1990;78:15–18.

28. King AC, Haskell WL, Young DR, Oka RK, Stefanick ML. Long-term effects of varying intensities and formats of physical activity on participation rates, fitness, and lipoproteins in men and women aged 50 to 65 years. Circulation 1995;91:2596–2604.

29. Gordon NF, Scott CB, Levine BD. Comparison of single versus multiple lifestyle interventions: are the antihypertensive effects of exercise training and diet-induced weight loss additive? Am J Cardiol 1997;79:763–767.

30. Centers for Disease Control and Prevention, National Center for Chronic Disease Prevention and Health Promotion. Surgeon General's Report on Physical Activity and Health. Atlanta: CDC, 1996.

31. American College of Sports Medicine. Guidelines for Exercise Testing and Prescription, 6th ed. Philadelphia: Lippincott Williams & Wilkins, 2000.

32. Centers for Disease Control and Prevention. Available at: http://www.cdc.gov/nccdphp/dnpa/physical/recommendations/adults.htm. Accessed October 20, 2005.

33. Pritchard JE, Nowson CA, Wark JD. A worksite program for overweight middle-aged men achieves lesser weight loss with exercise than with dietary change. J Am Diet Assoc 1997;97:37–42.

34. North American Association for the Study of Obesity. Available at: http://www.obesityonline.org/slides/slide01.cfm?tk=37&dpg=2. Accessed October 20, 2005.

35. Package insert. Meridia (sibutramine hydrochloride monohydrate). North Chicago, IL: Abbot Laboratories, December 2004.

36. United States Department of Agriculture. Available at: http://www.mypyramid.gov. Accessed October 20, 2005.

37. Ainsworth BE, Haskell WL, Leon AS, et al. Compendium of physical activities: classification of energy costs of human physical activities. Med Sci Sports Exerc 1993;25:70–80.

38. Ainsworth BE, Haskell MC, Whitt ML, et al. Compendium of physical activities: an update of activity codes and MET intensities. Med Sci Sports Exerc 2000;32(9 Suppl):S498–S516.

CHAPTER 4

Tobacco Cessation

OBJECTIVES

At the end of this chapter the reader should be able to:

1. Recall the prevalence of smoking among adults in the United States.
2. List the diseases and illnesses that can be caused by smoking.
3. Explain the causative effect of smoking on cardiovascular disease and cancer.
4. Outline the steps of a brief intervention for a patient who smokes cigarettes.
5. Develop a smoking-cessation plan for a patient ready to make a quit attempt.

OVERVIEW AND PREVALENCE

The act of smoking can be traced back in time for centuries. The hazardous effects of smoking, however, have only been known to be a public health concern for the past several decades. In 1964 the U.S. Surgeon General released the first report on smoking from the U.S. Department of Health, Education, and Welfare.[1] Interestingly, the conclusions of the Surgeon General's report 40 years later (and every report in between) are the same. The most recent report of the Surgeon General in 2004, entitled "The Health Consequences of Smoking," concluded that smoking is the single greatest cause of avoidable morbidity and mortality in the United States.[1]

Smoking was shown to be the number one actual cause of death in the United States in 1990 and in 2000.[2] Many times only the leading cause of death is reported, in which case, **cardiovascular disease** has been the leading cause of death in the United States for the past century.[3] But the actual cause of cardiovascular disease is attributable to smoking more often than any other cause.[2] In 2000, tobacco use was the actual cause of 18.1% of deaths.[2] To give some perspective, the number two actual cause of death in 2000 was poor diet and physical inactivity accounting for 16.6% of deaths, followed by alcohol consumption (3.5%) and microbial agents (3.1%).[2] In addition, the societal cost of tobacco-related death and disease is approximately $100 billion per year.

In 2000 the U.S. Department of Health and Human Services released national health objectives called Healthy People 2010.[4] One of the national health objectives is to decrease the prevalence of cigarette smoking to less than 12% among American adults.[4,5] In 2004 approximately 20.9% of U.S. adults were current smokers.[5] This represents 44.5 million Americans.[5] Of the current adult smokers in the United States, 81.3% (36.1 million) smoke every day, and among these individuals, 40.5% (14.6 million) report that they had stopped smoking at least 1 day in the previous 12 months because they were trying to quit.[5]

Population subgroups indicate that men (23.4%) smoke more than women (18.5%) and that persons older than 65 years had the lowest prevalence of smoking (8.8%) among U.S. adults in 2004.[5] Native Americans have the highest prevalence of smoking (33.4%), followed by non-Hispanic whites (22.2%) and non-Hispanic blacks (20.2%).[5] Those racial or ethnic populations with the lowest prevalence of smoking are Asians (11.3%) and Hispanics (15.0%). Smoking prevalence is also related to education and income. Generally, the prevalence of smoking decreases with increasing years of education, and there is a higher prevalence of smoking among those individuals who live below the poverty level (29.1%) as compared with those who live above the poverty level (20.6%).[5]

Although the percentage of U.S. adults who smoked in 2004 was far from the national health objective goal, the prevalence of adult smokers is decreasing. In 2003 and 2002 the percentage of smokers was 21.6% and 22.5%, respectively, compared with 20.9% in 2004.[5] In addition, the prevalence of adult heavy smokers (≥25 cigarettes per day) has decreased from 19.1% in 1993 to 12.1% in 2004.[5] In 2004 the mean number of cigarettes smoked per day among U.S. adults was 16.8 (18.1 for men and 15.3 for women), which was down compared with 1993 when U.S. adult smokers averaged 19.6 cigarettes per day (21.3 for men and 17.8 for women).[5] More than 70% of all current smokers have expressed a desire to stop smoking.

SMOKING-RELATED DISEASES

As stated above, smoking is the number one actual cause of death in the United States. Smoking, however, leads not only to death but to much comorbidity as well. Table 4-1 provides a list of diseases and illnesses from the U.S. Surgeon General's 2004 report in which smoking has been identified as a cause. Cardiovascular disease and **cancer** are the top two killers among Americans.[2] Below is a brief description of the physiologic effects of smoking on the progression of these two diseases.

Cardiovascular Disease and Smoking

It has been known for several decades that smoking is associated with cardiovascular disease (CVD). A hypothesis of the relationship between smoking and injury to the heart in the form of atherosclerosis was first proposed in the mid 1970s.[1,6,7] It is now known that smoking affects the functionality of several aspects of the cardiovascular system. Some of these aspects include the endothelial cells of the vessel walls, platelet function, inflammation, lipids and lipid metabolism, and increased oxygen demand of the heart.[1]

The underlying physiologic process of most clinically significant diseases of the heart and peripheral vasculature is the development of atherosclerosis.[1] **Atherosclerosis**

TABLE 4–1	Smoking-Related Diseases and Illnesses

Disease Category	Disease
Cardiovascular	Abdominal aortic aneurysm Atherosclerosis Cerebrovascular disease Coronary heart disease
Cancer	Bladder Cervical Esophageal Kidney Laryngeal Leukemia Lung Oral Pancreatic Stomach
Respiratory	Chronic obstructive pulmonary disease Pneumonia Respiratory effects in utero Respiratory effects in childhood and adolescence Respiratory effects in adulthood Other respiratory effects
Reproductive	Fetal deaths and stillbirths Fertility Low birth weights Pregnancy complications
Others	Cataracts Diminished health status/morbidity Hip fractures Low bone density Peptic ulcer disease

Source: U.S. Department of Health and Human Services. The health consequences of smoking. A report of the Surgeon General. Atlanta: U.S. Department of Health and Human Services, Centers for Disease Control and Prevention, National Center for Chronic Disease Prevention and Health Promotion, Office of Smoking and Health, 2004.

is the process by which lipids are deposited on the inner layer of the arteries, and of the fibrosis and thickening of the arterial wall.[1] The lipids that are deposited on the arterial walls can grow and become advanced fibrotic lesions, which can block blood flow through the artery and become unstable.[1] Plaque that becomes unstable can then burst, causing a series of events that lead to thrombus development, which can then cause **myocardial infarction** or **stroke.**[1] A homeostatic balance must exist within the cardiovascular system to prevent a myocardial infarction or stroke. If one or more of the elements that helps to maintain cardiovascular homeostasis is disrupted, cardiovascular or cerebrovascular complications can occur. Smoking has been shown to disrupt the balance of several key elements involved in cardiovascular homeostasis.[1]

The **endothelium** is a monolayer of cells that lines the interior lumen of arteries. When these cells become damaged it is referred to as **endothelial dysfunction.** It is now well recognized that endothelial dysfunction plays a critical role in the early stages of atherosclerosis.[1,8,9] Smoking has been shown to change the endothelium, causing endothelial dysfunction. This has been reported in both adults and infants born to smoking mothers.[1,10–14] Smoking can also cause a dysfunctional endothelium to secrete growth factors and to stimulate the inflammatory process, leading to atherosclerosis.[1]

Smoking has also been shown to have direct effects on platelet activation and platelet adhesion, making smokers more susceptible to thrombosis.[1] Even non-smokers who are exposed to cigarettes through second-hand smoke can experience acute increases in platelet aggregation.[1,14] In addition, smoking induces a localized inflammatory response in the lungs and elevates inflammatory markers in the circulating blood, putting the smoker at increased risk for CVD.[1,15]

There is strong evidence that supports an association between smoking and adverse blood lipid levels.[1,16,17] A meta-analysis of 54 studies revealed that smokers have higher concentrations of **low-density lipoprotein (LDL)** and **very low-density lipoprotein (VLDL),** or the bad cholesterols, when compared with non-smokers.[17] In addition, smokers also have lower levels of **high-density lipoprotein (HDL),** or the good cholesterol, compared with non-smokers.[18] Smoking may also have a significant impact on lipid metabolism, which can also lead to atherosclerosis.[1]

With regard to cardiovascular hemodynamics, it is well known that cigarette smoking induces the release of the catecholamines, epinephrine and norepinephrine. Increased catecholamine levels are associated with an increased baseline heart rate, increased heart contractility, and increased vascular tone.[1,19] Smokers also experience a lower than expected heart rate in response to physical exercise, which is a marker that is associated with increased risk of myocardial infarction and heart arrhythmias, and an overall increased risk of mortality.[20] In addition, smoking acutely increases peripheral vascular resistance and blood pressure.[21,22] Each of these hemodynamic changes can lead to increased oxygen demand to the heart, causing the heart to not function optimally or leading to a myocardial infarction.

Cancer and Smoking

It was first reported in the Surgeon General's 1964 report that a causal relationship existed between smoking and lung cancer.[23] Since that time many reports have been published stating a causal relationship between smoking and several other types of cancers. The list of cancers caused by smoking includes bladder and kidney (renal cell, renal pelvis), esophagus, laryngeal, lung, oral cavity and pharyngeal, esophageal, cervical, gastric, pancreas, and acute myeloid leukemia.[1] In addition, there is evidence to suggest that smoking may lead to endometrial, colorectal, and liver cancers as well.[1]

It was first speculated in 1939 that smoking may cause lung cancer.[1] Forty years after smoking was first identified in the U.S. Surgeon General's report as directly causing lung cancer, however, it still remains the leading cause of cancer and of death from cancer today.[1] In 2003, lung cancer accounted for 28% of all cancer deaths in the United States with almost 172,000 new cases diagnosed that same year.[24] The survival rate of lung cancer is poor, with the 5-year survival rate at only 15% for all stages of lung cancer combined.[24]

In the past 50 years the amounts of nicotine and tar in cigarettes have decreased substantially according to regulations by the Federal Trade Commission. Unfortunately, the risk for lung cancer in smokers has not declined. Smoking causes genetic changes in the lung that ultimately lead to the development of lung cancer.[1] The four types of cancers that comprise greater than 90% of lung cancers are squamous cell carcinoma, adenocarcinoma, large cell carcinoma, and small cell undifferentiated carcinoma. The most common type of lung cancer in smokers among these is adenocarcinoma. It is important to note that even after many years of not smoking, the risk of lung cancer in smokers remains higher than in persons who have never smoked and will in fact never decline to that of persons who have never smoked.[1] Therefore, only prevention of smoking can stop the epidemic of lung cancer.[1]

SMOKING CESSATION IN CLINICAL PRACTICE

In 2000, the U.S. Department of Health and Human Services published a document entitled "Treating Tobacco Use and Dependence" that is to be used as clinical practice guidelines for smoking cessation.[25] The guidelines are a sponsored consortium of seven federal government and non-profit organizations and consist of 6,000 screened and reviewed articles published between 1975 and 1999 that serve as the basis for guideline data analysis and panel opinion. The guidelines were designed to assist clinicians, tobacco-dependence treatment specialists, healthcare administrators, insurers, and purchasers in delivering and supporting effective treatments for tobacco use and dependence.[25]

A key finding that is reported in the guidelines is that tobacco dependence is now increasingly recognized as a chronic disease.[25] This means that those patients who currently use tobacco or are former users typically require ongoing assessment and repeated interventions. Patients who are successful at quitting their use of tobacco still require assessment and intervention much like patients with **hypertension** who have their blood pressure successfully controlled. Effective treatments are currently available that can produce long-term or even permanent abstinence.[25]

The guidelines strongly recommend that each patient seen by a clinician or healthcare provider, including a pharmacist, be assessed for their use of tobacco.[25] Patients willing to try to quit tobacco use should be provided with treatments identified as effective in the guidelines. Patients unwilling to try to quit tobacco use should be provided with a brief intervention designed to increase their motivation to quit. This recommendation stems from the evidence that there is a strong dose relationship between the intensity of tobacco-dependence counseling and its effectiveness.[25] The greater the number of healthcare providers who talk to a patient about stopping tobacco use and the greater the amount of time that is spent in the intervention, the more likely the patient is to quit.[25]

Data in the guidelines strongly indicate that effective tobacco-cessation interventions require a coordination of interventions.[25] Healthcare providers must have a systematic identification, assessment, and treatment process established to intervene with their patients. This process will be discussed below. In addition, the healthcare administrator, insurer, and purchaser must foster and support tobacco intervention as an integral element of healthcare delivery. Healthcare administrators and insurers should ensure that clinicians and providers have the necessary training and support, and receive necessary reimbursement to achieve consistent and effective interventions with tobacco users.[25] This aspect of the tobacco-cessation process will not be discussed in this chapter but is discussed in detail in the "Treating Tobacco Use and Dependence" guidelines if the reader would like more information.[25]

Rx for Change: Clinician-Assisted Tobacco Cessation

Rx for Change: Clinician-Assisted Tobacco Cessation is a tobacco-cessation education program that was first developed in 1999 to address an identified need to enhance the tobacco-cessation education of pharmacists. The Rx for Change program has since expanded and is currently adapted for use by students and licensed clinicians in all health professional disciplines and is anchored in the "Treating Tobacco Use and Dependence" guidelines discussed above. The teaching strategies for the program include a preclass assigned reading, lecture with animated PowerPoint slides, videotape (an introductory videotape segment, videotaped counseling sessions, and trigger tapes), a hands-on workshop with the pharmaceutical aids for cessation, and role-playing with case scenarios. The program has been shown to be very successful in the pharmacy and non-pharmacy education setting, and many U.S. pharmacy schools have adopted this program as a means for teaching students about tobacco cessation. The Rx for Change program is highly recommended, and more information can be found at the Rx for Change website: http://rxforchange.ucsf.edu/.

The Benefits of Quitting

Nicotine is the substance in cigarettes that causes smokers to crave or become addicted to smoking. Nicotine, however, is not the only thing that gets put into the body of smokers when they light up. There are more than 4,000 chemicals in cigarette smoke.[1] Some of the same chemicals that are in cigarette smoke are also in wood varnish, the insect poison DDT, arsenic, nail polish remover, and rat poison. In addition, the ashes, tar, gases, and other poisons that are in cigarettes can cause great damage to the body over time, especially to the heart and lungs.[1] Smoking cigarettes also makes it harder for the smoker to taste and smell things and to fight off infections.

Secondhand smoke is also dangerous. Secondhand smoke can cause cancer, breathing problems, and heart disease in non-smokers.[1] It can also cause those who breathe it to get more colds and flus and to even die younger than those who do not breathe secondhand smoke. Women who smoke while they are pregnant are at increased risk for miscarriages. Their babies are at increased risk for being born underweight, are more likely to die from sudden infant death syndrome (SIDS), and are more irritable. They get sick more often, are more likely to have **asthma** and ear and lung infections like pneumonia, and are more likely to have learning problems.[26]

Because smoking causes so much damage to the body, it is no surprise that quitting has great benefits. Here are a few benefits that occur when a smoker quits: *20 minutes after quitting,* heart rate begins to drop, putting less load on the heart; *12 hours after quitting,* the carbon monoxide level in the blood drops to normal; *2 to 3 months after quitting,* circulation improves and lung function increases; *1 to 9 months after quitting,* coughing and shortness of breath decrease, the cilia (tiny hairlike structures that move mucus out of the lungs) regain normal function in the lungs, which increases their ability to handle mucus, clean the lungs, and reduce the risk of infection; *1 year after quitting,* the excess risk of **coronary heart disease** is half that of a current smoker's risk; *5 to 15 years after quitting,* stroke rate is reduced to that of a lifetime non-smoker; *10 years after quitting,* lung cancer death rate is about half that of a current smoker and the risk of cancer of the mouth, throat, esophagus, bladder, cervix, and pancreas decreases; and *15 years after quitting,* the risk of coronary heart disease is that of a non-smoker's risk.[16]

Quitting can also have a significant personal financial impact. For example, people who smoke one pack per day at a rate of $5 per pack can save $35 per week, $150 per month, $1,820 per year, $18,200 after 10 years, and $36,400 after 20 years of quitting. These savings will differ based on cigarette prices and the number of cigarettes smoked per day, but showing this information to patients contemplating quitting can be a useful motivational tool.

Identification and Assessment of Tobacco Use Through Brief Intervention

There are two types of interventions that a healthcare professional can provide to patients who use tobacco. They are a brief intervention or an intensive intervention. Brief interventions can be provided by any healthcare provider but are most relevant to primary care providers such as pharmacists, physicians, nurses, dentists, and respiratory therapists who are bound by time constraints.[25] The guidelines state that a wide variety of providers can implement brief interventions, and these techniques have evidence to show that they are effective.[25] The main strategy is to provide at least a brief intervention to all tobacco users at each clinical visit. Each time the patient visits the pharmacist, physician, dentist, or other healthcare professional, an intervention should be made as to his or her smoking status.

This first step in treating patients who smoke and use tobacco is to identify the users. Effectively doing this important step can set the stage for a successful intervention with an individualized treatment plan.[25] Screening patients for current or former tobacco use will result in one of four answers: (1) the patient never regularly used tobacco; (2) the patient is currently using tobacco and is now willing to make a quit attempt; (3) the patient is currently using tobacco but is not willing to make a quit attempt at this time; and (4) the patient once used tobacco but has since quit.[25] Strategies for treating tobacco dependence in each of these patients (except for patients who have never regularly used tobacco) will be discussed in detail below. Figure 4-1 depicts an algorithm for treating tobacco use.

Smokers Willing to Make a Quit Attempt

There are five major steps involved in a brief intervention with a patient. These steps are referred to as the "5 A's" and are listed in Table 4-2. These strategies are designed to be brief, requiring 3 minutes or less of direct healthcare provider time.[25]

The first step is to **A**sk the patient if he or she currently uses or formerly used tobacco.[25] In the pharmacy or the clinic, this question can be incorporated into drug counseling or on a document in which other patient information is recorded.

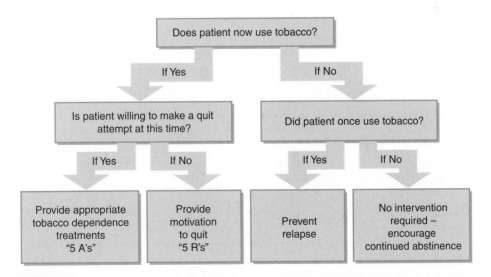

FIGURE 4–1   Algorithm for treating tobacco use. (*Source:* Fiore MC, Bailey WC, Cohen SJ, et al. Treating Tobacco Use and Dependence. Clinical Practice Guideline. Rockville, MD: U.S. Department of Health and Human Services, Public Health Service, June 2000.)

TABLE 4–2   The "5 A's" for Brief Intervention

ASK about tobacco use	Identify and document tobacco use status for every patient at every visit.
ADVISE to quit	In a clear, strong, and personalized manner urge every tobacco user to quit.
ASSESS willingness to make a quit attempt	Is the tobacco user willing to make a quit attempt at this time?
ASSIST in quit attempt	For the patient willing to make a quit attempt, use counseling and pharmacotherapy to help him or her quit.
ARRANGE follow-up	Schedule follow-up contact, preferably within a week after the quit date.

Source: Fiore MC, Bailey WC, Cohen SJ, et al. Treating Tobacco Use and Dependence. Clinical Practice Guideline. Rockville, MD: U.S. Department of Health and Human Services, Public Health Service, June 2000.

The next step is to **A**dvise or strongly urge all smokers and tobacco users to quit.[25] The harmful effects of smoking should be communicated in a manner clear to the patient and in a strong, firm, and supportive voice to let the patient know that it is important to quit and that you are there to help. It is also important to personalize the conversation in a way that makes it important for the patient to quit because of specific health conditions, family history, or impact on children and others in the household.[25]

Third, **A**ssess the patient's willingness to make a quit attempt at this time.[25] This can be anytime within the next 30 days but ideally within the next 2 weeks. If the patient is willing to make a quit attempt at this time, provide assistance (discussed in Step 4). If the patient will participate in intensive treatment, deliver such treatment or refer him or her to an intensive intervention. Intensive treatment will be discussed later.

The fourth step is to **A**ssist or help the patient with a quit plan.[25] This can be accomplished through several strategies. Among these strategies are the following: (1) setting a quit date (ideally within the next 2 weeks); (2) telling family, friends, and coworkers about quitting and requesting understanding and support; (3) anticipating challenges and identifying barriers to the quit attempt, especially during the critical first few weeks, and including nicotine withdrawal symptoms; (4) removing tobacco products from the environment and avoiding smoking in places where much time is spent (e.g., work, home, car); (5) providing supplementary materials for the patient to use as a reference that is culturally, racially, educationally, and age appropriate; (6) recommending appropriate counseling; and (7) recommending the use of approved pharmacotherapy, except in special circumstances.[25]

Behavioral Counseling   Behavioral counseling is an important part of a smoking-cessation program. Evidence in the guidelines states that more-intense and longer-lasting interventions are more likely to help patients to become and remain smoke-free.[25] Even interventions lasting fewer than 3 minutes have been shown to be effective. A general overview of patient counseling strategies is listed in Table 4-3.

There are three types of counseling that have been shown to be especially effective and should be used in all patients attempting tobacco cessation.[25] The first type is called "practical counseling." In this type of counseling the clinician provides recommenda-

TABLE 4–3   Brief Intervention Patient Counseling Strategies to "Assist" a Quit Attempt

Action	Strategies for Implementation
Provide practical counseling (problem solving/training)	1. Abstinence—Total abstinence is essential. "Not even a single puff after the quit date." 2. Past quitting experience—Review past quit attempts including identification of what helped during the quit attempt and what factors contributed to relapse. 3. Anticipate triggers or challenges in upcoming attempt—Discuss challenges and triggers and how patient will overcome them. 4. Alcohol—Because alcohol can cause relapse, the patient should consider limiting or abstaining from alcohol while quitting. 5. Other smokers in the household—Quitting is more difficult when there is another smoker in the household. Patients should encourage housemates to quit with them or not to smoke in their presence.
Provide intratreatment social support	Provide a supportive clinical environment while encouraging the patient in his or her quit attempt. "My office staff and I are available to assist you."
Help patient obtain extratreatment social support	Help patient develop social support for his or her quit attempt in his or her environments outside of treatment. "Ask your spouse or partner, friends, and coworkers to support you in your quit attempt."

Source: Fiore MC, Bailey WC, Cohen SJ, et al. Treating Tobacco Use and Dependence. Clinical Practice Guideline. Rockville, MD: U.S. Department of Health and Human Services, Public Health Service, June 2000.

tions that can assist the patient to solve problems that may hinder the quit attempt.[25] These include recognizing situations such as events or activities that can increase the risk of smoking or relapse. Examples of these situations are drinking alcohol, being under time pressure, and being around other smokers. This type of counseling also offers coping skills such as learning to anticipate and avoid temptation, participating in lifestyle changes that reduce stress, suggestions that improve quality of life or produce pleasure, and learning cognitive and behavioral activities to cope with smoking urges. In addition, practical counseling provides patients with basic information about smoking and successful quitting, such as telling patients that any smoking (even a single puff) increases the likelihood of a full relapse, and examples of withdrawal symptoms, and tells patients that withdrawal typically peaks within 1 to 3 weeks after quitting.[25]

Another type of counseling is called intratreatment social support. This type of counseling deals with establishing a culture of smoking cessation within the clinic or pharmacy.[25] The environment should be one that encourages patients to quit, communicates caring and concern, and encourages the patient to talk about the quitting process. Patients should be asked how they feel about quitting, what their reasons are for quitting, and what concerns and worries they have about quitting.[25]

The third type of counseling is the extratreatment social support. This type of counseling trains the patient to seek support from others outside the clinic or pharmacy.[25] Patients can be shown videos that model support skills, practice requesting social support from family, friends, and coworkers, and establish a smoke-free home. In addition, the healthcare provider can arrange outside support by mailing letters or calling others who support the patient and inviting them to the cessation session.[25]

Pharmacotherapy   There are nine different pharmacotherapy agents that are considered to be effective for smoking cessation.[25] Seven of these agents are considered first-line medications with the remaining two as second-line agents. The guidelines recommend that a pharmacotherapy agent be used in all patients attempting to quit smoking except in the presence of special circumstances.[25] The guidelines list special circumstances as patients with medical contraindications, those smoking fewer than 10 cigarettes per day, women who are pregnant or breastfeeding, and adolescent smokers.[25] Healthcare providers should encourage every smoker to use pharmacotherapies endorsed by the guidelines and explain how these medications increase smoking-cessation success and reduce withdrawal symptoms.[25]

All seven first-line agents are approved by the U.S. Food and Drug Administration (FDA) for smoking cessation and include bupropion SR, nicotine gum, nicotine inhaler, nicotine nasal spray, nicotine patch, nicotine lozenge, and verenicline.[25] There are currently not enough data to suggest a rank order of these first-line agents. Healthcare providers must choose an agent based on patient preference and previous experience (positive or negative), patient characteristics (e.g., history of depression, concerns of weight gain), contraindications, and provider familiarity with the agents.[25] Patients concerned about weight gain may want to try bupropion SR and nicotine-replacement therapies (especially nicotine gum) as they have been shown to delay, but not prevent, weight gain.[25] Other lifestyle modifications such as exercise and calorie reduction have been shown to be effective to prevent weight gain and can be used in patients who are attempting to quit smoking. Patients with a history of depression should try bupropion SR as a first-line agent as it appears to be effective in this population. In addition, there is evidence that combining the nicotine patch with either nicotine gum or nicotine nasal spray increases the long-term abstinence rates over those produced by a single form of nicotine-replacement therapy.[25]

Drug Interactions With Smoking

Pharmacists are accustomed to looking for drug interactions in their patients' drug regimens. Pharmacists, however, may not be aware that certain drugs interact with tobacco smoke.[27] More than 4,000 chemicals exist in a cigarette. This results in many opportunities for drug interactions with these chemicals. Some of the substances in tobacco smoke that can cause drug interactions include nicotine, carbon monoxide, acetone, pyridine, benzene, and heavy metals such as cadmium.[27] It is believed, however, that these chemicals are responsible for only a few of the drug interactions that exist with smoking.[27]

Most of the drug interactions with tobacco smoke are related to a chemical produced from the incomplete combustion of tobacco that occurs while smoking.[27] The chemical is polycyclic aromatic hydrocarbons (PAHs), and it is reported to cause drug interactions by inducing the hepatic cytochrome P450 microsomal enzymes CYP1A1, CYP1A2 and, possibly, CYP2E1.[27] These result in a pharmacokinetic interaction between certain medications and tobacco smoke.[27]

Several medications and drug classes have been identified as having significant interactions with tobacco smoke. These include benzodiazepines, β-blockers, caffeine, chlorpromazine, clozapine, flecainide, fluvoxamine, haloperidol, heparin, insulin, mexiletine, olanzapine, opioids (propoxyphene, pentazocine), propranolol, oral contraceptives, tacrine, and theophylline.[27] The drug interactions that have been identified as being the most clinically significant are those with caffeine, fluvoxamine, olanzapine, oral contra-ceptives, tacrine, and theophylline.[27]

In addition, a more recently released human insulin inhalation powder with the brand name of Exubera (Pfizer Labs) has a significant interaction with cigarette smok-ing.[28] In smokers, the systemic insulin exposure of Exubera is two to five times higher than in non-smokers, increasing the patient's risk for hypoglycemia. As a result, Exubera is contraindicated in patients who smoke or who have discontinued smoking less than 6 months before starting the drug.[28]

The drug interaction with oral contraceptives is particularly important to note because of the potential effects of smoking and taking oral contraceptives concur-rently. The interaction is pharmacodynamic in nature, and the concomitant use increases the risk for cardiovascular adverse events.[27] As a result, women who smoke and use oral contraceptives are at even greater risk for stroke, myocardial infarction, and thromboembolism aside from the increased risk of smoking itself.[27] In addition, the risk of these adverse events significantly increases in women who are both older than 35 years of age and who smoke more than 15 cigarettes per day.[27]

When counseling patients regarding smoking cessation, it is important to also edu-cate them on the drug interactions that may exist with the medications that they are taking. Female patients older than age 35, taking oral contraceptives, and smoking more than 15 cigarettes per day should be particularly educated about the increased risk for cardiovascular events that are in addition to all the other health risks associated with smoking. Pharmacists are ideally positioned and qualified to offer this type of counseling to patients.

Second-line pharmacotherapy agents include clonidine and nortriptyline and should be considered for patients unable to use first-line medications because of contra-indications or for patients for whom first-line agents are not helpful.[25] Nortriptyline can also be used in patients with a history of depression, but it is important to monitor the side effects of both nortriptyline and clonidine if these agents are used.[25] Table 4-4 lists pharmacotherapy agents that can be used for smoking cessation.

The fifth and final step in the brief intervention is to **A**rrange follow-up contact with the patient. Follow-up appointments with patients can be done either in person or via tele-phone.[25] The guideline reports that telephone counseling has been shown to be an effec-tive method of assisting patients in the smoking-cessation process. Follow-up contact should occur soon after the quit date, preferably during the first week. A second follow-up contact is recommended within the first month, and further contact should be con-ducted as needed.[25]

Actions taken during follow-up appointments include congratulating the patient for success, or reviewing circumstances that have caused the patient to resume using tobacco.[25] Patients who resume tobacco use can be counseled on recommitting to total abstinence and reminded that a lapse can be used as a learning experience. Other topics that can be discussed at follow-up appointments include identifying problems already encountered and challenges in the immediate future, assessing pharmacother-apy use and problems, and considering use or referral to more intensive treatment.[25]

Smokers Unwilling to Make a Quit Attempt

Many times patients who smoke will not be willing to make a quit attempt at the present time for several reasons. Clinicians should intervene with these patients to try to motivate

TABLE 4–4   Pharmacotherapy Agents for Smoking Cessation

Drug	Precautions or Contraindications	Side Effects	Dosage	Duration	Availability
First-line Agents (approved by the FDA for smoking cessation)					
Bupropion SR	History of seizure and eating disorder	Insomnia Dry mouth	150 mg every morning for 3 days, then 150 mg twice daily (begin 1–2 weeks before quit)	7–12 weeks Maintenance up to 6 months	Zyban (Rx only)
Nicotine gum		Mouth soreness Dyspepsia	1–24 cigarettes per day = 2 mg gum (up to 24 pieces/day) 25+ cigarettes per day = 4 mg gum (up to 24 pieces/day)	Up to 12 weeks	Nicorette, Nicorette Mint (OTC only)
Nicotine inhaler		Local irritation to mouth and throat	6–16 cartridges per day	Up to 6 months	Nicotrol inhaler (Rx only)
Nicotine nasal spray		Nasal irritation	8–40 doses per day	3–6 months	Nicotrol NS (Rx only)
Nicotine patch		Local skin reaction Insomnia	21 mg/24 hr 14 mg/24 hr 7 mg/24 hr 15 mg/16 hr	4 weeks then 2 weeks then 2 weeks 8 weeks	NicoDerm CQ (OTC only) Generic patches (Rx and OTC) Nicotrol (OTC only)
Nicotine lozenge		Mouth soreness Throat irritation Hiccups Heartburn or indigestion	2 mg or 4 mg (up to 20 pieces per day)	12 weeks	Commit (OTC only)

TABLE 4–4   Pharmacotherapy Agents for Smoking Cessation (*Continued*)

Drug	Precautions or Contraindications	Side Effects	Dosage	Duration	Availability
Varenicline	Combination therapy with nicotine patch	Nausea Sleep disturbance Headaches Abnormal dreams Constipation	1 mg twice daily following 1 week of a titration schedule of: Days 1–3: 0.5 mg once daily Days 4–7: 0.5 mg twice daily Day 8–end of treatment: 1 mg twice daily	Begin treatment 1 week before stop date and continue for 12 weeks. If successful, an additional 12 weeks is recommended.	Chantix (Rx only)
Second-line agents (not FDA approved for smoking cessation)					
Clonidine	Rebound hypertension	Dry mouth Drowsiness Dizziness Sedation	0.15–0.75 mg per day	3–10 weeks	Oral clonidine-generic Catapres (Rx only) Transdermal Catapres (Rx only)
Nortriptyline	Risk of arrhythmias	Sedation Dry mouth	75–100 mg per day	12 weeks	Nortriptyline HCl-generic (Rx only)

Rx, prescription; OTC, over-the-counter.
Source: Fiore MC, Bailey WC, Cohen SJ, et al. Treating Tobacco Use and Dependence. Clinical Practice Guideline. Rockville, MD: U.S. Department of Health and Human Services, Public Health Service, June 2000.

them to make a future quit attempt. The guideline offers the use of the "5 R's," which are designed to motivate smokers who are unwilling to quit at this time.[25] The "5 R's" are relevance, risk, rewards, roadblocks, and repetition.[25] Smokers may be unwilling to quit because of misinformation, concern about the effects of quitting, or demoralization because of previous unsuccessful quit attempts. Therefore, after **A**sking about tobacco use, **A**dvising the smoker to quit, and **A**ssessing the willingness to quit, the guideline recommends providing the "5 R's" motivational intervention.[25] The "5 R's" are summarized in Table 4-5.

Preventing Relapse in Former Smokers

As stated earlier, smoking should be viewed as a chronic disease. Even when patients have successfully made a quit attempt, follow-up is still required to prevent relapse. Most

TABLE 4–5   The "5 R's" of Motivational Intervention

Relevance	Encourage the patient to indicate why quitting is personally relevant to his or her life. This can include health status or risk, family or social situation, age, gender, prior quitting experience, personal barriers to cessation.
Risks	Ask the patient to identify potential negative consequences to tobacco use. The clinician can highlight those that are relevant to the patient. Examples include: Acute risks: shortness of breath, exacerbation of asthma, harm to pregnancy, impotence, infertility, and increased serum carbon monoxide. Long-term risks: Heart attacks and strokes, lung and other cancers, chronic obstructive pulmonary disease, long-term disability, and need for extended care. Environmental risks: Increased risk of lung cancer and heart disease in spouses; higher rates of smoking in children of tobacco users; increased risk of low birth weight, sudden infant death syndrome, asthma, middle ear disease, and respiratory infections in children of smokers.
Rewards	Ask the patient to identify potential benefits of stopping tobacco use. Some examples of rewards are improved health; food will taste better; improved sense of smell; saving money; feeling better about yourself; home, car, clothing, breath will smell better; can stop worrying about quitting; setting a good example for children; having healthier babies and children; not worrying about exposing others to smoke; feeling better physically; performing better on fitness activities; reduced wrinkling or aging of skin.
Roadblocks	Ask the patient to identify barriers to quitting and note elements of treatment (problem solving, pharmacotherapy) that could address these barriers. Typical barriers might include withdrawal symptoms, fear of failure, weight gain, lack of support, depression, enjoyment of tobacco.
Repetition	The Guideline recommends that the motivational intervention be repeated every time an unmotivated patient visits the pharmacy or clinic setting. Tobacco users who failed in previous attempts should be told that most people make repeated attempts to quit before they are successful.

Source: Fiore MC, Bailey WC, Cohen SJ, et al. Treating Tobacco Use and Dependence. Clinical Practice Guideline. Rockville, MD: U.S. Department of Health and Human Services, Public Health Service, June 2000.

relapses occur soon after the patient quits smoking.[25] Some patients, however, may relapse months or even years after quitting. Therefore, it is important that all clinicians work to prevent relapse by maintaining contact with those patients who have quit.

There are two types of programs recommended in the guidelines for preventing relapse. The first type is a minimal or brief program and the second is a more intensive program.[25] The brief program is intended to be an intervention encounter that is done every time the healthcare provider sees the patient. Congratulatory comments and strong encouragement to remain abstinent are the goal of brief interventions. In addition, to foster active discussion the provider should ask the patient open-ended questions about how smoking cessation has helped him or her. The provider should also inquire about any problems the patient may be having and offer solutions to prevent relapse.[25]

A more intensive relapse-prevention program may be necessary for patients who are experiencing specific problems and who require more time in resolving these problems.[25] Such problems can include a lack of support for cessation, negative mood or depression, strong or prolonged withdrawal symptoms, weight gain, or flagging motivation and feeling deprived.[25] The healthcare provider should reassure the patient that what he or she is experiencing is common and help the patient resolve the problems or refer the patient to a specialist. Patients with depression and prolonged withdrawal symptoms may need to be referred to a physician for adjustment in drug therapy. Patients experiencing weight gain can be recommended to begin an exercise program, eat a healthy and well balanced eating plan, and take medications known to delay weight gain such as bupropion SR or nicotine gum.[25] In any case, the most important aspect of relapse prevention is contact with the patient.

Identification and Assessment of Tobacco Use Through Intensive Intervention

Up to this point in the chapter, much of the discussion has focused on brief interventions with patients. Brief interventions work well for healthcare providers on a tight time schedule, such as pharmacists, because they generally can be completed in a short period.[25] Some providers, however, may want to offer intensive intervention programs. Intensive interventions are appropriate for any tobacco user willing to use them.[25] Evidence shows that intensive interventions are more effective than brief interventions and should be used whenever possible (e.g., available resources, patient is willing).[25] There are six main components of an intensive intervention: assessment, program clinicians, program intensity, program format, type of counseling and behavioral therapies, and pharmacotherapy.[25] Each of these components will be discussed below.

Proper assessment of a patient should be made to ensure that the tobacco user is willing to make a quit attempt using an intensive treatment program.[25] Other assessments can be performed as well to provide information useful in counseling. Such assessments can include level of stress and presence of comorbidities.

Multiple types of healthcare providers can be used in intensive interventions to offer more effective treatments.[25] One strategy could be to have a medical or healthcare professional, such as a pharmacist, talk with patients about health risks with smoking and benefits associated with smoking cessation, as well as counseling regarding smoking-cessation medications. A non-medical clinician could then deliver additional psychosocial or behavioral interventions.[25]

Strong evidence shows that a dose–response relationship between the intensity of the smoking-cessation program and quitting success does exist.[25] The guidelines recommend that intensive programs consist of a minimum of four sessions and the duration of each session be at least 10 minutes in length. The total contact time with the patient for all sessions combined should be at least 30 minutes in length.[25]

The program format can consist of either individual or group counseling. In addition, proactive telephone counseling has been shown to be effective in smoking cessation and can be used as well.[25] Likewise, self-help material can be distributed to participants, and follow-up assessment interventions measuring participant success should be performed.[25]

Counseling and behavioral therapies should involve practical counseling to solve specific patient problems and to teach coping skills as discussed above. Intratreatment and extratreatment social support should also be used in the intensive program as was discussed in the brief intervention program. The intensive intervention program can expand on and spend more time with these social support systems compared with the brief intervention program.[25]

Pharmacotherapy used in the intensive intervention program is the same as discussed above in the brief intervention program. Clinicians in either intervention program should explain how these medications increase smoking-cessation success and reduce withdrawal symptoms.[25] As with all medications, special care should be taken to make sure patients are taking medications that are appropriate for their specific needs and in conjunction with all other medications taken by the patient.

SMOKING CESSATION IN PHARMACY PRACTICE

A smoking-cessation program can work into a pharmacy practice setting very nicely. In a community pharmacy setting, patients can be asked whether they smoke each time drug counseling takes place. In addition, flyers and advertisements can be placed around the pharmacy alerting customers of the smoking-cessation services that the pharmacy offers. It is important that the pharmacy have a private counseling area to conduct smoking-cessation services. In a hospital setting, pharmacists can also be effective at talking to patients about smoking cessation, especially with regard to the effectiveness of the medications that can be used.

Below is a sample patient of a smoking-cessation program incorporated into a pharmacy practice community setting.

PATIENT ATTEMPTING TO QUIT SMOKING

L.B. is a 37-year-old white female who comes to the pharmacy today as a new patient filling a new prescription for a lipid-lowering agent to treat her newly diagnosed hypercholesterolemia. L.B. has no other medical history, no family history of hyperlipidemia, and no heart disease or cancer history. She has normal body weight and is married with three young children. While counseling L.B. on her new medication, the pharmacist asks her whether she currently smokes. L.B. states that she has smoked approximately 20 cigarettes per day for the past 20 years. The pharmacist tells her that he would like to ask her more questions regarding her smoking habits and begins with the "5 A's" of a brief intervention, which is documented as such:

BRIEF SMOKING CESSATION DOCUMENTATION

Patient information:
Name: L.B. Date: January 27
Height: 5′4″ Weight: 122 lb Age: 37 years
Comorbidities: Hypercholesterolemia
Medications: Lipitor 20 mg daily, Ortho Tri-Cyclen daily
Family history: None
Smoking history: 20 cigarettes per day for 20 years

ASK	Current smoker, never has tried a quit attempt.
ADVISE	Statement was made to L.B. that even though she did not have other significant health issues, smoking can increase the risk for hypercholesterolemia, heart attack, stroke, and thromboembolism. She is especially at risk because she is older than 35 years, smokes more then 15 cigarettes per day, and is taking oral contraceptive medication. Also, smoking can impact the health of her children and spouse. L.B. was informed that the pharmacist and pharmacy staff could assist her if she would like to quit.
ASSESS	L.B. states that her husband is not a smoker and has asked her to quit on several occasions. L.B. states that she is now willing to make a quit attempt and will participate in the brief intervention program that the pharmacy offers.

ASSIST	A quit date was set for 1 week from today (February 3). L.B. was advised to tell her family, friends, and coworkers that she was quitting and to ask for their support.

L.B. was advised to remove all tobacco products from her home, car, office, and any other place she might have them. In addition, she was advised to have her house and car cleaned to remove smoky odors and establish a "clean or fresh start" to her quit attempt.

Counseling advice consisted of telling L.B. to:

- Not smoke even a single puff after the quit date.
- Avoid personal trigger situations by not eating lunch in the cafeteria and abstaining from alcohol for several weeks.
- Avoid time pressures and stress at work and home by being well organized.
- Learn to anticipate and avoid temptation.
- Exercise by walking with a partner on most days of the week to decrease weight gain and to feel good about herself.
- Talk about the quitting process, such as reasons for quitting and concerns and worries about quitting.

Pharmacotherapy recommendation:

- Nicotine gum 2 mg, up to 24 pieces per day as needed. This is available over the counter and has been shown to delay weight gain, which L.B. is concerned about. Counsel L.B. about side effects of mouth soreness and dyspepsia.

ARRANGE	A follow-up phone call was arranged for the day before the quit date (February 2) and 1 week after the quit date (February 10).

Long-term follow-up should continue with L.B. and can be conducted via telephone and when she comes to the pharmacy to fill her prescription. If L.B. fails at the quit attempt, she should be reassured that she can still be successful at quitting in the future and the failed attempt can be used as a learning experience. L.B.'s physician should also be contacted by the pharmacist so he or she can give L.B. support and guidance in the quitting process.

Tobacco dependence is a chronic disease that deserves attention and treatment from all healthcare providers, including pharmacists. Many effective treatments are available, including several medication options that should be used in all eligible patients. Pharmacists are in an ideal position to screen patients who are current and past smokers and to offer treatment within the pharmacy or refer the patient to other treatment centers. Preventing disease through smoking-cessation programs should be a priority for all healthcare providers as smoking cessation has been shown to decrease the risk for cardiovascular disease and many types of cancers. Even if a pharmacy does not have an active smoking-cessation program, it is the responsibility of the pharmacist, as a healthcare provider, to screen all patients for smoking status and willingness to quit and to refer, educate, and motivate patients to make a quit attempt.

REFERENCES

1. U.S. Department of Health and Human Services. The health consequences of smoking. A Report of the Surgeon General. Atlanta: U.S. Department of Health and Human Services, Centers for Disease Control and Prevention, National Center for Chronic Disease Prevention and Health Promotion, Office of Smoking and Health, 2004.
2. Mokdad AH, Marks JS, Stroup DF, Gerberding JL. Actual causes of death in the United States, 2000. JAMA 2004;291:1238–1245.

3. American Heart Association. Heart Disease and Stroke Statistics—2006 Update. Available at: http://american-heart.org/downloadable/heart/113535864858055-1026_HS_Stats06book.pdf. Accessed January 28, 2006.

4. U.S. Department of Health and Human Services. Healthy People 2010: Understanding and Improving Health, 2nd ed. Washington, DC: US Department of Health and Human Services, 2000. Available at http://www.healthypeople.gov/.

5. CDC. Cigarette smoking among adults—United States, 2004. MMWR Morb Mortal Wkly Rep 2005;54:1121–1124.

6. Ross R, Glomset J. The pathogenesis of atherosclerosis (first of two parts). N Engl J Med 1976;295:369–377.

7. Ross R, Glomset J. The pathogenesis of atherosclerosis (second of two parts). N Engl J Med 1976;295:420–425.

8. Ross R. The pathogenesis of atherosclerosis: a perspective for the 1990s. Nature 1993;362:801–809.

9. Ross R. Atherosclerosis—an inflammatory disease. N Engl J Med 1999;340:115–126.

10. Asmussen I, Kjeldsen K. Intimal ultrastructure of human umbilical arteries: observations on arteries from newborn children of smoking and nonsmoking mothers. Circ Res 1975;36:579–589.

11. Asmussen I. Ultrastructure of human umbilical arteries from newborn children of smoking and nonsmoking mothers. Acta Pathol Microbiol Immunol Scand Sect A Pathol 1982;90:375–383.

12. Asmussen I. Ultrastructure of the umbilical artery from a newborn delivered at term by a mother who smoked 80 cigarettes per day. Acta Pathol Microbiol Immunol Scand Sect A Pathol 1982;90:397–404.

13. Pittilo RM. Cigarette smoking and endothelial injury: a review. Adv Exp Med Biol 1990;273:61–78.

14. Davis JW, Shelton L, Eigenberg DA, Hignite CE, Watanabe IS. Effects of tobacco and nontobacco cigarette smoking on endothelium and platelets. Clin Pharmacol Ther 1985;37:529–533.

15. Freidman GD, Siegelaub AB, Seltzer CC, Feldman R, Collen MF. Smoking habits and the leukocyte count. Arch Environ Health 1973;26:137–143.

16. U.S. Department of Health and Human Services. The Health Benefits of Smoking Cessation. Surgeon General's Report on Smoking and Health. Atlanta: U.S. Department of Health and Human Services, Public Health Service, Centers for Disease Control and Prevention, Center for Chronic Disease Prevention and Health Promotion, Office of Smoking and Health, 1990. DHHS Publication No. (CDC) 90-8416.

17. Craig WY, Palomaki GE, Haddow JE. Cigarette smoking and serum lipid and lipoprotein concentrations: an analysis of published data. BMJ 1989;298:784–788.

18. Krupski WC. The peripheral vascular consequences of smoking. Ann Vasc Surg 1991;5:291–304.

19. Benowitz NL. Drug therapy: pharmacologic aspects of cigarette smoking and nicotine addiction. N Engl J Med 1988;319:1318–1330.

20. Lauer MS, Francis GS, Okin PM, Pashkow FJ, Snader CE, Marwick TH. Impaired chronotropic response to exercise stress testing as a predictor of mortality. JAMA 1999;281:524–529.

21. Cryer PE, Haymond MW, Santiago JV, Shah SD. Norepinephrine and epinephrine release and adrenergic mediation of smoking-associated hemodynamic and metabolic events. N Engl J Med 1976;295:573–577.

22. Koch A, Hoffmann K, Steck W, et al. Acute cardiovascular reactions after cigarette smoking. Atherosclerosis 1980;35:67–75.

23. U.S. Department of Health, Education, and Welfare. Smoking and Health: Report of the Advisory Committee to the Surgeon General of the Public Health Service. Washington, D.C.: U.S. Department of Health, Education, and Welfare, Public Health Service, 1964. PHS Publication No. 1103.

24. American Cancer Society. Cancer Facts and Figures, 2003. Atlanta: American Cancer Society, 2003.

25. Fiore MC, Bailey WC, Cohen SJ, et al. Treating Tobacco Use and Dependence. Clinical Practice Guideline. Rockville, MD: U.S. Department of Health and Human Services, Public Health Service, June 2000.

26. U.S. Department of Health and Human Services. Women and Smoking. A Report of the Surgeon General. Rockville, MD: U.S. Department of Health and Human Services, Public Health Service, Office of the Surgeon General, 2001.

27. Corelli RL, Suchanek Hudmon K. Tobacco use and dependence. In: Koda-Kimble MA, ed. Applied Therapeutics: The Clinical Use of Drugs, 8th ed. Philadelphia: Lippincott Williams & Wilkins, 2005;85:1–85.29.

28. Package Insert. Exubera (insulin human [rDNA origin]) Inhalation Powder. New York: Pfizer Labs, May 2006.

CHAPTER 5

Health Behavior Change

OBJECTIVES

At the end of this chapter the reader should be able to:

1. Recall the number of Americans who are fully adherent to the combination of recommendations for physical activity, fruit and vegetable intake, and smoking abstinence.
2. Explain the Health Belief Model, Transtheoretical Model of Change, the 5 A's Behavioral Intervention Protocol, and Social Cognitive Theory.
3. List patient-related and healthcare system and provider-related barriers to adherence.
4. List and explain several patient-related and program-related behavior changes strategies that can improve adherence.

IMPACT OF PATIENT NON-ADHERENCE

The study of behavior change is not a new concept in medicine and certainly not new to pharmacists. Counseling patients to take their medications properly is a hallmark of pharmacy practice and an area in which pharmacists have made significant contributions to overall patient care. Issues of non-adherence to medications remain, however, a significant problem in the United States and around the world. The World Health Organization (WHO) estimates that adherence to long-term therapy for those with chronic diseases averages only 50%.[1] In the United States, approximately 125,000 deaths are a result of medication non-adherence annually.[2] In addition, up to 11% of hospital and 40% of nursing home admissions are attributed to the lack of adherence to medication therapy.[2] The cost of medication non-adherence is also significant. It is estimated that the direct and indirect cost of medication non-adherence in the United States is approximately $100 billion per year.[2–4]

Pharmacists must always be acutely aware of medication adherence problems that may arise with their patients. Similarly, pharmacists who counsel patients about lifestyle modifications such as smoking cessation, physical activity, and proper nutrition must also make a concerted effort to focus on patient adherence. Overall patient adherence rates for physical activity and proper nutrition are even lower than those reported for medication adherence.

Physical inactivity, unhealthy food consumption, and smoking are identified as the three leading health behaviors that contribute the most to the prevalence of **coronary heart disease (CHD)** in the United States.[5] Recommendations for each of these behaviors have been established and are discussed in previous chapters in this book. It is reported that 75% of the U.S. population adheres to recommendations not to smoke.[5,6] In addition, 25% adheres to physical activity recommendations, and only 20% of the U.S. population adheres to the recommendations for fruit and vegetable intake.[5,7,8] Studies have shown that the lowest incidence of CHD occurs in patients who adhere to multiple risk-reducing behaviors.[5,9] Therefore, patients who can adhere to smoking cessation, physical activity, and proper nutrition recommendations at the same time are most likely to have the lowest incidence of CHD. Adherence, however, to multiple risk-reducing behaviors such as these is known to be low.[5]

In one particular study, researchers took data from the 2000 Behavioral Risk Factor Surveillance System (BRFSS) to study adherence rates of the U.S. population to the combination of recommendations for physical activity, fruit and vegetable intake, and smoking abstinence.[5,10] On studying a final sample of 38,851 subjects, overall only 5.1% of Americans without CHD and 7.2% of Americans with CHD fully adhered to all three health behaviors.[5] Characteristics of fully adherent patients with and without CHD tended to be female, older in age (>45 years), with higher education (>high school) and higher income (>$50,000).[5]

There cannot be enough emphasis placed on program adherence when working with patients to modify their lifestyle behaviors. Adherence is truly the rate-limiting step to disease prevention. A pharmacist or other healthcare professional can design the perfect risk-reduction program that incorporates physical activity, proper nutrition, weight loss, and smoking cessation that is ideal for a particular patient, but if the patient does not participate in the behavior change, the program will not work and is a waste of time, energy, and resources for both practitioner and patient. Therefore, a fundamental step to designing a disease-prevention program is to outline strategies to improve the adherence to that program. This chapter will focus on behavior change models and behavior change strategies that will enhance disease-prevention program adherence.

BEHAVIOR CHANGE THEORIES AND MODELS

The following section will summarize several theories that attempt to explain the complex process of behavior change. These theories can not only provide a framework for understanding the behavior change process but also provide guidance to healthcare professionals to help their patients obtain their program goals.[11] Several behavior change theories exist. This chapter, however, will only review a few that have been frequently applied to disease-prevention models.

Many of the theories have similar components. One of the fundamental components of behavior change is the theory of **self-efficacy.** This concept states that for patients to make change they must believe in themselves and have confidence that they can execute the desired behavior.[12] In addition, the patient should be at the center of the behavior change process. Effective communication, intervention, and follow-up that is appropriate for each individual patient is at the heart of successful behavior change.

These concepts should be evaluated and discussed with all patients when designing a disease-prevention program.

Health Belief Model

The Health Belief Model was designed to predict and explain why certain individuals engage in disease-prevention practices and others do not.[11,13,14] The general theory says that people make health decisions based on their readiness to take action along with the threat or consequences of not taking action.[11] The Health Belief Model theorizes that four main components serve to explain whether a patient will take action to prevent disease. Individuals must:

1. Believe that they are susceptible to a certain disease.
2. Believe the consequences of the disease are serious enough to warrant taking preventive action.
3. Perceive that the actions taken have benefits.
4. Believe that the barriers that are involved with making the change (e.g., cost, inconvenience, pain, risk of embarrassment) are not too great and can be successfully overcome.[11,12]

The key to this model (as with other models) is good communication with the patient. Giving proper information from credible sources and discussing this information with patients on multiple occasions are good techniques to convince patients to make a change.

Transtheoretical Model of Change

The Transtheoretical Model of Change is sometimes also called the stages for motivational readiness for change.[11] This model is used many times to describe the stages of change for patients with regard to an exercise or tobacco-cessation program.[11,12] The model theorizes that patients move through a series of five stages on their way to becoming and remaining physically active, in the case of establishing an exercise program. The first stage is called the precontemplation stage. When patients are in this stage they are not thinking about or considering a change to become physically active. The stages then progress through the contemplation stage (thinking about making a change), to the preparation stage (making preparations to change), to the action stage (implementing the change), and finally to the maintenance stage (maintaining the change).[12]

The key to using this theory in practice is to first assess the patient's stage and then try to educate and persuade the patient to move toward the action and maintenance stages.[12] For example, if a patient is in the contemplation stage but has many barriers that prohibit physical activity, the pharmacist can help the patient to work through the barriers and move to the next stage of preparing for the change.

5 A's Behavioral Intervention Protocol

The 5 A's Behavioral Intervention Protocol is a series of five steps that the healthcare practitioner uses to get a patient to change behavior. The five steps consist of the following:[12]

1. Addressing the issue
2. Assessing the patient
3. Advising the patient
4. Assisting the patient
5. Arranging follow-up

This method of changing behavior has been shown to be effective when applied with skill and consistency. The 5 A's protocol is most often used in smoking-cessation programs and is discussed and applied in Chapter 4 of this book.

Social Cognitive Theory

The Social Cognitive Theory fits nicely into the concept of adopting new lifestyle change behaviors as it provides a framework for understanding, predicting, and changing human behavior.[15] The theory identifies human behavior as a continual interaction between one's environment, one's behaviors, and one's own personal factors.[15] Fundamental beliefs of this theory state that human behavior and behavior change (important for our discussion) depend on observing the behaviors of others, the potential for self-directed changes in behavior, and a process of self-reflection. At the core of the Social Cognitive Theory is the concept of self-efficacy. The theory states that self-efficacy provides a foundation for human motivation, well-being, and personal accomplishment. Individuals who believe that their actions can produce an outcome that they desire are motivated to continue in that behavior.[15]

The Social Cognitive Theory is useful for healthcare practitioners because it can help explain and justify behaviors and techniques for patients who are trying to quit smoking, exercise more, eat more healthful foods, and lose weight. Techniques such as modeling successful behavior, self-monitoring with a contract that a patient has with himself or herself or with others, and setting up a rewards system are explained in the Social Cognitive Theory as effective toward successful health behavior change. Knowing the concepts of this theory can help pharmacists and other healthcare professionals understand why their patients behave as they do.

BARRIERS TO ADHERENCE

Inherent to any kind of behavior change are barriers. Behavior change barriers can be as individual as the patient and can range from simple to complex. A key component to program adherence is the ability to identify and overcome barriers that prohibit participation in the recommended activities. Some potential barriers can be identified before beginning a program, and others will not become known until the patient attempts to engage in the activities. In either case, patients should be counseled to the fact that everyone has certain individual barriers that may cause setbacks. Barriers will need to be discussed at the beginning of the program and continually addressed during the program maintenance phase. Patients need not be discouraged by their barriers but should learn from them to prevent future setbacks. Barriers to adherence can be grouped into those related to the patient and those related to the healthcare system and provider.

Patient-Related Barriers

During the past couple of decades the U.S. government and other organizations such as the American Heart Association have developed and publicized campaigns that have attempted to educate the American population about healthy behaviors. As a result, many people know that smoking abstinence, physical activity, healthy food consumption, and maintaining a healthy body weight are important for overall good health. For example, it may be difficult to find someone in America who does not know that smoking can have harmful health effects or that exercise has health benefits. Yet, only 5% of the U.S. population without CHD adheres to the combination of smoking abstinence, adequate fruit and vegetable intake, and adequate physical activity.[5] The reasons for low adherence to healthy behaviors can be as complex and individualistic as the patients themselves.

Barriers to healthy behaviors that are related to the patients themselves can range from financial, to poor health literacy, to logistic and motivational issues. In addition, a positive social support system that consists of family members, friends, and coworkers appears to greatly benefit program adherence and ultimately program success. Table 5-1 lists possible barriers to program adherence.

Financial barriers appears to be a key deterrent to adherence.[2] Financial barriers can be related to a lack of healthcare insurance, limited access to healthcare in general, or difficulty paying for items needed for a disease-prevention program.[2] For example, consuming foods such as fresh fruits and vegetables is more expensive and less convenient than purchasing processed, high-fat foods that are easily accessible and cheaper to buy. Also, memberships to fitness clubs and clothing such as proper footwear can be expensive when beginning an exercise program.

A study on medication adherence showed that higher copayments lead to reduced adherence and poorer adverse health outcomes.[2,16-18] If patients are willing to stop taking medications as a result of financial barriers, they may also be non-adherent to

---

TABLE 5–1   **Program Adherence Barriers**

Patient related

Financial

Poor health literacy

Motivation level

Logistic issues
   Perceived lack of time
   Poor access to proper food
   Poor access to exercise facilities
   Lack of childcare for young parents while exercising
   Poor weather conditions during certain times of the year (winter)

Poor access to healthcare facilities and healthcare providers

Lack of social support system

Medical factors prohibiting participation

Healthcare system and provider related

Lack of time to work with patients

Little or no reimbursement

Lack of support staff to assist the provider

Lack of training and knowledge in the area of disease prevention

Professional attitude

   Lack of realization that disease prevention is a responsibility of <u>ALL</u> healthcare providers including pharmacists

State pharmacy practice regulations

Source: American Pharmacists Association. Enhancing Patient Adherence: Proceedings of the Pinnacle Roundtable Discussion. American Pharmacists Association Highlights Newsletter 2004;7(4):1–12.

lifestyle-related changes when financial issues arise. Discussing financial barriers and devising a plan to overcome these barriers before beginning a disease-prevention program are important to giving the program the best possible chance for success and overall high adherence rates.

Health literacy is the ability to read, understand, and use health information.[2] Poor health literacy has become a major reason for healthcare non-adherence in America. The Institute of Medicine has estimated that nearly half of all Americans (90 million people) have poor health literacy.[2,19] More than 300 studies confirm that health-related materials distributed to patients cannot be understood by most of the people for whom they are intended.[2,19] Obtaining adequate health literacy in all patients should be a goal for all healthcare providers whether the patients are learning about the medications they take or lifestyle modifications they should perform. Pharmacists and other healthcare professionals should communicate simply, clearly, and frequently with patients to ensure they understand the health information in the way that it is intended.[2]

Healthcare System- and Provider-Related Barriers

In the past there has been a tendency to focus only on the patient-related factors that affect adherence and ignore those factors that are related to the providers themselves or the healthcare system in general.[1,2] Program adherence should be viewed as a shared responsibility by both the patient and provider, as well as the system. Simply providing patients with written information about the actions they are to perform and then solely blaming them for non-adherence is not acceptable. Proper healthcare involves quality patient education. To provide quality patient education, providers need to have proper training and be reimbursed for their actions. Reimbursing pharmacists only for dispensing medications does not promote adequate patient counseling and can lead to non-adherence. State pharmacy practice regulations can have a major impact on counseling levels.[2] Changes in state practice acts to require more face-to-face patient counseling could play a role in improving patient adherence as well as proper medication usage.[2] Pharmacist and other healthcare providers should be advocates for healthcare system changes that promote more face-to-face contact with patients and for the financial reimbursements of such care.

BEHAVIOR CHANGE STRATEGIES

Several behavior change strategies are available for use to improve adherence when designing a disease-prevention program. Some of the strategies are specific to the patient (patient-related) and some are specific to the program or provider (program-related). The strategies that are appropriate for each individual patient should be used as needed as not all patients will require all of the patient-related and program-related strategies. Tables 5-2 and 5-3 provide a list of examples with a description of patient-related and program-related behavior change strategies, respectively.[20–22]

In addition to the specific strategies listed in Tables 5-2 and 5-3, healthcare practitioners can help patients improve adherence rates by being good problem solvers. Likewise, patients can also be taught to problem solve with a few suggestions from their healthcare provider. Providers and patients must first identify the problem and then generate possible solutions to each of the problems.[23] The next step is to evaluate the positives and negatives of each solution and rank them from least practical to most practical.[23] Finally, try out a solution to see whether it works while remaining flexible to other

TABLE 5–2	Patient-Related Strategies to Improve Adherence

Strategy	Description
Patient-centered approach	Successful adherence programs are grounded in a trusting relationship between the patient and the provider, the integration of adherence into the care plan, and a provider skilled in communication and behavior modification techniques.
Trust building	Patients who trust their provider are more likely to be adherent to the program and also more likely to trust themselves and their ability to be successful in the program.
Communication	Poor health literacy is a major problem in the United States. Effective communication with patients can help them understand their health conditions, recommendations to improve their health, and consequences of non-adherence. Genuine interest, empathy, and active listening are important traits of effective communication. Assessing the effectiveness of communication through asking the patient open-ended questions can help better understand what the patient does and does not understand.
Interest and empathy	These are important techniques for effectively communicating with patients and building trust.
Active listening	Practitioners who only offer advice and do not give patients a chance to talk are not effectively communicating. Active listening means the practitioner is engaged in what the patient is saying and willing to make program adjustments based on the patient's needs.
Log books	Patients who keep a daily log of physical activity and food consumption may be more likely to modify their behaviors. Patients often do not realize the total amount of food they are consuming in a day or the amount of a single type of food (e.g., candy, chips). Writing it down can make this more obvious to patients. Likewise, patients can use a pedometer along with their physical activity log to keep track of daily or weekly activity. This can sometimes motivate patients to maintain a certain level of activity.
Patient self-efficacy	Patients must truly believe in themselves when making behavior changes. If patients think they can do it, they are more likely to be successful. Effectively communicating with patients to assess their self-efficacy is important. In addition, continual empathy, encouragement, and troubleshooting the patient's barriers are needed for program success.
Modifying patient beliefs	Knowledge alone is not enough to be able to change behavior. Patients not only must understand how they can change their behavior but also must truly believe they need to change to decrease health risks and believe they can be successful at modifying their behavior.

Sources: American Pharmacists Association. Enhancing Patient Adherence: Proceedings of the Pinnacle Roundtable Discussion. American Pharmacists Association Highlights Newsletter 2004;7(4):1–12; and Whiteley JA, Lewis B, Napolitano MA, Marcus BH. Health counseling skills. In: Kaminsky LA, et al., eds. ACSM's Resource Manual for Guidelines for Exercise Testing and Prescription, 5th ed. Baltimore: Lippincott Williams & Wilkins, 2006:588–597.

TABLE 5–3   Program-Related Strategies to Improve Program Adherence

Strategy	Description
Simplicity	Lifestyle modification programs need to be easy to understand and implement for patients to be adherent. Programs that are complex can be discouraging for patients and often lead to non-adherence and program failure. For most patients it may be a good idea to try and implement only one or two modifications at a time. For example, a patient who is obese, smokes, is sedentary, and has a poor diet may not be successful if the program tries to change all these behaviors at the same time. One option can be to choose the behavior that poses the most immediate risk (i.e., smoking) first, followed by other modifications at a later time. Or, first choose a behavior that the patient has the best chance at being successful at modifying. This way the patient can realize success, which may motivate him or her to try other behavior modifications.
Convenience	A program designed to fit the current lifestyle of the patient will have a greater chance of success. Modifying a patient's lifestyle is the goal, rather than completely changing the patient's lifestyle. This means that no one program is right for all patients and an individual approach works best.
Goal setting	Setting realistic and attainable goals is a hallmark to program success. Goals should be measurable and easily understood for patients. Short-term goals are important to achieve relatively quick success while also keeping the long-term goals in mind.
Enjoyment	Choose activities and foods that the patient enjoys and that are also appropriate for achieving the program goals.
Variety	To prevent boredom, which often leads to non-adherence, a variety of activities and foods should be chosen based on what the patient prefers.
Rewards and incentives	Rewards and incentives for achieving goals are important to maintaining an adequate motivation level. Rewards should be something that is of value to the patient and can range from small to large.
Self-management	The program should be simple enough that the patient has the ability to self-manage issues that arise in-between visits with the practitioner. Changes to activities and food consumption that may arise because of vacations, illness, and so forth should be simple enough for the patients to problem-solve alone. This empowers patients to be an advocate for their own healthcare.
Frequent contact	Studies have shown that patients who have frequent contact with their providers have greater adherence. Contacts may be more frequent toward the beginning of the program and less frequent during the maintenance phase when patients can more effectively self-manage their program.
Social support	Supportive family, friends, and coworkers are important to the success and adherence of any behavior change program. It is a good idea for the pharmacist to counsel the people in the support system, especially the family, in addition to the patient in most instances.

TABLE 5–3   Program-Related Strategies to Improve Program Adherence (*Continued*)

Strategy	Description
Cost and time of implementation	Cost and implementation time are major factors to program adherence. Working within the patient's budget and time constraints to develop creative ways to become physically active and to eat healthy are challenging to the practitioner, but very rewarding and conducive to program adherence.
Multidisciplinary approach	No healthcare practitioner should work alone. Each discipline has unique skills that can enable patients to produce better health outcomes. Referring patients to other providers who are more knowledgeable and skilled should be viewed as collaborative partnerships that are best for the patient and not as a failure of any one practitioner. In addition, patients who hear the same message about positive health behaviors from multiple providers are more likely to change behavior.
Leading by example	Pharmacists and all healthcare providers should not only talk to their patients about positive health behaviors, but should engage in them also. Patients are more likely to accept changing their health behaviors if they know that the practitioner thinks that it is important enough to participate in also.
Evaluating adherence	Like all measures of health, adherence levels should be evaluated during each patient's visit to the pharmacy. Dialogue regarding adherence can expose barriers, which can then be resolved during that visit. Adherence rates can be recorded along with other health measures at each visit.

Source: Dunn AL, Chambliss HO. Psychopathology. In: Kaminsky LA, et al., eds. ACSM's Resource Manual for Guidelines for Exercise Testing and Prescription, 5th ed. Baltimore: Lippincott Williams & Wilkins, 2006:581–587.

solutions.[23] Practitioners and patients should then reflect back about the problem to see whether the problem was positively influenced by the solution.[23] By doing this method of problem solving, practitioners and patients can better understand current patient behavior and learn from it should future problems arise. If problems become difficult to solve, practitioners and patients should consult other practitioners and patients in similar situations, remember what problem-solving methods have worked in the past, and use coping skills instead of giving up.[23]

Motivational Counseling

Motivation can often be a barrier to participating in positive health behaviors. Healthcare practitioners can perform brief motivational interviewing approaches as a method of assessing and encouraging patients to become more motivated. Motivational interviewing was first used in patients who abuse alcohol and tobacco as a means to make positive behavior changes.[24] These methods can also be used for patients who are advised to eat a more healthful diet and increase physical activity levels. Key components to brief motivational counseling include acknowledging, normalizing, and gently working through a patient's ambivalence toward positive lifestyle behaviors; emphasizing the patient's freedom to make the choice not to participate in positive behaviors while also encouraging change and accepting responsibility for not changing behavior; and encouraging the patient to evaluate the pros and cons of continuing the pattern of unhealthy behavior versus adopting positive lifestyle changes.[24] Motivating a patient who is unmotivated to change behavior can be difficult. Effective communication that builds trust between the patient and the practitioner is important. Pharmacists and other healthcare practitioners should understand that increasing motivation levels may take time, and several counseling sessions may be required to see positive changes. Pharmacists can address motivation for making positive changes at the same time drug counseling is done when the patient visits the pharmacy for prescription refills.

PROGRAM ADHERENCE AND PHARMACY PRACTICE

Adherence is not a new concept for pharmacists as medication adherence is something that pharmacists strive for in their patients every day. The same techniques and strategies that are used to enhance medication adherence can also be used to improve adherence to healthy eating, physical activity, weight control, and smoking abstinence. At the forefront of adherence improvement should be a patient-centered approach to healthcare. A patient-centered adherence program has three key components: a trusting relationship between the patient and the pharmacist and other healthcare practitioners; an integration of adherence into the overall care plan of the patient; and pharmacists and other healthcare professionals who are competent in behavior modification and patient communication skills.[2] Patients view pharmacists as trusted, caring, and compassionate healthcare providers. Pharmacists who exemplify these qualities can earn the trust of their patients so that patients can be open and honest with not only the pharmacist as their provider but with themselves.[2]

Link Between Depression and Non-Adherence

According to the World Health Organization, major depression ranks as the second most significant disease burden in the world behind **ischemic heart disease.**[22,25] Approximately 13 million American adults currently suffer from depression each year, and Americans have a 16% lifetime prevalence of a major depressive disorder.[22,26] Depression has been shown to be a cause of non-adherence, but the link between the two may often go unrecognized.[2]

When looking at medication adherence, studies show that patients who are depressed are less likely than non-depressed patients to adhere to their drug therapy, even for medications that are not related to depression.[27] Patients who have depression in addition to diseases such as **diabetes mellitus,** HIV/AIDS, and **cardiovascular disease** are less likely to take any of their medications when compared with patients who do not have depression.[27–30] Additionally, studies have shown that treating depression with antidepressants can have a positive effect on medication adherence for all diseases that the patient may have.[2] In another study, pharmacists showed that patients who took more than 50% of their antidepressant medication had significantly higher rates of adherence to medications to treat their **hypertension, dyslipidemia,** and diabetes compared with patients who took less than 50% of their antidepressant medication.[2]

If patients who are depressed become less adherent to taking their medications, it is likely that they will also become non-adherent to healthy lifestyle behaviors. For these reasons it is important to be able to detect signs and symptoms of major depression when working with patients. Psychological symptoms include a depressed mood, reduced interest or pleasure in activities that were once enjoyable, feelings of guilt, hopelessness, and worthlessness, and recurrent suicidal thoughts.[2] Other physically related symptoms include sleep disturbances, appetite and weight changes, attention or concentration difficulties, decreased energy, and unexplained fatigue and psychomotor disturbances.[2]

The link between depression and non-adherence emphasizes the importance of good communication and quality patient counseling. Pharmacists can recognize symptoms of depression in patients who have become non-adherent and refer them to their primary care physician for further evaluation. Detecting depression can help reduce the risks associated with hypertension, hyperlipidemia, diabetes, and other diseases by improving medication adherence rates as well as lifestyle behavior adherence rates.

The Asheville Project is a landmark pharmaceutical care program that has been able to show several positive clinical, humanistic, and economic outcomes as a result of pharmacist-managed care of patients with diabetes and **asthma**.[31–34] One of the hallmarks of the project was that pharmacists were able to spend one-on-one time counseling patients (30-minute sessions on one day each month) and were reimbursed for doing so. Pharmacists participating in the study reported that the face-to-face patient contact was very successful toward building the trust of the patient.[2] Study results demonstrated that the patients who receive more personal and intensive treatment from pharmacists show positive clinical outcomes, financial benefits, and overall better adherence rates.[31–34]

The pharmacy profession is a key player at improving adherence in the healthcare system. Pharmacists generally have frequent contact with patients in which effective communication and trust building can occur. Continuing to work toward getting financial reimbursement for these services is important as trusting relationships take time to develop. Offering quality healthcare services through more frequent face-to-face contact with patients is realistic and affordable as demonstrated in the Asheville Project. Pharmacists should be advocates for this type of healthcare by continually seeking reimbursement for clinical services.

REFERENCES

1. World Health Organization. Adherence to Long-Term Therapies: Evidence for Action. Geneva: World Health Organization, 2003. Available at: http://www.who.int/chronic_conditions/adherencereport/en/. Accessed March 2, 2006.
2. American Pharmacists Association. Enhancing Patient Adherence: Proceedings of the Pinnacle Roundtable Discussion. American Pharmacists Association Highlights Newsletter 2004;7(4):1–12.
3. Medication compliance aids. Available at: http://www.lifeclinic.com/focus/blood/supply_aids.asp. Accessed March 2, 2006.
4. American Pharmacists Association. Medication Compliance-Adherence-Persistence (CAP) Digest. Washington, D.C.: American Pharmacists Association, 2003.

5. Miller RR, Sales AE, Kopjar B, Fihn SD, Bryson CL. Adherence to heart-healthy behaviors in a sample of the U.S. population. Prev Chronic Dis April 2005. Available at: http://www.cdc.gov/pcd/issues/2005/apr/04_0115.htm. Accessed March 2, 2006.

6. Centers for Disease Control and Prevention. Cigarette smoking among adults—United States, 1999. MMWR Morb Mortal Wkly Rep 2001;50:869–873.

7. Centers for Disease Control and Prevention. Increasing physical activity. A report on recommendations of the Task Force on Community Preventive Services. MMWR Recomm Rep 2001;50(RR-18):1–14.

8. Li R, Serdula M, Bland S, Mokdad A, Bowman B, Nelson D. Trends in fruit and vegetable consumption among adults in 16 states: Behavioral Risk Factor Surveillance System, 1990–1996. Am J Public Health 2000;90:777–781.

9. Stampfer MJ, Hu FB, Manson JE, Rimm EB, Willett WC. Primary prevention of coronary heart disease in women through diet and exercise. N Engl J Med 2000;343:16–22.

10. Centers for Disease Control and Prevention. Behavioral Risk Factor Surveillance System. Technical information and data—2000. Atlanta: Centers for Disease Control and Prevention, 2003 (Jan 3).

11. Napolitano MA, Lewis B, Whiteley JA, Marcus BH. Principles of health behavior change. In: Kaminsky LA, et al., eds. ACSM's Resource Manual for Guidelines for Exercise Testing and Prescription, 5th ed. Baltimore: Lippincott Williams & Wilkins, 2006:545–557.

12. Lorish CD, Gale JR. Facilitating adherence to healthy lifestyle behavior changes in patients. In: Shepard KF, Jensen GM, eds. Handbook of Teaching for Physical Therapists, 2nd ed. Boston: Butterworth Heinnemann, 2002:351–385.

13. Becker MH, ed. The health belief model and personal health behavior. Health Educ Monogr 1974;2:324–508.

14. Rosenstock IM, Strecher VJ, Becker MH. Social learning theory and the health belief model. Health Educ Q 1988;15:175–183.

15. Pajares F. Overview of social cognitive theory and of self-efficacy. Available at: http://www.emory.edu/EDUCATION/mfp/eff.html. Accessed July 9, 2006.

16. Harris Interactive. Multi-tier co-pays and the chronically ill. Available at: http://www.npcnow.org/newsroom/factsheets/PDFs/Multi-tier_Co-pays_Chronically_Ill.pdf. Accessed March 2, 2006.

17. Harris Interactive. Out of pocket costs are a substantial barrier to prescription drug compliance. Available at: http://www.harrisinteractive.com/news/newsletters/healthnews/HI_HealthCareNews2001Vol1_iss32.pdf. Accessed March 2, 2006.

18. Harris Interactive. The impact of tiered co-pays: a survey of patients and pharmacists. Research Report. September 2003. Available at: http://www.npcnow.org/resources/PDFs/Co-payStudyFinal.pdf. Access March 2, 2006.

19. Institute of Medicine. Health Literacy: A Prescription to End Confusion. Washington, D.C.: National Academies Press, 2004.

20. Whiteley JA, Lewis B, Napolitano MA, Marcus BH. Health counseling skills. In: Kaminsky LA, et al., eds. ACSM's Resource Manual for Guidelines for Exercise Testing and Prescription, 5th ed. Baltimore: Lippincott Williams & Wilkins, 2006:588–597.

21. Atreja A, Bellam N, Levy SR. Strategies to enhance patient adherence: making it simple. Medscape General Medicine 2005;7(1). Available at: http://www.medscape.com/viewarticle/498339. Accessed March 2, 2006.

22. Dunn AL, Chambliss HO. Psychopathology. In: Kaminsky LA, et al., eds. ACSM's Resource Manual for Guidelines for Exercise Testing and Prescription, 5th ed. Baltimore: Lippincott Williams & Wilkins, 2006:581–587.

23. Jensen GM, Lorish CD, Shepard KF. Understanding and influencing patient receptivity to change: the patient-practitioner collaborative model. In: Shepard KF, Jensen GM, eds. Handbook of Teaching for Physical Therapists, 2nd ed. Boston: Butterworth Heinnemann, 2002:323–350.

24. King AC, Martin JE, Castro C. Behavioral strategies to enhance physical activity participation. In: Kaminsky LA, et al., eds. ACSM's Resource Manual for Guidelines for Exercise Testing and Prescription, 5th ed. Baltimore: Lippincott Williams & Wilkins, 2006:572–580.

25. American Psychiatric Association: Diagnostic and Statistical Manual of Mental Disorders, 4th ed. Washington, D.C.: American Psychiatric Association, 1994.

26. Kessler BC, Berglund P, Demler O, et al. The epidemiology of major depressive disorder: Results from the National Comorbidity Survey Replication (NCS-R). JAMA 2003;289:3095–3105.

27. McKellar JD, Humphreys K, Piette JD. Depression increases diabetes symptoms by complicating patients' self-care adherence. Diabetes Educ 2004;30:485–492.

28. Bangsberg DR. Optimizing HIV therapy for patients with comorbidities: depression treatment to improve HIV treatment outcomes. Available at: http://www.aafmed.com/comor/depression.html. Accessed March 3, 2006.

29. Turner BJ. Factors effecting adherence in HIV-infected patients. Available at: http://www.medscape.com/viewarticle/412897_7. Accessed March 3, 2006.
30. Carter S, Taylor D. A Question of Choice—Compliance in Medication Taking, 2nd ed. London: Medicines Partnership, October 2003. Available at: http://www.medicines-partnership.org/our-publications. Accessed March 3, 2006.
31. Cranor CW, Christensen DB. The Asheville Project: short-term outcomes of a community pharmacy diabetes care program. J Am Pharm Assoc 2003;43:149–159.
32. Cranor CW, Christensen DB. The Asheville Project: factors associated with outcomes of a community pharmacy diabetes care program. J Am Pharm Assoc 2003;43:160–172.
33. Cranor CW, Bunting BA, Christensen DB. The Asheville Project: long-term clinical and economic outcomes of a community pharmacy diabetes care program. J Am Pharm Assoc 2003;43:173–184.
34. Bunting BA, Cranor CW. The Asheville Project: Long-term clinical, humanistic, and economic outcomes of a community-based medication therapy management program for asthma. J Am Pharm Assoc 2006;46:133–147.

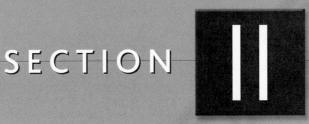

SECTION II

Chronic Diseases

INTRODUCTION

Section I provides basic background information on the lifestyle modification strategies of proper nutrition, physical activity, weight control, tobacco cessation, and health behavior change. Section II will now apply that background information to patients with specific chronic diseases. Chapters in this section may be read either in the order in which they are presented or read out of order. The 13 chapters in Section II do not build on each other, but rather are a practical application of the information covered in Chapters 1–5. These chapters begin by briefly explaining the epidemiology and pathophysiology of the disease state and are meant to complement information that the student pharmacist or practicing pharmacist has already obtained from other courses or experiences.

Each of the chapters in Section II is similarly structured and contains five tables (with the exception of Chapters 6 and 12) in consistently titled categories that are modified relative to the subject matter. This allows the reader to develop a consistent pattern of critical thinking when designing wellness programs for virtually any disease state. Additionally, each chapter in Section II concludes with a case study that is germane to the information presented in that chapter. Approximately one half of the case studies in Section II are relevant to providing primary prevention lifestyle modification strategies to patients with certain risk factors, while the other half of the case studies are geared toward designing a wellness plan for the secondary prevention of disease for patients with existing chronic diseases. This allows the reader ample opportunities to practice both primary and secondary prevention strategy wellness plans. The answers to the case studies are provided in Appendix C. The approach of these chapters lends well toward an understanding and application of the material that builds skills, rather than memorization.

Hypertension

At the end of this chapter the reader should be able to:

1. Explain the health risks associated with hypertension.
2. Summarize the treatment options available for hypertension.
3. Describe the adoption of the Dietary Approaches to Stop Hypertension (DASH) eating plan.
4. Suggest appropriate exercises for patients with prehypertension and hypertension.
5. Formulate a basic nutrition and exercise program for a patient with hypertension.

OVERVIEW OF HYPERTENSION

Hypertension is a disease that is commonly undertreated in the United States. Unfortunately, many patients, and perhaps even some healthcare providers, underestimate the significance of untreated and mismanaged hypertension. Because patients usually do not "feel bad" when they have high blood pressure, they can mistakenly interpret this lack of symptoms as a sign of unimportance. Pharmacists are ideally positioned within the community to educate the public about the importance of hypertension and the significant impact that it can have on the incidence of cardiovascular disease and overall health. This chapter will discuss the health risks associated with hypertension and present ways to treat and prevent high blood pressure through lifestyle modifications.

PREVALENCE, ECONOMIC COSTS, AND HEALTH RISKS ASSOCIATED WITH HYPERTENSION

Hypertension (high blood pressure) is defined as having one of three criteria: (1) having a **systolic blood pressure** of 140 mm Hg or higher or a **diastolic blood pressure** of 90 mm Hg or higher; (2) taking antihypertensive medication; or (3) being told at least twice by a physician or other healthcare professional that you have hypertension.[1,2] **Prehypertension** is defined as having a systolic pressure of 120 to 139 mm Hg, or a diastolic pressure of 80 to 89 mm Hg in addition to not taking antihypertensive medication and having not been told by a physician or other healthcare professional that you have hypertension.[1,2]

In 2002, 32.3% of Americans had high blood pressure and 31% of Americans had prehypertension.[1,3] Of those people with high blood pressure, 34% are on medication and have it under control; 25% are on medication but do not have their high blood pressure under control; 11% are not on medication; and 30% do not know they have high blood pressure.[1] Therefore, of the 65 million Americans with high blood pressure, nearly 66% (42.9 million Americans) either do not know they have high blood pressure or do not have it under control.[1,2] In addition, the prevalence of hypertension increases with advancing age.[2] The lifetime risk of hypertension is reported to be approximately 90% for men and women who were non-hypertensive at 55 or 65 years old, respectively, and survive to age 80 to 85 years.[2,4]

Worldwide, as many as 1 billion individuals have hypertension with approximately 7 million deaths per year attributed to high blood pressure.[5] The World Health Organization reports in 2002 that having a systolic blood pressure greater than 115 mm Hg was the number one attributable risk for death throughout the world.[1,5] It was responsible for 49% of **ischemic heart disease** and 62% of cerebrovascular disease, and precedes congestive heart failure in 91% of patients.[1,2,5] The estimated direct and indirect cost associated with hypertension in the United States in 2005 was $59.7 billion.[1]

PATHOPHYSIOLOGY AND ETIOLOGY OF HYPERTENSION

The Seventh Report of the Joint National Committee of Prevention, Detection, Evaluation, and Treatment of High Blood Pressure (JNC 7) (http://www.nhlbi.nih.gov/guidelines/hypertension/index.htm) is considered the hypertension treatment guidelines to be used by healthcare professionals.[2] JNC 7 provides classifications for persons with high blood pressure. The classifications are noted in Table 6-1. For patients to be placed into a category they must have two or more seated and properly measured blood pressure readings that are averaged together from two or more office visits.[2] Prehypertension is not considered a disease category, but rather a marker to identify patients who are at a greater risk of developing hypertension. Patients in this category should be alerted by their healthcare professional of their high risk for developing hypertension and be encouraged to provide strategies to prevent or delay the disease from occurring.[2]

Hypertension can be classified into two types: **essential hypertension** and secondary hypertension.[2] Essential hypertension occurs in 90% of all patients with high blood pressure, and secondary hypertension makes up the remaining 10%.[6–8] Secondary causes of hypertension are also called "identifiable causes" and can range from drug-induced or drug-related to chronic kidney disease.[7] Essential hypertension, the most common type of hypertension, has no identifiable causes. Many factors, however, play a role in the development of essential hypertension such as genetics, **obesity,** sodium

TABLE 6–1	Classification of Blood Pressure for Adults			
Classification	**Systolic Blood Pressure (mm Hg)**		**Diastolic Blood Pressure (mm Hg)**	
Normal	<120	AND	<80	
Prehypertension	120–139	OR	80–89	
Stage 1 hypertension	140–159	OR	90–99	
Stage 2 hypertension	≥160	OR	≥100	

Source: U.S. Department of Health and Human Services, National Institutes of Health, National Heart, Lung, and Blood Institute. The seventh report of the Joint National Committee on Prevention, Detection, Evaluation and Treatment of High Blood Pressure. JNC 7 Express. Accessed at http://www.nhlbi.nih.gov/guidelines/hypertension/express.pdf on August 2, 2006.

consumption, and others.[2,6–8] These factors can lead to hypertension by affecting **cardiac output** or peripheral resistance.[6] The identifiable causes and other causes playing a role in essential hypertension are listed in Table 6-2.

Patients who have hypertension are at a significantly increased risk of developing **cardiovascular disease.** The relationship between high blood pressure and cardiovascular disease is a direct correlation and is independent of other risk factors.[2,8] Starting with a systolic blood pressure of 115 mm Hg, the risk of cardiovascular disease doubles with every 20-mm Hg incremental increase. Likewise, starting with a diastolic blood pressure of 75 mm Hg, the risk of cardiovascular disease doubles with every 10-mm Hg incremental increase. This emphasizes the point that patients are at risk if either the systolic OR the diastolic blood pressure is increased rather than both having to be increased for the patient to be at risk. In addition, individuals with prehypertension are at a significantly greater risk for a cardiovascular event compared with individuals with normal blood pressure.[2,9] It is also important to note that accumulating evidence shows that an elevated diastolic blood pressure (≥90 mm Hg) is a more potent cardiovascular risk factor than systolic blood pressure for those younger than 50 years old.[2] However, an elevated systolic blood pressure (≥140 mm Hg) for those older than 50 years is a more reliable predictor for cardiovascular disease than is diastolic blood pressure.[2] As the incidence of hypertension increases with advancing age, the focus should be on controlling systolic blood pressure for the majority of patients with hypertension.

Hypertension also increases the risk of several other diseases. The diseases resulting from high blood pressure are often referred to as target organ damage.[2] It is important that healthcare professionals clinically assess patients with hypertension for evidence of target organ damage that may be a result of uncontrolled hypertension.[2] These diseases are listed in Table 6-3.

HYPERTENSION DISEASE PREVENTION AND TREATMENT

The ultimate goal of blood pressure management is the reduction of cardiovascular and renal morbidity and mortality. The systolic blood pressure goal is 140 mm Hg or less, whereas the diastolic blood pressure goal is 90 mm Hg or less.[2,10] Patients with hypertension and diabetes or renal disease should obtain a treatment goal of 130/80 mm Hg or less.[2,11,12] These treatment goals are associated with a decrease in cardiovascular disease complications.[2]

TABLE 6–2   **Causes of Hypertension**

Identifiable Causes (Secondary Hypertension)

Chronic kidney disease
Coarctation of the aorta
Cushing's syndrome and other glucocorticoid excess states including chronic steroid therapy
Obstructive uropathy
Pheochromocytoma
Primary aldosteronism and other mineralocorticoid excess states
Renovascular hypertension
Sleep apnea
Thyroid or parathyroid disease
Drug-induced or drug-related
    Non-adherence
    Inadequate dose
    Inappropriate combination
    Excess alcohol intake
    Non-steroidal anti-inflammatory drugs (NSAIDs)
    Cyclo-oxygenase 2 inhibitors (COX 2 inhibitors)
    Cocaine, amphetamines, other illicit drugs
    Sympathomimetics (decongestants, anorectics)
    Oral contraceptive hormones
    Adrenal steroid hormones
    Cyclosporine and tacrolimus
    Erythropoietin
    Licorice (including some chewing tobacco)

Factors Contributing to Essential Hypertension

Genetic
Obesity
Sodium consumption
Renin-angiotensin-aldosterone system
Natriuretic peptide system
Homocysteine
Uric acid

Source: U.S. Department of Health and Human Services, National Institutes of Health, National Heart, Lung, and Blood Institute. The seventh report of the Joint National Committee on Prevention, Detection, Evaluation and Treatment of High Blood Pressure. JNC 7 Express. Accessed at http://www.nhlbi.nih.gov/guidelines/hypertension/express.pdf on August 2, 2006.

The adoption of a healthy lifestyle is of critical importance for the prevention of hypertension as well as the management of those with high blood pressure. The components of lifestyle modification listed in the JNC 7 guidelines are weight reduction, adopting the DASH eating plan, reduction of dietary sodium intake, **physical activity,** and moderating alcohol consumption.[2] Each of these components can have an impact on reducing systolic blood pressure when adopted. Table 6-4 lists the approximate systolic blood pressure reductions resulting from the adoption of each lifestyle component. In addition, adopting these components can not only reduce blood pressures but they can also delay the incidence of hypertension, enhance antihypertensive drug efficacy, and decrease cardiovascular risk independent of changes

TABLE 6–3	Disease Outcomes Resulting From Hypertension

Brain
  Stroke
  Transient ischemic attack
  Dementia
Eyes
  Retinopathy
Heart
  Left ventricular hypertrophy
  Angina
  Prior myocardial infarction
  Prior coronary revascularization
  Heart failure
Kidney
  Chronic kidney disease
  Peripheral vasculature
  Peripheral arterial disease

Source: U.S. Department of Health and Human Services, National Institutes of Health, National Heart, Lung, and Blood Institute. The seventh report of the Joint National Committee on Prevention, Detection, Evaluation and Treatment of High Blood Pressure. JNC 7 Express. Accessed at http://www.nhlbi.nih.gov/guidelines/hypertension/express.pdf on August 2, 2006.

in blood pressure readings.[2] This is important to note because, as stated above, the ultimate goal in blood pressure management is reducing the risk for cardiovascular and renal morbidity and mortality. In addition, smoking cessation is an important component for the overall reduction of cardiovascular risk and is strongly encouraged as a lifestyle modification.[2]

The JNC 7 guidelines recommend that every individual with a blood pressure classification of prehypertension or hypertension participate in lifestyle modification activities. This includes 28% of American adults (59 million) who have prehypertension and 32% of American adults (65 million) with hypertension.[1] Therefore 60% of adults in the United States (124 million individuals) should currently be participating in lifestyle modification activities as recommended by the JNC 7 guidelines.

TABLE 6–4	Systolic Blood Pressure Reductions Resulting From the Adoption of Healthy Lifestyle Changes

Lifestyle Modification	Systolic Blood Pressure Reduction
Body weight reduction	5–20 mm Hg per 10 kg of weight loss
Adopting the DASH eating plan	8–14 mm Hg
Restricting dietary sodium	2–8 mm Hg
Physical activity	4–9 mm Hg
Moderating alcohol consumption	2–4 mm Hg

Source: U.S. Department of Health and Human Services, National Institutes of Health, National Heart, Lung, and Blood Institute. The seventh report of the Joint National Committee on Prevention, Detection, Evaluation and Treatment of High Blood Pressure. JNC 7 Express. Accessed at http://www.nhlbi.nih.gov/guidelines/hypertension/express.pdf on August 2, 2006.

The JNC 7 guidelines offer several recommendations to improve patient adherence to antihypertensive therapy regardless of the regimen. Many health behavior models report that the best and most effective therapy can be implemented, but it will only work if the patient is motivated to take the medication and participate in the healthy lifestyle activities. Therefore, several strategies must be used to improve patient motivation, which foster positive experiences, trust, good communication, and empathy. Table 6-5 lists several strategies for healthcare professionals to use while treating patients with hypertension that promote a final outcome of patient adherence to their specific regimen.

Treatment for hypertension involves proper prescriptions of lifestyle modifications with or without adequate antihypertensive drug doses or drug combinations. Many patients will be able to achieve effective blood pressure control with lifestyle modification and a single blood pressure medication. However, the majority of patients (two thirds) who have hypertension will require two or more antihypertensive drugs.[2] Many drugs are currently available for treating hypertension. Table 6-6 lists commonly used antihypertensive agents.

Nutrition and Hypertension

Recommendations for proper nutrition for patients with hypertension are well established, evidence based, and very specific. Research studies have shown that eating patterns can have a significant influence on blood pressure. Certain components in some food have been shown to increase blood pressure whereas other food types have been shown to decrease blood pressure.

Two landmark studies published in the late 1990s and early 2000s lay the foundation for setting the dietary guidelines portion of JNC 7.[13,14] The dietary recommendations have come to be collectively known as the DASH (Dietary Approaches to Stop Hypertension) eating plan. The first study, published in 1997, randomized 459 adults with high blood pressure (<160/80–95 mm Hg) to one of three eating plans for 8 weeks.[13] The first group ate a diet similar to what many Americans consume in fats, carbohydrates, protein, **cholesterol,** fiber, potassium, magnesium, and calcium. The second group ate a plan similar to what many Americans consume in fats, carbohydrates, protein, and cholesterol but consumed a higher amount of fruits and vegetables. This allowed them to have more fiber, potassium, magnesium, and calcium in their diet. The third group consumed a combination regimen that had the same amounts of fiber, potassium, magnesium, and calcium as in group two by increasing their fruits and vegetables, but also consumed less saturated fat and cholesterol. The study was designed to keep all groups the same for sodium intake (3,000 mg/day) and all study participants' body weight constant.[13]

The results of this study showed that after 8 weeks of being on the eating plan high in fruits and vegetables and low in saturated fat and cholesterol, study participants decreased systolic and diastolic blood pressures by 5.5 and 3.0 mm Hg, respectively, compared with the eating plan that was typical of an American diet ($P < 0.001$ for each).[13] In addition, those participants who had hypertension (≥140/90 mm Hg) before the study experienced an even greater reduction in blood pressure (11.4 and 5.5 mm Hg, $P < 0.001$ for each) compared with the typical American diet.[13] It should also be noted that those participants who did not have hypertension before the study (<140/90 mm Hg) also experienced a significant reduction in blood pressure compared with those who consumed the typical American diet (3.5 mm Hg, $P < 0.001$; and 2.1 mm Hg, $P = 0.003$).[13]

TABLE 6–5   Program Adherence Recommendations for Patients With Hypertension

Provide empathetic reinforcement

Adopt an attitude of concern, hope, and interest in the patient's future

Provide positive feedback

Schedule more frequent appointments for patients who are not achieving their blood pressure goals

Provide clinical awareness and monitoring

Be willing to change unsuccessful regimens to ones that will succeed

Anticipate adherence problems for young men

Encourage patients to bring in all medications (prescription, over-the-counter, herbal) to rule out medication causes of elevated blood pressure

Recognize depression and other psychiatric illnesses and manage appropriately

Organize care-delivery systems

Schedule next appointment before patient leaves office or pharmacy

Use appointment reminders and contact patients to confirm appointments

Follow up with patients who miss appointments

Offer patient education about treatment

Assess patient's understanding, acceptance, and willingness to treat their diagnosis of hypertension

Discuss patient concerns and clarify misunderstandings

Tell the patients what their blood pressure reading is and provide a written copy

Come to a mutual agreement for a blood pressure goal

Emphasize the importance of blood pressure control and the need to continue treatment

Collaborate with other healthcare professionals

Use complementary skills of other healthcare providers

Refer selected patients for more intensive counseling

Individualize the regimen

Include the patient in the decision-making

Simplify the regimen as much as possible

Incorporate the treatment into the patient's daily lifestyle

Agree on realistic short-term and long-term goals

Encourage self-monitoring with validated blood pressure devices, food and exercise diary

Minimize cost of therapy

Promote social support systems

Involve caring family members with the patient's permission

Suggest common interest group activities such as a walking group

Source: U.S. Department of Health and Human Services, National Institutes of Health, National Heart, Lung, and Blood Institute. The seventh report of the Joint National Committee on Prevention, Detection, Evaluation and Treatment of High Blood Pressure. JNC 7 Express. Accessed at http://www.nhlbi.nih.gov/guidelines/hypertension/express.pdf on August 2, 2006.

The second study involved 412 participants who consumed either the typical American diet or the DASH eating plan as described above and then were followed for 30 days at each of three sodium levels.[14] The three sodium levels were a higher intake of 3,300 mg/day (typical of an American diet); intermediate intake of 2,400 mg/day (recommended daily allowance by the U.S. Food and Drug Administration [FDA]); and

TABLE 6–6	Drug Classes of Commonly Used Antihypertensive Agents

Thiazide diuretics
Loop diuretics
Potassium-sparing diuretics
Aldosterone receptor blockers
β-Blockers
β-Blockers with intrinsic sympathomimetic activity
Combined α-blockers and β-blockers
Angiotensin-converting enzyme inhibitors
Angiotensin II antagonists
Calcium-channel blockers
α_1-Blockers
Central α_2 agonists and other centrally acting drugs
Direct vasodilators

Source: U.S. Department of Health and Human Services, National Institutes of Health, National Heart, Lung, and Blood Institute. The seventh report of the Joint National Committee on Prevention, Detection, Evaluation and Treatment of High Blood Pressure. JNC 7 Express. Accessed at http://www.nhlbi.nih.gov/guidelines/hypertension/express.pdf on August 2, 2006.

a lower intake of 1,500 mg/day. The results showed that the lower the sodium intake, the lower the blood pressures regardless of the eating plan. However, at each sodium level, blood pressure was lower on the DASH eating plan compared with the other eating plan. The greatest reduction in blood pressure was seen when participants consumed the DASH eating plan along with 1,500 mg of sodium/day.[14] Compared with those consuming the typical American diet with the highest sodium intake, those consuming the DASH eating plan with the lowest sodium intake experienced a 7.1-mm Hg decrease in blood pressure in those without hypertension and an 11.5-mm Hg decrease in blood pressure in those with hypertension.[14]

As a result of these two studies, the current dietary recommendations for those with high blood pressure are to decrease salt and sodium intake regardless of other aspects of dietary intake.[15] In addition and as equally important, individuals with high blood pressure should consume a diet that is high in fiber, calcium, potassium, and magnesium and low in saturated fat and cholesterol.[15] Specific details of the DASH eating plan are listed in Tables 6-7 and 6-8.

In both of these trials, body weight remained constant throughout the study period.[13,14] As discussed earlier, reducing body weight decreases systolic blood pressure from 5 to 20 mm Hg per 10 kg of body weight lost. This reduction is in addition to blood pressure reductions experienced from the DASH eating plan as well as other lifestyle modifications listed in Table 6-4. Therefore, the greatest reductions in blood pressure will be experienced by participating in multiple lifestyle modifications.

The PREMIER trial implemented weight loss, sodium reduction, increased physical activity, and limited alcohol intake and adopted the DASH eating plan in 269 patients with above-normal blood pressures (>120/80 mm Hg).[16] The results of this trial found that a comprehensive lifestyle modification program can improve the likelihood of obtaining an optimal blood pressure (<120/80 mm Hg) by 35%.[16] In addition, this study also showed that insulin sensitivity can be significantly improved in those implementing multiple lifestyle interventions.[17]

TABLE 6–7   Dietary Recommendations for Patients With Hypertension

Nutrients	Nutrient Target
Fat (% of total kcal)	27%
Saturated	6%
Monounsaturated	13%
Polyunsaturated	8%
Carbohydrates (% of total kcal)	55%
Protein (% of total kcal)	18%
Cholesterol	150 mg/day
Fiber	31 g/day
Potassium	4,700 mg/day
Magnesium	500 mg/day
Calcium	1,240 mg/day
Sodium	1,500 mg/day

Source: U.S. Department of Health and Human Services, National Institutes of Health. Facts about the DASH eating plan. Publication No. 03-4082, May 2003.

TABLE 6–8   The DASH Eating Plan

Food Group	Daily Servings	Nutrients Included	Examples
Grains	7–8	Fiber	Whole-wheat bread, pita bread, oatmeal, unsalted popcorn and pretzels
Vegetables	4–5	Fiber, potassium, magnesium	Tomatoes, potatoes, carrots, green peas, green beans, sweet potatoes
Fruits	4–5	Fiber, potassium, magnesium	Bananas, grapes, oranges, orange juice, melons, peaches, raisins, strawberries
Low-fat or fat-free dairy products	2–3	Protein, calcium	Fat-free (skim) or low-fat (1%) milk, fat-free or low-fat regular or frozen yogurt
Meats, poultry, and fish	2 or less	Protein and magnesium	Lean cuts of meat, poultry without skin, not prepared by frying
Nuts, seeds, and dry beans	4–5	Protein, fiber, magnesium, potassium	Almonds, mixed nuts, peanuts, walnuts, sunflower seeds
Fats and oils	2–3	None	Soft margarine, vegetable oils like olive, corn, canola, and safflower
Sweets	5 per week	None	Sugar, jelly, hard candy, fruit punch, sorbet

Source: U.S. Department of Health and Human Services, National Institutes of Health. Facts about the DASH eating plan. Publication No. 03-4082, May 2003.

Physical Activity and Hypertension

In 2004 the American College of Sports Medicine (ACSM) released a position paper regarding exercise and hypertension.[18] As was previously known for years, but further clarified with greater evidence in the new position paper, high blood pressure can be prevented and treated with physical activity. It is thought that blood pressure decreases in response to chronic endurance exercise are related to a decrease in total peripheral resistance (TPR).[18] Reductions in TPR are associated with increases in blood vessel diameter. The ability of blood vessels to increase to a larger size during and after exercise is a structural adaptation resulting from training that results in lower peripheral resistance. This then leads to lower systolic and diastolic blood pressures. There also may be genetic factors that affect blood pressure adaptations after endurance exercise training.[18]

Exercise training implemented as a method to prevent the onset of hypertension was shown to be successful in several studies. The ACSM reports that white men who engage in higher levels of physical activity and achieve greater fitness have a lower incidence of developing high blood pressure compared with white men who do not engage in regular **physical fitness.**[18] This is true even when factors such as age, body fat, and initial blood pressure are ruled out as possible contributing factors. There are very few studies in women and minority populations with regard to preventing hypertension with exercise. Therefore, the roles of gender and ethnicity are currently unknown.[18]

The amount of evidence supporting increased physical activity for the treatment of high blood pressure is strong. Several meta-analyses of randomized controlled trials have been published.[18] Most of the study participants in these trials were men with a median age of 45 years. The exercises included in the studies were mostly walking, jogging, running, and cycling. The median duration of the studies was 16 weeks with two thirds of the studies using a training frequency of three times per week for a median of 40 minutes per training session. The intensity of the training sessions ranged from 30 to 90% maximal capacity.[18]

In three meta-analyses, which included 29, 44, and 54 trials, systolic blood pressure (SBP) and diastolic blood pressures (DBP) decreased on average 4.7/3.1 mm Hg, 3.4/2.4 mm Hg, and 3.8/2.8 mm Hg, respectively, compared with baseline blood pressures.[18] Study participants who had high blood pressure before being studied reduced their SBP/DBP by 7.4/5.8 mm Hg, which was statistically significant.[18] Those who did not have high blood pressure before being tested showed a lesser blood pressure response of 2.6/1.8 mm Hg, but this response was also statistically significant.[18] Other studies have also shown that average 24-hour blood pressures are reduced as a result of exercise training. In addition, blood pressure and heart rate during exercise tend to be lower in individuals who are trained versus those who are untrained.[18]

Therefore, the ACSM states that both hypertensive and non-hypertensive individuals can significantly lower resting blood pressure through dynamic aerobic exercise and that individuals with high blood pressure will experience a greater response compared with normotensive individuals.[18] The optimal training frequency, intensity, time, and type of exercise needed to lower blood pressure are still unclear. Many studies have been completed that show varying results. The ACSM position stand has compiled all the available data and offered recommendations. These recommendations are evidence based and are listed in Table 6-9. In addition to aerobic activity, resistance training has also been shown to reduce blood pressure in both hypertensive and normotensive individuals. A meta-analysis including 320 subjects revealed that chronic resistance training reduced both SBP and DBP by 3 mm Hg.[19] Therefore, the ACSM recommends resistance training as an adjunct activity to aerobic exercise to treat and prevent high blood pressure.

TABLE 6–9	Physical Activity Recommendations for Patients With Hypertension
Exercise Variable	**Recommendation**
Goals	Lower or control systolic and diastolic blood pressures, decrease risk for cardiovascular disease, stroke, and renal disorders, increase caloric expenditure, increase peak workload and endurance
Type	Aerobic exercises (large muscle activities) such as walking, jogging, running, cycling, or individual aerobic exercise preference Resistance training can be adjunctive to aerobic exercises
Intensity	Moderate-intensity endurance activity
Duration	30 minutes or more continuous or intermittent exercise per day
Frequency	Most, preferably all, days of the week
Lifestyle activity	Increase overall daily activities through increasing the duration of activities of daily living (e.g., walking the dog, taking stairs, yard work, household duties)

PHARMACY PRACTICE APPLICATION

Pharmacists have been involved in treating patients with hypertension for several years. Much has been published showing how pharmacists can have a positive impact in blood pressure management. Pharmacists have helped patients control their blood pressure in settings such as nursing homes, outpatient clinics, in-patient hospitals, community pharmacies, and community health centers in both rural and metropolitan areas.

Pharmacists encounter patients with high blood pressure in almost every setting in which they work. Measuring blood pressure is a skill that pharmacists can master and use as part of screening patients for cardiovascular and stroke risks. Knowing a patient's blood pressure is useful information when advising patients regarding disease prevention. As stated earlier, 124 million Americans have either prehypertension or hypertension and can benefit from lifestyle modification strategies offered by pharmacists. Screening patients for increased blood pressure can be done in almost any pharmacy setting because of the high exposure pharmacists have with patients. Pharmacists can be a valuable resource for hypertension prevention and management.

Prehypertension

Prehypertension is a new category for the JNC 7 guidelines, compared with previous versions of the guidelines. It is defined as having a systolic blood pressure of 120 to 139 mm Hg or a diastolic blood pressure of 80 to 89 mm Hg. According to JNC 7, prehypertension is not a disease category, but rather a designation to identify individuals who are at high risk of developing hypertension.[2]

Since the release of the JNC 7 guidelines in 2003, much has been written about the significance and health risks associated with prehypertension. Nearly one third of the American population has prehypertension.[2] It is reportedly associated with an increased prevalence of having other risk factors. In fact, those who have prehypertension are 1.65 times more likely to have at least one other risk factor for cardiovascular disease or **stroke**.[3,20,21]

People with prehypertension are significantly more likely to have higher amounts of proinflammatory mediators such as C-reactive protein, tumor necrosis factor-α, amyloid-α, and homocysteine levels in their blood compared with people with blood pressures less than 120/80 mm Hg.[22] It has also been shown in one study that Japanese men with prehypertension are at an increased risk for coronary **atherosclerosis** compared with those with a blood pressure of less than 120/80 mm Hg.[23] In addition, data pooled together from nine long-term cohort studies involving a total of more than 81,000 individuals showed that both whites and blacks with prehypertension have twice the risk of stroke compared with those with lower blood pressures.[24] Prehypertension has been shown, however, to not be associated with an increased risk of cardiovascular disease mortality or total mortality as an independent risk compared with those of normal blood pressure.[25]

JNC 7 reports that the importance of knowing whether an individual has prehypertension is significant because it can alert both the healthcare practitioner and the patient of the condition and then early intervention can be undertaken.[2] Individuals with prehypertension are not candidates for drug therapy but should be informed of the significance of prehypertension and firmly encouraged to participate in lifestyle modifications to prevent the onset of hypertension and to lower their risk for cardiovascular disease and stroke.[2] Lifestyle modifications are of the utmost importance for the 59 million Americans who have prehypertension and pose an excellent point of intervention for pharmacists and other healthcare providers to talk with patients about diet, exercise, weight loss and maintenance, and other lifestyle modifications.

CASE STUDY

M.M. is a 64-year-old white male with a medical history of hypertension for 10 years and hyperlipidemia for 8 years who comes to your pharmacy for refills of his medication. For the past 10 years he has been able to manage his blood pressure with hydrochlorothiazide 12.5 to 25 mg daily and his hyperlipidemia with simvastatin 20 mg daily without regard to his lifestyle. He is 5′8″ tall, weighs 240 lb, is sedentary with a body mass index (BMI) of 36 kg/m², and follows no specific eating plan but does frequently eat fast food. He does not drink alcohol or use tobacco. His most recent lipid panel (4 weeks ago) revealed total cholesterol 162, low-density lipoprotein (LDL) 98, high-density lipoprotein (HDL) 47, and triglycerides 132. He just came from his physician's office to your pharmacy with a prescription for metoprolol 50 mg daily because his blood pressure averaged 194/88 mm Hg in his previous two visits. He seems very concerned about managing his blood pressure.

After visiting with M.M. he states that he is interested in adopting lifestyle modifications such as diet, exercise, and weight loss. Results from a 3-day dietary analysis were as follows:

Total caloric intake per day = 3,900 calories
Carbohydrates = 48% of total calories
Monounsaturated fats = 13% of total calories
Polyunsaturated fats = 8% of total calories
Saturated fats = 16% of total calories
Total fats = 37% of total calories

Protein = 15% of total calories
Total dietary cholesterol = 300 mg
Fiber = 9 g
Calcium = 450 mg/day
Potassium = 1,700 mg/day
Magnesium = 165 mg/day
Sodium = 3,000 mg/day

Case Activities

1. *Write an SOAP note for M.M.*
2. *Write short-term and long-term dietary and exercise goals for M.M.*
3. *Write an exercise prescription and dietary suggestions for M.M.*

REFERENCES

1. American Heart Association. Heart Disease and Stroke Statistics—2005 Update. Dallas: American Heart Association, 2005.
2. Chobanian AV, Bakris GL, Black HR, et al. Seventh report of the Joint National Committee on Prevention, Detection, Evaluation, and Treatment of High Blood Pressure. Hypertension 2003;42:1206–1252.
3. Greenland KJ, Croft JB, Mensah GA. Prevalence of heart disease and stroke risk factors in persons with pre-hypertension in the United States, 1999–2000. Arch Intern Med 2004;164:2113–2118.
4. Vasan RS, Beiser A, Seshadri S, et al. Residual lifetime risk for developing hypertension in middle-aged women and men: the Framingham Study. JAMA 2002;287:1003–1010.
5. World Health Report 2002: reducing risks, promoting healthy life. Geneva: World Health Organization, 2002. Available at: http://www.who.int/whr/2002. Accessed February 8, 2007.
6. Carter BL, Zillich AJ. Management of hypertension. Pharmacotherapy Self-Assessment Program. American College of Clinical Pharmacy, 2004:129–164.
7. Carter BL, Saseen JJ. Hypertension. In: Dipiro JT, ed. Pharmacotherapy: A Pathophysiologic Approach, 5th ed. New York: McGraw-Hill, 2002:157–183.
8. Saseen JJ, Carter BL. Essential Hypertension. In: Koda-Kimble MA, ed. Applied Therapeutics: The Clinical Use of Drugs, 8th ed. Philadelphia: Lippincott Williams & Wilkins, 2005:14.1–14.46.
9. Vasan RS, Larson MG, Leip EP, et al. Impact of high-normal blood pressure on the risk of cardiovascular disease. N Engl J Med 2001;345:1291–1297.
10. Last JM, Abramson JH. A Dictionary of Epidemiology, 3rd ed. New York: Oxford University Press, 1995.
11. American Diabetes Association. Treatment of hypertension in adults with diabetes. Diabetes Care 2003;26: S80–S82.
12. National Kidney Foundation Guideline. K/DOQI clinical practice guidelines for chronic kidney disease: evaluation, classification, and stratification. Kidney Disease Outcome Quality Initiative. Am J Kidney Dis 2002;39:S1–S246.
13. Appel LJ, Moore TJ, Obarzanek E, et al. A clinical trial of the effects of dietary patterns on blood pressure. N Engl J Med 1997;336:1117–1124.
14. Sacks FM, Svetkey LP, Vollmer WM, et al. Effects on blood pressure of reduced dietary sodium and the dietary approaches to stop hypertension (DASH) diet. N Engl J Med 2001;344:3–10.
15. U.S. Department of Health and Human Services, National Institutes of Health. Facts about the DASH eating plan. Publication No. 03-4082, May 2003.
16. Appel LJ, Champagne CM, Harsha DW, et al. Effects of comprehensive lifestyle modification on blood pressure control: main results of the PREMIER clinical trial. JAMA 2003;289:2083–2093.
17. Ard JD, Grambow SC, Liu D, Slentz CA, Kraus WE, Svetkey LP. The effect of the PREMIER interventions on insulin sensitivity. Diabetes Care 2004;27:340–347.
18. Pescatello LS, Franklin BA, Fagard R, et al. American College of Sports Medicine position stand. Exercise and hypertension. Med Sci Sports Exerc 2004;36:533–553.
19. Kelley GA, Kelley KS. Progressive resistance exercise and resting blood pressure. A meta-analysis of randomized controlled trials. Hypertension 2000;35:838–843.

20. Wang Y, Wang QJ. The prevalence of prehypertension and hypertension among US adults according to the New Joint National Committee Guidelines. New challenges of an old problem. Arch Intern Med 2004;164: 2126–2134.

21. Russell LB, Valiyeva E, Carson JL. Effects of prehypertension on admissions and deaths. A simulation. Arch Intern Med 2004;164:2119–2124.

22. Chrysohoou C, Pitsavos C, Panagiotakos DB, Skoumas J, Stefanadis C. Association between prehypertension status and inflammatory markers related to atherosclerotic disease: the ATTICA Study. Am J Hypertens 2004;17:568–573.

23. Washio M, Tokunaga S, Yoshimasu K, et al. Role of prehypertension in the development of coronary atherosclerosis in Japan. J Epidemiol 2004;14:57–62.

24. Lackland DT. Black Pooling Project (American Stroke Association International Stroke Conference, New Orleans, LA). Feb 2, 2005.

25. Mainous AG, Everett CJ, Liszka H, King DE, Egan BM. Prehypertension and mortality in a nationally representative cohort. Am J Cardiol 2004;94:1496–1500.

CHAPTER 7

Dyslipidemia

OBJECTIVES

At the end of this chapter the reader should be able to:

1. Explain the health risks and pathophysiology associated with dyslipidemia.
2. Summarize the importance of treating dyslipidemia in relation to cardiovascular disease prevention.
3. List the components included in therapeutic lifestyle changes for the treatment and prevention of dyslipidemia.
4. Describe the important components of proper nutrition for patients with dyslipidemia.
5. Suggest appropriate exercises for patients with dyslipidemia.
6. Formulate a basic nutrition and exercise program for patients with dyslipidemia.

OVERVIEW OF DYSLIPIDEMIA

Drugs to control dyslipidemia are among those that are most commonly dispensed from U.S. pharmacies. As a result, pharmacists are in constant contact with patients who currently have dyslipidemia, or who may be at risk for developing dyslipidemias. Because dyslipidemia has been closely linked with coronary heart disease, it is important for pharmacists to have a good understanding of appropriate drug therapy, as well as lifestyle strategies that help control and prevent dyslipidemia. This chapter will discuss the risks associated with dyslipidemia and present ways to treat and prevent dyslipidemia that decrease the incidence of coronary heart disease.

HEALTH RISKS AND ECONOMIC COSTS ASSOCIATED WITH DYSLIPIDEMIA

Coronary heart disease (CHD) is the number one cause of death in the United States.[1] It is reported that nearly 1 million Americans experience a CHD event annually, of which 40% are fatal.[1] In addition, direct medical costs for the diagnosis and management of **cardiovascular disease** are approximately $100 billion per year.[1]

One of the major risk factors for CHD is hyperlipidemia. Approximately 18% of Americans have a blood **cholesterol** level considered to be too high.[2] The most cost-effective approach to the treatment of CHD is through population interventions like dietary modifications, **exercise,** and weight control combined with smoking avoidance and cessation.[1]

In 2001 the Third Report of the National Cholesterol Education Program's (NCEP) Expert Panel on Detection, Evaluation, and Treatment of High Blood Cholesterol in Adults (Adult Treatment Panel III, or ATP III) was published (http://www.nhlbi.nih.gov/guidelines/).[1] High blood cholesterol has been shown to cause atherosclerotic plaque to accumulate in the coronary arteries, leading to the development of coronary heart disease (CHD). The focus of the NCEP ATP III guidelines is on short-term prevention of **acute coronary syndromes** as well as the need for long-term prevention of coronary **atherosclerosis.** In 2004, an update to the NCEP ATP III guidelines was published, which placed greater importance on treating high-risk CHD patients more aggressively.[3]

The clinical management of lifestyle therapies in the NCEP ATP III guidelines has been called therapeutic lifestyle changes (TLC). The components of lifestyle therapy have been chosen based on their ability to lower both serum cholesterol and the risk for coronary heart disease. It is a multifactorial lifestyle approach in which patients participate in several, if not all, of the TLC components.[1] Interventions included in TLC therapy are (1) reduced intake of saturated fats and cholesterol, (2) therapeutic dietary options for enhancing low-density lipoprotein (LDL) cholesterol lowering (i.e., plant stanols or sterols and increased viscous [soluble] fiber), (3) weight reduction, and (4) increased regular **physical activity.**

PATHOPHYSIOLOGY OF DYSLIPIDEMIA

Dyslipidemia, by definition, is a combination of increased blood lipid levels and lipoprotein concentrations and can be caused by environmental, genetic, and pathologic risk factors.[4] Environmental risk factors causing dyslipidemia are listed in Table 7-1.

The major blood lipids involved in dyslipidemia are **cholesterol, triglycerides,** and phospholipids.[5] Cholesterol is an important and needed component for maintaining normal physiologic functioning. It is an essential precursor for steroid hormones and bile acid formation as well as an important component for maintaining the integrity of cell membranes. Dietary cholesterol contributes relatively little to the total serum cholesterol levels.[4-6] Approximately 90% of serum cholesterol is derived from cholesterol synthesis by the body. The rate-limiting step for cholesterol biosynthesis involves the conversion of 3-hydroxy-3-methylglutarate–coenzyme A (HMG-CoA) to mevalonate via the enzyme HMG-CoA reductase. Excess serum levels of total cholesterol have been shown to contribute to coronary artery plaque formation and are often referred to as hypercholesterolemia.[4-6] The NCEP ATP III guidelines recommend that serum total cholesterol levels be less than 200 mg/dL.[1]

TABLE 7–1	Environmental Risk Factors Leading to Dyslipidemia

Overweight and obesity

Physical inactivity

Cigarette smoking

Excess alcohol intake

Diabetes mellitus

Hypothyroidism

Chronic renal failure

Nephrotic syndrome

Very high-carbohydrate diet

Pharmacologic therapy (corticosteroids, protease inhibitors, β-adrenergic blockers, estrogens, thiazide diuretics)

Source: National Institutes of Health, National Heart, Lung, and Blood Institute. Third report of the National Cholesterol Education Program (NCEP) Expert Panel on Detection, Evaluation, and Treatment of High Blood Cholesterol in Adults (Adult Treatment Panel III). NIH Publication No. 02-5215, September 2002.

Triglycerides consist of glycerol (triacylglycerol) that has been esterified with three **fatty acids** and are the main constituent of stored **energy** in adipose tissue.[5] Triglycerides can be derived from the diet as well as formed in the liver from newly synthesized fatty acids or fatty acids recycled from adipose tissue. Moderate elevations in serum triglyceride levels have been shown to contribute to the development of atherosclerosis, whereas severe increases can raise the risk for pancreatitis. The NCEP ATP III guidelines recommend that serum triglyceride levels be less than 150 mg/dL.[1] Elevated triglyceride concentrations are called hypertriglyceridemia, whereas the combination of elevated blood triglyceride and cholesterol concentrations is referred to as hyperlipidemia.

Phospholipids, although not directly contributory to the development of atherosclerosis, are essential for cholesterol and triglyceride transportation in the serum in the form of lipoproteins.[5] The major phospholipid is lecithin.

Elevated lipoprotein concentrations have also been shown to be atherogenic and contribute to overall dyslipidemia.[6] Lipoproteins can be separated into four major classifications based on molecular density:

■ **Chylomicrons** are triglyceride-rich lipoproteins formed in the intestine and found in the blood after a dietary intake high in fat. Chylomicron remnants are partially degraded chylomicrons and are thought to be atherogenic.

■ **Very low-density lipoprotein (VLDL)** is synthesized in the liver and is the primary transport mechanism for endogenous triglyceride.

■ **Low-density lipoprotein (LDL)** is the major cholesterol transport lipoprotein and is mostly derived from LDL catabolism and cellular synthesis. **Intermediate-density lipoprotein (IDL)** is a subfraction of LDL and is included in the LDL measurement in clinical practice.

■ **High-density lipoprotein (HDL)** performs reverse cholesterol transport by taking excess cholesterol from tissues, such as coronary arteries, to be metabolized.

Cholesterol and triglycerides circulate among the liver, intestines, and extrahepatic tissue via a transport system facilitated by serum lipoproteins.[4] Chylomicrons, VLDL, IDL, and LDL move lipids from the liver or intestines to the peripheral tissues like coronary arteries.[4-6] High-density lipoprotein, on the other hand, is involved in the opposite process of moving lipids from the peripheral tissues to the liver to be metabolized.

Therefore, to decrease the risks for CHD, elevated levels of triglycerides, LDL, and VLDL must be decreased while low levels of HDL should be increased. The NCEP ATP III guidelines recommend that serum HDL levels be no less than 40 mg/dL.[1] In addition, HDL cholesterol levels of 60 mg/dL or greater counts as a "negative" risk factor, which means its presence removes one of the patient's risk factors from the total count.[1]

DYSLIPIDEMIA DISEASE PREVENTION AND TREATMENT

The basic principles for prevention and treatment of dyslipidemia outlined in the NCEP ATP III guidelines and in the 2004 update support the idea that the intensity of therapy for patients is guided by the patient's risk for a CHD event.[1,3] As a result, those with a high and very high short-term CHD event risk receive the most intensive LDL-lowering therapy. Patients who have the greatest short-term risk are those who currently have established CHD disease along with multiple other risk factors such as **diabetes mellitus, metabolic syndrome,** or severe or poorly controlled CHD risk factors. Other CHD risk factors include **peripheral arterial disease,** abdominal aortic aneurysm, symptomatic carotid artery disease, or multiple risk factors that result in a 10-year risk for CHD of more than 20% according to the Framingham Heart Study.[1,3] Framingham risk scores can be estimated with worksheets provided with the NCEP ATP III guidelines. High-risk patients, those with existing CHD alone or multiple CHD risk factors, have an LDL-cholesterol goal of less than 100 mg/dL.[1,3] Patients in the very high-risk category have a treatment option of lowering LDL levels to less than 70 mg/dL.[3] Framingham risk scores can be calculated using Appendix A.

Moderately high-risk patients (two or more risk factors with a 10-year Framingham risk of 10 to 20%) have an LDL-cholesterol goal of less than 130 mg/dL with the optional goal of less than 100 mg/dL.[3] Moderate-risk patients (two or more risk factors with a 10-year Framingham risk of <10%) have an LDL-cholesterol goal of less than 130 mg/dL.[3] Those with 0 to 1 risk factors have an LDL-cholesterol goal of less than 160 mg/dL.[1,3]

The NCEP ATP III guidelines establish treatment strategies for obtaining optimal cholesterol goals. The first treatment priority for patients with high blood cholesterol is to lower LDL cholesterol.[1] The second treatment priority goal is to manage risk factors for metabolic syndrome and other lipid risk factors. The NCEP ATP III 2004 update placed even greater emphasis on TLC therapy. It states that all moderate- to very high-risk patients with CHD lifestyle risk factors must incorporate therapeutic lifestyle changes into their treatment strategies regardless of LDL levels. Low-risk patients not at their LDL goal should initiate a 3-month period of therapeutic lifestyle changes before assessing its effectiveness.[1] If the goal LDL cholesterol is not achieved, drug therapy may then be added while TLC therapies are continued.[1] ATP III emphasizes the initial use of dietary therapy to reduce cholesterol, with the addition of weight loss and increased exercise for patients with metabolic syndrome.[1]

It is estimated that patients who adhere to the NCEP ATP III dietary recommendations can experience a 20 to 30% reduction in LDL cholesterol lowering.[1] This effect can be even more pronounced with the addition of other TLC therapies. In addition, decreases in triglycerides and increases in HDL cholesterol can be seen by following the dietary recommendations and by increasing physical activity.

Unfortunately, many patients are unable to reach their LDL cholesterol goal through lifestyle modifications alone. Reasons for this include TLC therapy non-compliance and baseline LDL cholesterol that requires LDL lowering that is greater than what is capable with TLC therapy alone (i.e., 30%). Improving patient compliance to lifestyle changes is

TABLE 7–2   **Program Adherence Recommendations for Patients With Dyslipidemia**

1. Ensure the patient has a clear understanding of the TLC components and the importance of each
2. Explain that multiple adherence strategies work better than a single approach
3. Establish weekly contact with patients for the first 4 weeks of the program, then monthly thereafter, to continually assess the patient's progress and troubleshoot problems
4. Set achievable goals
5. Obtain baseline assessment of dietary intake
6. Institute a self-monitoring program such as keeping a log of food intake and exercise participation
7. Identify patient-specific barriers to the lifestyle changes
8. Distribute information that uses health messages associated with dyslipidemia that are easy to understand, interactive, and culturally sensitive
9. Design a program that is reasonable, gradual, and easily implemented

Source: National Institutes of Health, National Heart, Lung, and Blood Institute. Third report of the National Cholesterol Education Program (NCEP) Expert Panel on Detection, Evaluation, and Treatment of High Blood Cholesterol in Adults (Adult Treatment Panel III). NIH Publication No. 02-5215, September 2002.

similar to improving medication compliance.[1] Both medication compliance and lifestyle change compliance are important and complex topics that should be addressed with patients when initiating therapy.

Several program adherence strategies have been identified in the ATP III guidelines that have shown success in various studies.[7–9] A majority of the information comes from studies assessing weight-management therapy. In general, the literature emphasizes the importance of baseline assessment of dietary therapy as well as self-monitoring techniques of both dietary and exercise habits to improve program compliance.[1] In addition, offering health information that is culturally sensitive, interactive, and from reliable sources is important for improving adherence.[1] Suggestions to improve program adherence are listed in Table 7-2.

It is important to note that the 2004 NCEP ATP III update emphasizes that patients with moderate- to very high-risk dyslipidemia not at their respective LDL goal are recommended to begin pharmacotherapy along with TLC therapy.[3] Low-risk patients who are unable to obtain their LDL goal with TLC therapy alone are recommended to begin pharmacotherapy while continuing TLC therapy. Several pharmacotherapy agents exist to treat dyslipidemia. Pharmacotherapy drug classes are listed in Table 7-3.

TABLE 7–3   **Medications Used to Treat Dyslipidemia**

HMG-CoA reductase inhibitors (statins)

Bile acid sequestrants

Selective intestinal cholesterol absorption inhibitor

Fibric acid derivatives

Niacin

Plant sterols and stanols

HMG-CoA, 3-hydroxy-3-methylglutaryl–coenzyme A.

NUTRITION AND DYSLIPIDEMIA

Dietary modifications are the primary focus of the NCEP ATP III TLC therapy. The TLC diet is in general consistent with the Dietary Guidelines for Americans published by the U.S. Department of Agriculture and U.S. Department of Health and Human Services (http://healthierus.gov/dietaryguidelines/).[10] Lowering the LDL cholesterol is the first priority with diet modifications.[1] Once the patient has reached his or her LDL goal, emphasis on treating weight control and physical activity becomes the treatment priority.[1]

Lowering the LDL cholesterol through diet modifications can be accomplished most successfully by reducing the dietary intake of saturated fats, **trans fatty acids,** and cholesterol.[1,10] The NCEP ATP III guidelines recommend that total fat consumption should not exceed 25 to 35% of the total daily caloric intake.[1,10] Most of the fat **calorie** consumption should be obtained from **unsaturated fatty acids.**[1,10,11] **Polyunsaturated fats** and **monounsaturated fats** make up the total of unsaturated fatty acids and should represent approximately 10% and 20%, respectively, of the total daily caloric intake.[1,11] The remaining amount of fat intake (less than 7% of total calories) can come from saturated fats.[1,11] In addition, NCEP ATP III further recommends that 50 to 60% of total calories come from carbohydrate, 15% from protein, and a daily fiber intake should be 20 to 30 g.[1]

Saturated fats have proven to be closely associated with increases in total and LDL cholesterol.[1,11] Studies show that every 1% increase in calories of dietary saturated fatty acids correlates to a 2% increase in LDL cholesterol.[1,12,13] The opposite has also been shown to be true. Every 1% decrease in calories of dietary saturated fatty acids correlates to a 2% decrease in LDL cholesterol.[1,12–15] To limit the intake of saturated fatty acids, the American Heart Association recommends substituting unsaturated fatty acids in their place.[10,11] They have been shown to help reduce the amount of newly formed cholesterol and can help lower blood cholesterol levels when substituted for saturated fatty acids in the diet.[1,11] Monounsaturated fatty acids have also been shown to reduce blood cholesterol when consumed with a diet very low in saturated fats.[1,11]

A rise in LDL cholesterol levels has been associated with an increased dietary intake of *trans* fatty acids.[1,16–28] In addition, *trans* fatty acids have been associated with a higher risk for coronary heart disease.[1,29–32] It is recommended in NCEP ATP III to keep the intake of *trans* fatty acids low and to try to use liquid vegetable oil, soft margarine, and *trans* fatty acid-free margarine in place of stick margarine, butter, and shortening.[1]

The national average of dietary cholesterol intake in the U.S. is 256 mg/day.[1,33] Approximately one third of dietary cholesterol intake is obtained from the consumption of eggs.[1,34] It is recommended in the TLC diet that Americans consume an average of 200 mg or less of dietary cholesterol daily.[1] High consumptions of dietary cholesterol (10 mg/dL per 100 mg dietary cholesterol per 1,000 **kcal**) have been associated with an increased response in serum cholesterol.[1,35,36] In addition, higher intakes of dietary cholesterol have been associated with increases in LDL cholesterol, which then increases the risk for CHD.[1] Decreasing the intake of dietary cholesterol will decrease LDL cholesterol levels in most persons.[1]

Plant stanols and sterols are also recommended in ATP III to patients with high serum cholesterol because they have been shown to reduce LDL cholesterol levels.[1] Studies have shown that plant-derived stanols and sterol esters at dosages of 2 to 3 g/day lower LDL cholesterol levels by 6 to 15%, with a maximum LDL lowering effect occurring with 2 g/day.[1,37–43] Dietary consumption of plant stanols and sterols can be obtained from commercially available products containing plant sterols and stanols (i.e., margarines, juice).[1]

A summary of the dietary recommendations listed in the NCEP ATP III guidelines is provided in Table 7-4.

TABLE 7–4	Dietary Recommendations for Patients With Dyslipidemia
Nutrient	**Recommendation**
Total calories	Balance calorie intake with expenditure to obtain appropriate body weight
Carbohydrate[a]	50–60% of total calorie intake
Fiber	20–30 g/day
Protein	Around 15% of total calorie intake
Monounsaturated fat	Up to 20% of total calorie intake
Polyunsaturated fat	Up to 10% of total calorie intake
Saturated fat	Less than 7% of total calorie intake
Total fat	25–35% to total calorie intake
Dietary cholesterol	Less than 200 mg/day

Source: National Institutes of Health, National Heart, Lung, and Blood Institute. Third report of the National Cholesterol Education Program (NCEP) Expert Panel on Detection, Evaluation, and Treatment of High Blood Cholesterol in Adults (Adult Treatment Panel III). NIH Publication No. 02-5215, September 2002.
[a]Most carbohydrate intake should come from whole grains, fruits, and vegetables.

PHYSICAL ACTIVITY AND DYSLIPIDEMIA

In NCEP ATP III, the importance of regular physical activity is emphasized because of its benefits on the management of metabolic syndrome.[1] It is recommended in the NCEP ATP III guidelines that physical activity be introduced to hyperlipidemic patients when TLC therapy is initiated and that the concept be reinforced when the treatment emphasis shifts to metabolic syndrome management.[1] Increasing regular physical activity has been shown to reduce LDL, VLDL, and triglyceride levels and increase HDL cholesterol levels.[1,44–46] The purpose of promoting physical activity to patients with hypercholesterolemia is to promote energy balance to maintain a healthy body weight, reduce the risk for metabolic syndrome, and independently reduce the risk for coronary heart disease.[1,44–46]

Specific recommendations for physical activity are not outlined in ATP III, but it is noted that healthcare professionals are to refer to the U.S. Surgeon General's Report on Physical Activities published in 1996 (http://www.surgeongeneral.gov/).[45] The general recommendations made in the report emphasize moderate physical activity for 30 min/day on most, if not all, days of the week.[45] An emphasis should be placed on the amount of physical activity rather than the intensity of the activity as sedentary people should incorporate greater amounts physical activity into all aspects of daily life. Accumulating physical activity over the course of a day (i.e., walking 10 minutes at a time, several times a day) is also recommended as an effective alternative to a one-time exercise session, and may even lead to greater exercise adherence.[44,45] It is important to note that sedentary persons with preexisting disease, such as hypercholesterolemia, should start at lower levels of exercise intensity and gradually build up to the desired level of activity.[46]

For patients with hyperlipidemia, both aerobic and resistance-training exercises should be incorporated in the patient's disease risk-reduction program. Aerobic exercise should be incorporated to reduce the overall risk for coronary heart disease, and resistance-training exercises should be performed to enhance weight loss, if needed, and to reduce the risks associated with metabolic syndrome. Aerobic-type activities, among others, could include walking or jogging, bicycling, stairclimbing, dancing, basketball,

TABLE 7–5	Physical Activity Recommendations for Patients With Dyslipidemia
Goals	Promote healthy body weight Reduce risk of metabolic syndrome Reduce risk of CHD Decrease cholesterol and triglyceride concentrations
Type of activity	Large muscle activities (e.g., walking, jogging, bicycling, stairclimbing, dancing, basketball, volleyball, lawn mowing, gardening)
Intensity	Moderate level
Duration[a]	10–20 minutes (initially) 30–60 minutes (more advanced)
Frequency[a]	2–5 times per week (for initial 1–4 weeks) 6–7 times per week (after initial 4 weeks)
Lifestyle activity	Increase overall daily physical activities through taking stairs instead of elevators, parking further away in parking lots, walking the family pet, and so forth

Source: U.S. Department of Health and Human Services. Physical activity and health: a report of the Surgeon General. Atlanta: U.S. Department of Health and Human Services, Centers for Disease Control and Prevention, National Center for Chronic Disease Prevention and Health Promotion, 1996, 278 pages.
[a]Emphasize increasing duration rather than intensity.
CHD, coronary heart disease.

and volleyball, as well as lawn mowing and gardening. Resistance-training exercises can range from using stretch bands to weight-lifting exercises at a local health club. It is very important that the exercises recommended to patients are specific to their individual needs to optimize outcomes and adherence.[46]

Suggested exercise guidelines for patients with dyslipidemia are provided in Table 7-5.

PHARMACY PRACTICE APPLICATION

Pharmacists are well positioned to provide TLC pharmaceutical care to patients with hyperlipidemia for both treatment of LDL cholesterol and prevention of CHD. TLC therapy education can be offered to patients with hyperlipidemia simultaneously with drug therapy counseling. This can be incorporated in both the hospital and community-based pharmacy practices. Pharmacists practicing in the hospital setting can ensure that the drug therapy for each patient is appropriate and can introduce the concepts of TLC therapy and explain how these practices will assist the drugs they are taking and decrease the patient's risk for further CHD events. Pharmacists practicing in the community are in an ideal position to act as a resource of lifestyle therapy information for patient with dyslipidemia. Each time patients with dyslipidemia come to the pharmacy to refill their medications, the pharmacist can use this time to offer TLC therapy follow-up, counseling, and interventions. In addition, patients who obtain TLC therapy information from a variety of healthcare providers, including pharmacists, may be more likely to adhere to set TLC programs, which may lead to a greater reduction in CHD risk.[1]

In March 2000, a study conducted by the American Pharmacists Association assessing pharmaceutical care services in patients with hyperlipidemia was published (Project ImPACT: Hyperlipidemia).[47] Twenty-six community-based ambulatory care pharmacies from various settings in 12 states participated in the 24-month study. The objective of the study was to demonstrate whether pharmacists, in collaboration with patients and physicians, could have an impact on patient persistence and compliance with anti-hyperlipidemia drug therapy and enable patients to reach their National Cholesterol Education Program (NCEP) goals.[47]

Patient participants (N = 397) in the study were seen by the pharmacist at the initiation of the study, monthly for the first 3 months and then quarterly thereafter.[47] Pharmacist interventions with physicians were made regarding optimizing drug therapy that focused on achieving NCEP goals. The results of the study showed that medication persistence and compliance were 93.6% and 90.1%, respectively.[47] In addition, total cholesterol, triglyceride, HDL, and LDL levels improved significantly ($P < 0.001$) from baseline, and 63.5% of patients reached their NCEP goals at the end of the project.[47] The authors of the project concluded that pharmacists, working collaboratively with patients, physicians, and other healthcare providers, can provide an advanced level of care resulting in successful dyslipidemia management.[47] In addition to focusing on dyslipidemia drug therapy, added emphasis from pharmacists on TLC therapy may enhance NCEP goal achievement and further reduce the risks for CHD.

Muscle Pain With Exercise vs. Medication-Induced Myopathy

Occasionally questions arise with regard to the incidence of myopathy in physically active patients who are concomitantly taking lipid-lowering medication. It is well known that certain lipid-lowering medications (i.e., statins and fibric acids) can increase a patient's risk for myopathy. In addition, it has been shown that physically active individuals often experience muscle pain after strenuous activity. Therefore the question arises, do physically active, dyslipidemic patients who are also taking a statin drug (for example) have an even greater risk for myopathy than inactive patients on statin therapy?

The literature reports several studies and case reports indicating that persons taking statin drugs have a greater susceptibility to muscle injury.[48–54] One study concluded that lovastatin therapy exacerbated exercise-induced skeletal muscle injury.[48] Another study reported that lovastatin therapy plus exercise markedly increase creatine kinase (CK) levels in certain individuals.[50] A third study reported that 6 of 22 professional athletes with familial hypercholesterolemia followed for 8 years were unable to tolerate statin therapy.[54]

It is important to note that research in this area is limited. Although some research has concluded that exercisers taking statin drugs may be at greater risk for side effects, there are no definitive clinical conclusions. Therefore, it is still critical to stress the importance of physical activity to patients with dyslipidemia. It would, however, behoove the pharmacist to counsel dyslipidemic patients about the differences in myopathy and exercise-induced muscle soreness so that patients can differentiate the two should they experience symptoms.

Myopathy is generally associated with muscle aches, weakness, malaise, fever, and a CK level increase greater than 10 times the upper limit of normal.[55] Muscle soreness associated with myopathy is usually localized or can be widespread and can last days to weeks. Muscle soreness associated with physical activity, often referred to as delayed-onset muscle soreness or DOMS, is usually greatest 2 days after strenuous activity and lasts 3 to 4 days.[56] Like myopathy, soreness is usually localized but can be widespread and CK levels can increase, but most times not as significantly as with myopathy. In addition, DOMS is usually not accompanied by fever and malaise.[56]

CASE STUDY

A.A. is a 42-year-old male who enters your pharmacy for the first time with a prescription for simvastatin 20 mg daily. While assessing and counseling AA, you discover he is 5′ 10″ tall, weighs 210 lb, has a resting blood pressure of 124/78 mm Hg and a heart rate of 85 beats/min, is a non-smoker, drinks one alcoholic drink per week, maintains a sedentary lifestyle, and follows no specific diet. He is newly diagnosed with hyperlipidemia (total cholesterol = 265 mg/dL, LDL = 195 mg/dL, HDL = 35 mg/dL, triglycerides = 176 mg/dL) and has been provided no specific instructions with regard to lifestyle modification but does state that he is open to the idea of lifestyle modifications. Results of a 3-day dietary analysis were as follows:

Total caloric intake per day = 3,756 calories
Carbohydrates = 40% of total calories
Monounsaturated fats = 22% of total calories
Polyunsaturated fats = 13% of total calories
Saturated fats = 13% of total calories
Total fats = 48% of total calories
Protein = 12% of total calories
Total dietary cholesterol = 280 mg
Fiber = 20 g

Case Activities

1. *Write an SOAP note for A.A.*
2. *Write short- and long-term dietary and exercise goals for A.A.*
3. *Write an exercise prescription and dietary suggestions for A.A.*

REFERENCES

1. National Institutes of Health, National Heart, Lung, and Blood Institute. Third report of the National Cholesterol Education Program (NCEP) Expert Panel on Detection, Evaluation, and Treatment of High Blood Cholesterol in Adults (Adult Treatment Panel III). NIH Publication No. 02-5215, September 2002.
2. National Institutes of Health, Centers for Disease Control and Prevention. Available at: http://www.cdc.gov/nchs/data/hus/tables/2003/03hus067.pdf. Accessed July 22, 2004.
3. Grundy SM, Cleeman JI, Merz C, et al. Implications of recent clinical trials for the national cholesterol education program adult treatment panel III guidelines. Circulation 2004;110:227–239.
4. McKenney JM, Hawkins D. Handbook on the Management of Lipid Disorders, 2nd ed. St. Louis: National Pharmacy Cardiovascular Council, 2001:18–34.
5. Talbert RL. Hyperlipidemia. In: Dipiro JT, ed. Pharmacotherapy: A Pathophysiologic Approach, 6th ed. New York: McGraw-Hill, 2005:429–452.
6. White CM, McBride BF, Kalus JS. Pharmacotherapy Self Assessment Program, Cardiology, Dyslipidemias. Kansas City, MO: American College of Clinical Pharmacy, 2004:165–186.
7. National Institutes of Health. Clinical guidelines on the identification, evaluation, and treatment of overweight and obesity in adults. NIH Publication No. 98-4083, September 1998.
8. American College of Sports Medicine. ACSM's Guidelines For Exercise Testing and Prescription, 6th ed. Philadelphia: Lippincott Williams & Wilkins, 2000:3–32.
9. Pearson T, Kopin L. Bridging the treatment gap: improving compliance with lipid-modifying agents and therapeutic lifestyle changes. Prev Cardiol 2003;6:204–213.
10. U.S. Department of Agriculture and U.S. Department of Health and Human Services. Nutrition and your health: dietary guidelines for Americans, 5th ed. Home and Garden Bulletin no. 232. Washington, D.C.: U.S. Department of Agriculture, 2000, 44 pages.
11. American Heart Association. Delicious Decisions. Available at: http://www.deliciousdecisions.org/. Accessed March 23, 2004.
12. Kris-Etherton PM, Yu S. Individual fatty acid effects on plasma lipids and lipoproteins: human studies. Am J Clin Nutr 1997;65(Suppl 5):1628S–1644S.

13. Mensink RP, Katan MB. Effects of dietary fatty acids on serum lipids and lipoproteins: a meta-analysis of 27 trails. Arterioscler Thromb 1992;12:911–919.

14. Obarzanek E, Hunsberger SA, Van Horn L, et al. Safety of a fat-reduced diet: the Dietary Intervention Study in Children (DISC). Pediatrics 1997;100:51–59.

15. Niinikoski H, Lapinleimu H, Viikari J, et al. Growth until three years of age in a prospective, randomized trial of a diet with reduced saturated fat and cholesterol. Pediatrics 1997;99:687–694.

16. Lichtenstein AH, Ausman LM, Jalbert SM, Schaefer EJ. Effects of different forms of dietary hydrogenated fats on serum lipoprotein cholesterol levels. N Engl J Med 1999;340:1933–1940.

17. Judd JT, Clevidence BA, Muesing RA, Wittes J, Sunkin ME, Podczasy JJ. Dietary trans fatty acids: effects of plasma lipids and lipoproteins of healthy men and women. Am J Clin Nutr 1994;59:861–868.

18. Judd JT, Baer DJ, Clevidence BA, et al. Effects of margarine compared with those of butter on blood lipid profiles related to cardiovascular disease risk factors in normolipemic adults fed controlled diets. Am J Clin Nutr 1998;68:768–777.

19. Noakes M, Clifton PM. Oil blends containing partially hydrogenated or interesterified fats: differential effects on plasma lipids. Am J Clin Nutr 1998;68:242–247.

20. Aro A, Jauhiainen M, Partanen R, Salminen I, Mutanen M. Stearic acid, trans-fatty acids, and dairy fat: effects on serum and lipoprotein lipids, apolipoproteins, lipoprotein (a), and lipid transfer proteins in healthy subjects. Am J Clin Nutr 1997;65:1419–1426.

21. Almendingen K, Jordal O, Kierulf P, Sandstad B, Pedersen JI. Effects of partially hydrogenated fish oil, partially hydrogenated soybean oil, and butter on serum lipoproteins and Lp[a] in men. J Lipid Res 1995; 36:1370–1384.

22. Wood R, Kubena K, O'Brien B, Tseng S, Martin G. Effect of butter, mono- and polyunsaturated fatty acid-enriched butter, trans-fatty acid margarine on serum lipids and lipoproteins in healthy men. J Lipid Res 1993;34:1–11.

23. Wood R, Kubena K, Tseng S, Martin G, Crook R. Effect of palm oil, margarine, butter, and sunflower oil on the serum lipids and lipoproteins of normocholesterolemic middle-aged men. J Nutr Biochem 1993;4:286–297.

24. Nestel PJ, Noakes M, Belling GB, McArthur R, Clifton PM, Abbey M. Plasma cholesterol lowering potential of edible-oil blends suitable for commercial use. Am J Clin Nutr 1992;55:46–50.

25. Zock PL, Katan MB. Hydrogenation alternatives: effects of trans fatty acids and stearic acid versus linoleic acid on serum lipids and lipoproteins in humans. J Lipid Res 1992;33:399–410.

26. Katan MB, Zock, Mensink RP. Trans fatty acids and their effects on lipoproteins in humans. Ann Rev Nutr 1995;15:473–493.

27. Mensink RP, Katan MB. Effects of dietary trans fatty acids on high density and low density lipoprotein cholesterol levels in healthy subjects. N Engl J Med 1990;323:439–445.

28. Lichtenstein AH, Ausman LM, Carrasco W, Jenner JL, Ordovas JM, Schaefer EJ. Hydrogenation impairs the hypolipidemic effect of corn oil in humans: hydrogenation, trans fatty acids, and plasma lipids. Arterioscler Thromb 1993;13:154–161.

29. Willett WC, Stampfer MJ, Manson JE, et al. Intake of trans fatty acids and risk of coronary heart disease among women. Lancet 1993;341:581–585.

30. Pietinen P, Ascherio A, Korhonen P, et al. Intake of fatty acids and risk of coronary heart disease in a cohort of Finnish men: the Alpha-Tocopherol, Beta-Carotene Cancer Prevention Study. Am J Epidemiol 1997;145:876–887.

31. Hu FB, Stampfer MJ, Manson JE, et al. Dietary saturated fats and their food sources in relation to the risk of coronary heart disease in women. Am J Clin Nutr 1999;70:1001–1008.

32. Kromhout D, Menotti A, Bloemberg B, et al. Dietary saturated and trans fatty acids and cholesterol and 25 year mortality from coronary heart disease: the Seven Countries Study. Prev Med 1995;24:308–315.

33. Tippett KS, Cleveland LE. How current diets stack up: comparison of dietary guidelines. In: America's Eating Habits: Changes and Consequences. Washington, D.C.: United States Department of Agriculture, Economic Research Service, 1999:51–70.

34. Putnam J, Gerrior S. Trends in the U.S. food supply, 1970–1997. In: America's Eating Habits: Changes and Consequences. Washington, D.C.: United States Department of Agriculture, Economic Research Service, 1999:133–160.

35. Grundy SM, Barrett-Conner E, Rudel LL, Miettinen T, Spector AA. Workshop on the impact of dietary cholesterol on plasma lipoproteins and atherogenesis. Arteriosclerosis 1988;8:95–101.

36. National Research Council. Diet and health: implications for reducing chronic disease risk. Washington, D.C.: National Academy Press, 1989:171–201.

37. Hallikainen MA, Uusitupa MI. Effects of 2 low fat stanols ester containing margarines on serum cholesterol concentrations as part of a low fat diet in hypercholesterolaemic subjects. Am J Clin Nutr 1999;69:403–410.

38. Gylling H, Miettinen TA. Cholesterol reduction by different plant stanols mixtures and with variable fat intake. Metabolism 1999;48:575–580.

39. Gylling H, Radhakrishnan R, Miettinen TA. Reduction of serum cholesterol in postmenopausal women with previous myocardial infarction and cholesterol malabsorption induced by dietary sitostanol ester margarine: women and dietary sitostanol. Circulation 1997;96:4226–4231.

40. Hendriks HFJ, Weststrate JA, van Vliet T, Meijer GW. Spreads enriched with three different levels of vegetable oil sterols and the degree of cholesterol lowering in normocholesterolaemic and mildly hypercholesterolaemic subjects. Eur J Clin Nutr 1999;53:319–327.

41. Miettinen TA, Puska P, Gylling H, Vanhanen H, Vartianen E. Reduction of serum cholesterol with sitostanol ester margarine in a mildly hypercholesterolaemic population. N Engl J Med 1995;333:1308–1312.

42. Vanhanen HT, Blomqvist S, Ehnholm C, et al. Serum cholesterol, serum precursors, and plant sterols in hypercholesterolemic subjects with different apoE phenotypes during dietary sitostanol ester treatment. J Lipid Res 1993;34:1535–1544.

43. Vuorio AF, Gylling H, Turola H, Kontula K, Ketonen P, Miettinen TA. Stanol ester margarine alone with simvastatin lowers serum cholesterol in families with familial hypercholesterolemia caused by FH-North Karelia mutation. Arterioscler Thromb Vasc Biol 2000;20:500–506.

44. American College of Sports Medicine. ACSM's Guidelines For Exercise Testing and Prescription, 6th ed. Philadelphia: Lippincott Williams & Wilkins, 2000:3–32.

45. U.S. Department of Health and Human Services. Physical activity and health: a report of the Surgeon General. Atlanta, Georgia: U.S. Department of Health and Human Services, Centers for Disease Control and Prevention, National Center for Chronic Disease Prevention and Health Promotion, 1996. 278 pages.

46. Durstine JL, Moore GE. ACSM's Exercise Management for Persons with Chronic Diseases and Disabilities. Champaign, IL: Human Kinetics, 2003:142–148.

47. Bluml BM, McKenney JM, Cziraky MJ. Pharmaceutical care services and results in project ImPACT: hyperlipidemia. J Am Pharm Assoc 2000;40:157–165.

48. Thompson PD, Zmuda JM, Domalik LJ, Zimet RJ, Staggers J, Guyton J. Lovastatin increases exercise induced skeletal muscle injury. Metabolism 1997;46:1206–1210.

49. Smit JWA, De Bruin TWA, Eekhoff EMW, Glatz J, Erkelens DW. Combined hyperlipidemia is associated with increased exercise induced muscle protein release which is improved by triglyceride lowering intervention. Metabolism 1999;48:1518–1523.

50. Thompson PD, Gadaleta PA, Yurgalevitch PA, Cullinane E, Herbert P. Effects of exercise and lovastatin on serum creatine kinase activity. Metabolism 1991;40:1333–1336.

51. Thompson PD, Nugent AM, Herbert PN. Increases in creatine kinase after exercise in patients treated with HMG CoA reductase inhibitors. JAMA 1990;264:2992.

52. Walravens PA, Greene C, Frerman FB. Lovastatin, isoprenes, and myopathy. Lancet 1989;2:1097–1098.

53. Chrysanthopoulos C, Kounis N. Rhabdomyolysis due to combined treatment with lovastatin and cholestyramine. BMJ 1992;304:1225.

54. Sinzinger H, O'Grady J. Professional athletes suffering from familial hypercholesterolaemia rarely tolerate statin treatment because of muscular problems. Br J Clin Pharmacol 2004;57:525–528.

55. Bellosta S, Paoletti R, Corsini A. Safety of statins: focus on clinical pharmacokinetics and drug interactions. Circulation 2004;109(Suppl 3):III-50–III-57.

56. Cheung K, Hume PA, Maxwell L. Delayed onset muscle soreness: treatment strategies and performance factors. Sports Med 2003;33:145–164.

Coronary Heart Disease

OBJECTIVES

At the end of this chapter the reader should be able to:

1. Explain the risk associated with coronary heart disease.
2. Summarize the prevention and treatment options for coronary heart disease.
3. Describe appropriate nutritional strategies for patients with coronary artery disease.
4. Suggest appropriate exercises for patients with risk factors for coronary artery disease.
5. Formulate a basic nutrition, exercise, and smoking-cessation program for a patient at risk for developing coronary artery disease.

OVERVIEW OF CORONARY HEART DISEASE

Coronary heart disease (CHD), also called ischemic heart disease, is a complex disease process that ultimately results in an imbalance in the amount of oxygen that is available to supply the heart compared with the demand that the heart requires to function properly.[1] CHD pathogenesis can begin early in life but often presents in what is referred to as acute coronary syndrome (ACS).[1] Acute coronary syndrome can present in a number of emergent situations such as a myocardial infarction (MI) or heart attack, stable or unstable angina pectoris, and coronary artery vasospasm. In addition, CHD can cause other disease processes to occur such as heart failure, irregular heart rhythms, peripheral vascular disease (PVD), and stroke.[1]

Many times CHD can be confused with cardiovascular disease (CVD). Cardiovascular disease is a broader term used to describe illnesses associated with the heart or vasculature system. Among the most common types of CVD are CHD, ischemic stroke, heart failure, hypertension, peripheral arterial disease, rheumatic fever or rheumatic heart disease, and congenital cardiovascular defects.[2] Since 1900, CVD has been the number one killer in the United States each year except for 1918. In 2002, nearly 2,600 Americans died each day from CVD, which resulted in 38% of all deaths, or 1 of every 2.6 deaths.[2] Among the deaths associated with CVD, CHD accounted for most (53%) of the deaths, followed by stroke (18%), heart failure (6%), and hypertension (4%).[2]

PREVALENCE, ECONOMIC COSTS, AND HEALTH RISKS ASSOCIATED WITH CORONARY HEART DISEASE

CHD was prevalent in 13 million Americans in 2002, including 7.1 million Americans having experienced an MI.[2] The population with the greatest incidence of CHD is white males (8.9%) followed by black females (7.5%), black males (7.4%), Mexican-American males (5.6%), white females (5.4%), and Mexican-American females (4.3%).[2] In 2005, it was estimated that approximately 700,000 Americans would have a new coronary attack and that 500,000 would have a recurrent attack.[2] The average age of an American experiencing a first heart attack is 65.8 years for men and 70.4 years for women.[2] CHD caused one of every five deaths in the United States in 2002, which represents the single largest killer of American males and females. In addition, it is estimated that the direct and indirect costs associated with CHD in 2005 are $142 billion.[2]

PATHOPHYSIOLOGY OF CORONARY HEART DISEASE

The heart is a muscle with a primary responsibility of circulating blood and oxygen to the body. Unlike other types of muscle tissue in the body, the heart can only function when oxygen is continuously supplied.[3] Without a continuous supply of oxygen, the heart deteriorates and can no longer pump blood to the body.[3] **Ischemia** is a term used to describe a situation in which little or no blood flow is getting to the heart muscle.[1] **Angina pectoris** is a situation describing a decreased amount of blood perfusing the heart. Anginal symptoms are often characterized by discomfort in the chest, jaw, shoulder, back, and arm.[1] This can occur with **physical activity** and can sometimes be relieved by rest, in which case it is referred to as stable angina. If the anginal symptoms are not relieved by rest or change in intensity, frequency, and duration they are referred to as unstable angina. If the anginal symptoms worsen and are accompanied by specific changes in an electrocardiogram (ECG) that indicate very little or no blood flow to the heart, this condition is called an MI or heart attack.[1]

Angina and MI result from a process called **atherosclerosis,** which is a localized accumulation of blood fat (lipid) and fibrous tissue within the arteries. This process can occur in the heart, causing anginal symptoms, but can also occur in other arteries affecting the brain and lower extremities. Atherosclerosis involves the production of fatty streaks in the coronary arteries that eventually lead to a fibrous plaque formation in the lumen of the vessel.[4] If atherosclerotic plaque grows to the point of occluding greater than 50% of the arterial lumen, anginal symptoms can occur with physical activity as well as without activity as more of the lumen is taken up by the plaque.[1] When 95% or greater of the arterial lumen is occupied by plaque, coronary blood flow is functionally absent and results in an MI.[1] Most MIs, however, occur as a result of what is referred to as atherothrombosis. Atherothrombosis occurs as a result of rupture of the fibrous plaque. During this process the lipid core of the plaque leaks out into the lumen, causing a thrombosis to form, which can quickly break away from the site of the rupture.

TABLE 8–1   **Environmental Risk Factors Leading to Coronary Heart Disease**

Smoking
Hypertension
High total cholesterol
High LDL cholesterol (especially small, dense LDL)
Low HDL cholesterol
High triglycerides
Diabetes mellitus
Obesity or overweight
Physical inactivity
Emotional stress
Male gender
Increasing age (especially ≥45 years for men and ≥55 years for women)
Family history of CHD
High lipoprotein(a)
High homocysteine

Source: National Institutes of Health, National Heart, Lung, and Blood Institute. Third report of the National Cholesterol Education Program (NCEP) Expert Panel on Detection, Evaluation, and Treatment of High Blood Cholesterol in Adults (Adult Treatment Panel III). NIH Publication No. 02-5215, September 2002. CHD, coronary heart disease; HDL, high-density lipoprotein; LDL, low-density lipoprotein.

The thrombus then travels in the coronary vessel until it gets lodged because of the narrowing of the coronary vessels. This then inhibits blood flow to the heart tissue that is distal to the thrombus, causing an MI.

The formation of atherosclerotic plaque can begin very early in life but does not usually present itself in the form of symptoms and CHD until adults are middle aged or older.[5] Several risk factors can predispose individuals to the formation of plaque and eventually CHD. Many of these risk factors are preventable and modifiable through lifestyle modifications. A list of the risk factors leading to CHD is provided in Table 8-1. It should be noted that this list may not be complete as more studies and research data continually identify and confirm new causes.

Chronic Kidney Disease and Coronary Heart Disease

Chronic kidney disease (CKD) is a permanent loss of kidney function that results from structural kidney damage caused by either physical injury or other diseases.[6,7] The two most common diseases that cause CKD are **diabetes mellitus** and hypertension. It is estimated that 4.5% of U.S. adults have physiologic evidence of CKD and the rate of CKD has doubled between the years 1990 and 2000.[6] Chronic kidney disease can affect persons from any age, but most individuals with CKD are older than 60 years of age.[7] Some racial groups are at increased risk for CKD compared with others. African Americans, Native Americans, and Hispanic Americans are four times, three times, and two times, respectively, more likely to develop CKD compared with white Americans.[6] As CKD progresses to end-stage renal disease, the cost increases. It is estimated that the cost of dialysis in patients with end-stage renal disease is approximately $60,000 per patient per year.[7]

> Much of the focus on CKD centers on prevention strategies. Current prevention strategies include blood pressure control to a target of 130/80 mm Hg or lower; obtaining tight glycemic control in patients with diabetes; and using medications such as angiotensin-converting enzyme inhibitors (ACEIs) and angiotensin II receptor blockers (ARBs) in patients with diabetes and non-diabetic nephropathies.[8,9] Patients who have physiologic signs of decreased kidney function should also consume a low-protein diet.[6] Protein is broken down into waste products in the kidneys, and consuming too much protein can place undue stress on the kidneys and lead to a further decline in kidney function. Maintaining adequate nutritional amounts of protein while not overloading the kidney is important. Other strategies that are recommended to prevent CKD are adequate treatment of dyslipidemias, weight loss if necessary, smoking cessation, and anemia management.[8]
>
> Therefore, prevention of CKD and CHD are similar and center on proper blood pressure and glucose control, weight control, a healthy eating plan, and physical activity. Individuals at risk for CKD and CHD should work with their healthcare providers, including their pharmacist, to ensure they are doing all they can to prevent these diseases. Additionally, all healthcare providers should be aware of the prevention strategies that are effective in decreasing the risks for CKD and CHD.

CORONARY HEART DISEASE PREVENTION AND TREATMENT

Strategies for preventing CHD are approached in two separate ways, depending on the status of the patient. If the patient does not currently have CHD but does possess risk factors for CHD, primary prevention strategies are applied. If the patient currently has CHD (e.g., as a result of having an MI), the strategies turn to secondary prevention or an attempt to prevent a second heart attack. Many of the prevention strategies are similar with respect to lifestyle modification. However, drug therapy differs between primary and secondary prevention.

Primary Coronary Heart Disease Prevention

Pharmacists and virtually all other healthcare providers can encourage patients to participate in primary prevention strategies that decrease the risk for CHD. As stated above, many modifiable risk factors have been identified that contribute to the prevalence of CHD. Pharmacists are well positioned to address these issues with patients.

Tobacco use is the single largest preventable cause of disease and premature death in the United States.[10,11] Approximately 20% of cardiovascular disease deaths are caused by tobacco use, which includes about 148,000 deaths from active smoking with an additional 35,000 deaths from secondhand smoke.[12,13] The risk of cardiovascular disease death from smoking decreases by 50% after 1 year of smoking cessation.[14] In addition, lost productivity as a result of smoking-related cardiovascular disease was estimated to be approximately $35.6 billion in 2000.[11,15] Pharmacists who engage their patients in smoking-cessation programs can significantly decrease the risk for CHD in these patients.

Excess body weight is an independent risk factor for CVD. In addition, excess body weight can lead to other diseases that also increase CHD risk, such as hypertension, **dyslipidemia, type 2 diabetes mellitus,** and stroke.[12,16–21] Weight-loss programs and activities, even at modest levels, have been shown to decrease the risk for these diseases and therefore decrease the risk for CHD.[16,23–26] A sustained weight loss of 10% in individuals who are obese can significantly reduce the risk of CHD by 12 to 38 cases per 1,000 patients.[27]

Nutrition plays an important role not only in weight loss but also in controlling other risk factors for CHD such as hypertension and dyslipidemia. As discussed in other chapters in this book, a nutritionally balanced diet can help maintain a healthy weight and manage both hypertension and dyslipidemia.[10,11] Eating plans that consist of whole grains, fruits, and vegetables and that are high in fiber, calcium, and potassium and low in saturated fat and **cholesterol** are associated with decreased risk for CHD.[10,11,28] Refer to Chapter 1 for more detailed information.

Physical inactivity is an independent risk factor for CVD but can also contribute to increasing the incidence of other diseases such as type 2 diabetes, hypertension, dyslipidemia, and **obesity**.[10–12,28,29] It is well documented that increasing physical activity and the fitness levels of individuals decreases the risk for CHD.[12,30–33] The current recommendation for physical activity of 30 minutes per day on most days of the week has been documented to decrease the risk for CVD.[34] Pharmacists can design and monitor physical activity programs for physically inactive patients with primary prevention for CHD being the main goal of the program. Refer to Chapter 2 for more detailed information. In addition to emphasizing lifestyle modifications in patients at risk for CHD, pharmacists can also help patients monitor their blood pressure, blood lipids, blood glucose, and the medications associated with each.

Theoretically, almost all patients with whom a pharmacist comes in contact can be monitored for primary prevention of CHD. Working with "healthy" patients to avoid risk factors for CHD is at the heart of primary prevention and is an area that all healthcare providers, including pharmacists, should spend more time doing. Preventing weight gain in patients who are of normal body weight may be as important as helping patients who are obese lose weight. In addition, helping patients maintain physical activity and normal levels of blood pressure, blood lipids, and blood glucose are important concepts in the prevention of diseases.

Secondary Coronary Heart Disease Prevention

Approximately 70% of deaths from CHD and one half of MIs occur in patients with previously established CHD.[35,36] In addition, the likelihood of experiencing a fatal or nonfatal MI is about four to seven times higher in patients with CHD.[35] Therefore, instituting strategies for secondary CHD prevention is a major opportunity to reduce the risk for cardiovascular disease.[35]

The components or strategies for secondary CHD prevention are largely the same as those for primary CHD prevention with respect to lifestyle modifications. Smoking cessation, weight management, proper nutrition, and physical activity represent lifestyle strategies for patients with CHD. In addition, proper management of blood pressure, blood lipids, and blood glucose is also important in decreasing the further progression of CHD.[37] The specific recommendations for physical activity and **exercise** are different and require special attention in patients with CHD. Many times, patients with CHD are recommended to attend cardiac rehabilitation classes that offer special attention to their unique cardiac needs.

The American College of Cardiology and the American Heart Association (ACC/AHA) strongly recommend that all patients recovering from an MI exercise for a minimum of 30 minutes, preferably daily, but at least three to four times per week.[37] These patients are additionally recommended to supplement their scheduled physical activity program with increases in daily lifestyle activities.[37] It is also a recommendation from the ACC/AHA that, when available, patients with multiple modifiable risk factors or those with moderate to high risk participate in cardiac rehabilitation programs as they will receive supervised exercise training.[35] Cardiac rehabilitation is defined as "coordinated, multifaceted interventions designed to optimize a cardiac patient's physical, psychological, and social functioning, in addition to stabilizing, slowing, or even reversing the progression of the underlying atherosclerotic process, thereby reducing morbidity and mortality."[38,39]

Physical activity reduces symptoms in patients with cardiovascular disease and improves other cardiovascular disease risk factors.[35] Patients with cardiovascular disease often have unique needs and require special instructions with regard to strenuous activities such as heavy lifting, climbing stairs, yard work, and household activities.[35] Comprehensive cardiac rehabilitation offers information, instruction, and supervision about proper physical activity as well as cardiac risk factor modification, education, and counseling. These programs are designed to limit the physiologic and psychological effects of cardiac illness, reduce the risk for recurrent heart attacks, control cardiac symptoms, and stabilize and reverse the atherosclerotic process. In addition, the rehabilitation process enables patients to return to vocational activities more efficiently and effectively.[35,38]

Patients with moderate to severe CHD and patients who have experienced a heart attack or coronary artery bypass surgery should participate in a cardiac rehabilitation program.[37] It is beyond the scope of a pharmacist's training to be the sole physical activity counselor in patients acutely ill with CHD. The pharmacist's role in the secondary prevention of patients with CHD who have not yet attended a cardiac rehabilitation program is to encourage such participation and help monitor drug therapy associated with the disease. Treating patients with CHD is a team effort with all members of the healthcare team communicating effectively to ensure the optimal outcomes for the patient.

Drug Therapy

Drug therapy for primary CHD prevention in most patients is not needed unless patients have multiple risk factors or diabetes.[40] In such cases, aspirin or other antiplatelets or anticoagulants may be used. Patients who currently have CHD are recommended to take aspirin 75 to 325 mg daily unless contraindicated along with ACE-inhibitor and β-blocker therapy.[35,37] In addition, aggressive lipid lowering and control of hypertension and diabetes are recommended if warranted.[35,37] Table 8-2 lists medications used to treat patients with CHD.

TABLE 8–2 Medications Used to Treat Coronary Heart Disease

Antiplatelet drugs
Angiotensin-converting enzyme inhibitor
β-Blocker
Drugs to control hypertension (see Chapter 6)
Drugs to control dyslipidemia (see Chapter 7)
Drugs to control diabetes mellitus (see Chapter 12)

Behavior Therapy

Strategies to enhance program adherence for patients at risk for CHD and for those who currently have CHD largely focus around patient education. Most individuals who do not have CHD do not understand the importance of implementing strategies such as lifestyle modification. Many feel that there is nothing to treat as long as they do not feel bad or are not sick. Spreading the word about primary disease prevention can be a part of every healthcare provider's responsibilities. In addition, there is a lack of "visibility" and recognition by the public of the importance of cardiac rehabilitation services.[38] Pharmacists can support both primary and secondary CHD prevention by educating patients about their importance. The more education patients have regarding their health, even when they are not sick, the more informed their decision making can be. Table 8-3 lists program adherence recommendations for patients with CHD.

Getting Individuals to Participate

It is well established that lifestyle modifications such as smoking cessation, physical activity, weight loss, and proper nutrition decrease the risk for coronary heart disease (CHD) as well as diseases that can lead to CHD such as hypertension, dyslipidemia, diabetes mellitus, obesity, and others.[41] So the big question that needs to be answered is, "If these lifestyle changes are so good for you, why is it sometimes difficult to get individuals to participate?" The answer to this question is not well known. Research into behavioral strategies and techniques to increase participation in physical activity and other lifestyle modifications among those of young age to old age is lacking and not well understood.[41] For example, many individuals still perceive exercise as an "all or none" type of activity like smoking cessation rather than an implementation of incremental behavioral changes. It is well established that even modest changes in physical activity levels can yield significant benefits in improving health and preventing disease.[42] Therefore, more work needs to be done in the area of health promotion for whole populations of people at the school, work site, and community levels rather than at the individual patient level.[41] In addition to this, legislative policy changes that promote healthy behaviors need to be expanded.[41]

Much research has been conducted in the area of community interventions that increase physical activity and promote health. The Task Force on Community Preventive Services (within the U.S. Department of Health and Human Services) has conducted a systematic review of community interventions that aim to increase physical activity.[43] Conclusions from this review resulted in the task force recommending six community-wide interventions that have been shown through research to increase physical activity levels.[43] The six interventions included (1) community-wide campaigns that were large scale and highly visible; (2) prompts (called point-of-care prompts) that encourage people to use stairs instead of elevators or escalators; (3) increasing physical education programs in schools; (4) social support systems such as an exercise partner, buddy system, or exercise group; (5) behavioral change programs that are individually specific; and (6) creation of or access to places for physical activity.[41,43]

Pharmacists, as one of the most visible healthcare professionals, can play an important role in the implementation of interventions such as these. Pharmacists are viewed as a trusted leader in healthcare and should use this image to promote health. Pharmacists and all healthcare professionals should be viewed not only as "disease healers" but also as "disease preventers." Increasing the public's knowledge of the skills of a pharmacist in the area of disease prevention and heath promotion is an important step for the profession of pharmacy as it continues to evolve in its role in public health.

TABLE 8–3 Program Adherence Recommendations for Patients With Coronary Heart Disease

Patient education about prevention and treatment

Ensure the patient has a clear understanding of the disease-prevention components and the importance of each

Multiple adherence strategies work better than a single approach

Weekly contact with patients for the first 4 weeks of the program, then monthly thereafter, to continually assess the patient's progress and troubleshoot problems

Set achievable goals

Obtain baseline assessment of dietary intake

Institute a self-monitoring program such as keeping a log of food intake and exercise participation

Identify patient-specific barriers to the lifestyle changes

Design a program that is reasonable, gradual, and easily implemented

Source: National Institutes of Health, National Heart, Lung, and Blood Institute. Third report of the National Cholesterol Education Program (NCEP) Expert Panel on Detection, Evaluation, and Treatment of High Blood Cholesterol in Adults (Adult Treatment Panel III). NIH Publication No. 02-5215, September 2002.

NUTRITION AND CORONARY HEART DISEASE

Proper nutrition for patients with CHD and for those at risk for developing CHD is the same. The goal is to adopt the necessary dietary changes to decrease the risk for CHD. The dietary recommendations discussed in the National Cholesterol Education Program, Adult Treatment Panel III Guidelines (NCEP ATP III) (http://www.nhlbi.nih.gov/guidelines/) and those discussed in the Seventh Report of the Joint National Committee of Prevention, Detection, Evaluation, and Treatment of High Blood Pressure (JNC 7) (http://www.nhlbi.nih.gov/guidelines/) as well as the Dietary Guidelines for Americans 2005 (http://www.healthierus.gov/dietaryguidelines/) are recommended by the ACC/AHA for the treatment and prevention of CHD.[10,11,28,35,37] The recommendations stated in each of these guidelines are largely the same, with a primary focus on promoting health and reducing the risk for CHD and other chronic diseases by lowering **low-density lipoprotein** cholesterol (LDL) and blood pressure. The overarching themes are to eat fewer calories, be more physically active, and make wiser food choices.[28]

The NCEP ATP III guidelines focus a great deal on decreasing the risk of CHD by lowering LDL cholesterol. Lowering the LDL cholesterol through dietary modifications can most successfully be accomplished by reducing the dietary intake of saturated fats, *trans* **fatty acids,** and cholesterol.[10,44] The NCEP ATP III guidelines recommend that total fat consumption should not exceed 25 to 35% of the total daily caloric intake.[10,44] Most of the fat calorie consumption should be obtained from **unsaturated fatty acids.**[10,44,45] Polyunsaturated fats and monounsaturated fats make up the total of unsaturated fatty acids and should represent approximately 10% and 20%, respectively, of the total daily caloric intake.[10,45] The remaining amount of fat intake (less than 7% of total calories) can come from saturated fats.[10,45] In addition, NCEP ATP III further recommends that 50 to 60% of total calories come from carbohydrates, 15% from protein, and daily fiber intake should be 20 to 30 grams.[10]

Chapters 1, 6, and 7 discuss in further detail specific information regarding dietary modifications for patients at risk for developing CHD. Refer to these chapters for further detail. Table 8-4 lists dietary recommendations for the treatment and prevention of CHD.

TABLE 8–4	Dietary Recommendations for Patients With Coronary Heart Disease
Nutrient	**Recommendation**
Total calories	Balance calorie intake with expenditure to obtain appropriate body weight
Carbohydrate[a]	50–60% of total calorie intake
Fiber	20–30 g/day
Protein	Around 15% of total calorie intake
Monounsaturated fat	Up to 20% of total calorie intake
Polyunsaturated fat	Up to 10% of total calorie intake
Saturated fat	Less than 7% of total calorie intake
Total fat	25–35% of total calorie intake
Dietary cholesterol	Less than 200 mg/day

[a]Most carbohydrate intake should come from whole grains, fruits, and vegetables.
Source: U.S. Department of Health and Human Services, U.S. Department of Agriculture. Dietary Guidelines for Americans 2005. HHS Publication number: HHS-ODPHP-2005-01-DGA-A. Available at: http://healthierus.gov/dietaryguidelines. Accessed on August 3, 2006.

PHYSICAL ACTIVITY AND CORONARY HEART DISEASE

It is well established that regular amounts of aerobic physical activity produce cardiovascular changes that increase exercise capacity, endurance, and **muscular strength.**[46] Regular exercise also prevents the incidence of CHD and helps to decrease the symptoms associated with cardiovascular disease.[46] In addition, exercise can decrease the risk for and aid in controlling chronic diseases that can lead to CHD such as obesity, type 2 diabetes, hypertension, and dyslipidemia, as well as other diseases such as **osteoporosis,** depression, breast cancer, and colon cancer.[41,46–51] As a result, the American Heart Association has released a scientific statement that suggests all healthcare professionals promote increased physical activity among their patients.[46]

The evidence supporting the incorporation of increased physical activity among all individuals in an effort to decrease the risk of CHD is strong. Several prospective epidemiologic studies have supported the causal relationship between exercise and lower rates of CHD.[30,32,46,52,53] These studies show that individuals who participate in physical activity generally experience a CHD rate that is half that of sedentary individuals. Therefore, it is clear that primary CHD prevention strategies must incorporate increased physical activity as part of a disease prevention plan. The current recommendations by the AHA (http://www.americanheart.org/presenter.jhtml?identifier=1200013), Centers for Disease Control and Prevention (CDC) (http://www.cdc.gov/nccdphp/dnpa/physical/recommendations/index.htm), and the American College of Sports Medicine (ACSM) (http://www.acsm.org/) state that individuals should engage in 30 minutes or more of moderate intensity physical activity on most (preferably all) days of the week.[46,54–57] Table 8-5 lists exercise recommendations for patients with CHD.

Use of physical activity in treating patients with CHD has been studied for several years. Several meta-analyses have concluded that comprehensive, exercise-based cardiac rehabilitation reduces mortality rates, especially cardiac mortality rates, in patients after a heart attack.[42,46,58,59] Other studies show that exercise training improves tolerance to physical activity in patients with stable angina as a result of reductions in heart rate and blood pressure as well as improved oxygen delivery to the myocardium.[46] Likewise,

TABLE 8–5 Physical Activity Recommendations for Patients With Coronary Heart Disease

Exercise Variable	Recommendation
Goals	Decrease risk for CHD and CVD
	Decrease risk factors for CHD and CVD such as elevated blood pressure, insulin resistance and glucose intolerance, elevated triglyceride concentrations, low HDL-C concentrations, obesity, stroke, myocardial function
	Increase exercise peak workload and endurance
Type	Aerobic exercises (large muscle activities) such as walking, jogging, running, cycling, or individual aerobic exercise preference
	Resistance training can be adjunctive to aerobic exercises
Intensity	Moderate-intensity endurance activity
Duration	30 minutes or more continuous or intermittent exercise per day
Frequency	Most, preferably all, days of the week
Lifestyle activity	Increase overall daily activities through increasing the duration of activities of daily living (e.g., walking the dog, taking stairs, yard work, household duties)

Source: U.S. Department of Health and Human Services. Physical activity and health: a report of the Surgeon General. Atlanta: U.S. Department of Health and Human Services, Centers for Disease Control and Prevention, National Center for Chronic Disease Prevention and Health Promotion, 1996.
CHD, coronary heart disease; CVD, cardiovascular disease; HDL-C, high-density lipoprotein cholesterol.

exercise training has been shown to improve aerobic capacity and quality of life in patients who have undergone coronary revascularization through coronary artery bypass surgery or percutaneous interventions.[46]

As stated earlier, patients with existing CHD should perform exercise under supervision of a cardiac rehabilitation facility as these patients may pose additional risks while exercising compared with individuals without CHD.[46] Vigorous physical activity increases the risk for sudden cardiac death and MI in patients previously diagnosed with CHD.[46] Atherosclerotic CHD is the most frequent cause of exercise-related cardiac events. Therefore, the incidence of exercise-related cardiac events is higher among patients with atherosclerotic CHD compared with those individuals without CHD. The incidence of cardiac arrest, non-fatal myocardial infarction, and death is approximately 1 for every 117,000, 220,000, and 750,000 patient-hours of participation, respectively.[46,60] It is noted that the reason for the low ratio of cardiac arrest to death is related to the availability of acute medical care. Therefore, individuals with a diagnosis of CHD are recommended to exercise in a supervised cardiac rehabilitation facility.[46]

PHARMACY PRACTICE APPLICATION

Applying CHD prevention strategies to pharmacy practice is rich with potential. Many of the patients who pharmacists see each day possess any number of the diseases that can lead to CHD and many may already have CHD and be in need of secondary prevention strategies. In addition, individuals currently living without disease should incorporate primary prevention strategies as they have been shown to be effective at decreasing the risk factors leading to CHD. Pharmacists are in an excellent position within the community to promote prevention strategies. Those who work in community pharmacies have much exposure to the public and are easily accessible. Those who work in pharmacies that are located in grocery stores are in a particularly good position as they are able to offer nutrition services that take patients around the store to show them examples of healthy and unhealthy food choices. Pharmacists who work in hospital or inpatient settings, especially those with coronary care units, can promote healthy lifestyle behaviors along with appropriate drug therapy and compliance to patients with existing CHD. These patients may be acutely interested in health promotion topics if they are currently being treated for a coronary event.

An excellent example of how pharmacists can be effective in CHD prevention and medication therapy management has been shown in patients with dyslipidemia.[61] Project ImPACT: Hyperlipidemia was a community-based, ambulatory pharmacy-based project with the objective to demonstrate whether pharmacists, in collaboration with patients and physicians, could have an impact on patient persistence and compliance with antihyperlipidemia drug therapy and enable patients to reach their National Cholesterol Education Program (NCEP) goals.[61] Pharmacists managed both lifestyle behaviors and hyperlipidemia medication. The results of the study showed that medication persistence and compliance were 93.6% and 90.1%, respectively.[61] In addition, total cholesterol, **triglyceride, high-density lipoprotein (HDL)**, and LDL levels improved significantly ($P < 0.001$) from baseline, and 63.5% of patients reached their NCEP goals at the end of the project.[61]

The AHA Scientific Statement for healthcare professionals recommends that all healthcare providers support the implementation and maintenance of exercise programs for their patients across the lifespan.[46] This statement could be taken further to include other lifestyle modification strategies such as smoking cessation, weight loss, proper nutrition, and behavior modification. The AHA Scientific Statement continues to state that healthcare providers should use their influence within the community to promote healthy behaviors and advocate change that promotes active and healthy living. In addition, all healthcare providers should themselves participate in physical activity and abstain from tobacco use to act as a role model within the community and to understand the issues involved with maintaining lifelong physical activity and positive healthy behaviors.[46]

CASE STUDY

J.L. is a 46-year-old Hispanic male who came to your pharmacy with his wife because she wanted to participate in your pharmacy's health promotion and wellness services. During your discussions with J.L.'s wife, J.L. comments that he is in fine health despite his wife's encouragement that he should also join the program with her. J.L. states that he stays active with his job as a construction worker, is not overweight, and does not need the program but fills out the paperwork at the request of his wife. J.L.'s health history reveals that he is 5' 8" tall and weighs 160 lb and does not take prescription medications but does occasionally take ibuprofen for "aches and pains." He is a current smoker of one pack per day for the past 30 years and drinks about five beers per week. J.L.'s father had his first heart attack at the age of 54 years and died of a second heart attack at the age of 62. His mother is still living at age 66 years with chronic illnesses. A recent physical examination that was required for his job revealed a fasting glucose of 98 mg/dL, glycosylated hemoglobin A (HbA$_{1c}$) of 5.3%, and a lipid panel that showed total cholesterol of 155, LDL-cholesterol of 110, HDL-cholesterol of 23, and triglycerides at 235, a resting blood pressure of 118/76 mm Hg, and a heart rate of 72 beats/min. J.L. follows no specific diet and does not participate in planned *physical activity outside of the activity he gets from working. J.L. agrees to keep a dietary analysis log with his wife for 4 days and agrees to wear a pedometer for a week to measure his daily activity at work.*

The results of his daily activity pedometer readings showed an average of 8,650 steps per day. Results from a 4-day dietary analysis were as follows:

Average total caloric intake per day = 1,634 calories
Carbohydrates = 54% of total calories
Monounsaturated fats = 16% of total calories
Polyunsaturated fats = 12% of total calories
Saturated fats = 10% of total calories
Total fats = 38% of total calories
Protein = 8% of total calories
Total dietary cholesterol = 150 mg
Fiber = 12 g
Calcium = 502 mg/day
Potassium = 1,534 mg/day
Magnesium = 202 mg/day
Sodium = 3,250 mg/day

Case Activities

1. *Write an SOAP note for J.L.*
2. *List J.L.'s risk factors for CHD and determine whether intervention is needed.*
3. *If needed, design a program that includes nutrition, exercise, and smoking-cessation counseling for J.L. that will decrease his risk for CHD.*

REFERENCES

1. Talbert RL. Ischemic Heart Disease. In: Dipiro JT, ed. Pharmacotherapy: A Pathophysiologic Approach, 6th ed. New York: McGraw-Hill, 2005:261–290.
2. American Heart Association. Heart Disease and Stroke Statistics—2005 Update. Dallas: American Heart Association, 2005.
3. Trujillo TC, Nolan PE. Ischemic heart disease: anginal syndrome. In: Koda-Kimble MA, ed. Applied Therapeutics: The Clinical Use of Drugs, 8th ed. Philadelphia: Lippincott Williams & Wilkins, 2005:17.1–17.33.
4. Franklin BA. Myocardial infarction. In: Durstine JL, ed. ACSM's Exercise Management for Persons with Chronic Diseases and Disabilities, 2nd ed. Champaign, IL: Human Kinetics, 2003:24–31.
5. Kavey REW, Daneils SR, Lauer RM, Atkins DL, Hayman LL, Taubert K. American Heart Association guidelines for primary prevention of atherosclerotic cardiovascular disease beginning in childhood. Circulation 2005;107:1562–1566.
6. National Institute of Diabetes and Digestive and Kidney Diseases. Chronic kidney disease: a family affair. National Institute of Diabetes and Digestive and Kidney Diseases, National Institutes of Health. NIH publication no. 05-5391. March 2005. Available at: http://niddk.nih.gov/kudiseases/pubs/chronickidneydiseases/index.htm. Accessed April 12, 2006.
7. Painter P. Exercise and patients with end-stage renal disease. In: Kaminsky LA, et al., eds. ACSM's Resource Manual for Guidelines for Exercise Testing and Prescription, 5th ed. Baltimore: Lippincott Williams & Wilkins, 2006:480–488.
8. Schoolwerth AC, Engelgau MM, Hostetter TH, et al. Chronic kidney disease: a public health problem that needs a public health action plan. Prev Chronic Dis April 2006. Available at: http://www.cdc.gov/pcd/issues/2006/apr/05_0105.htm. Accessed April 12, 2006.
9. de Jong PE, Brenner BM. From sedentary to primary prevention of progressive renal disease: the case for screening for albuminuria. Kidney Int 2004;66:2109–2118.
10. National Institutes of Health, National Heart, Lung, and Blood Institute. Third report of the National Cholesterol Education Program (NCEP) Expert Panel on Detection, Evaluation, and Treatment of High Blood Cholesterol in Adults (Adult Treatment Panel III). NIH Publication No. 02-5215, September 2002.

11. Chobanian AV, Bakris GL, Black HR, et al. Seventh report of the Joint National Committee on Prevention, Detection, Evaluation, and Treatment of High Blood Pressure. Hypertension 2003;42:1206–1252.

12. Eyre HE, Kahn R, Robertson RM, ACS/ADA/AHA Collaborative Writing Committee. Preventing cancer, cardiovascular disease and diabetes. A common agenda for the American Cancer Society, the American Diabetes Association, and the American Heart Association. Circulation 2004;109:3244–3255.

13. Centers for Disease Control and Prevention. Smoking-attributable mortality, morbidity, and economic costs (SAMMEC): adult SAMMEC and maternal and child health (MCH) SAMMEC software. Available at: http://apps.nccd.cdc.gov/sammec. Accessed November 17, 2005.

14. US Department of Health and Human Services. The health benefits of smoking cessation: a report of the Surgeon General. Rockville, MD: US Department of Health and Human Services, Public Health Services, Centers for Disease Control, Center for Chronic Disease Prevention and Health Promotion, Office of Smoking and Health, 1990. Available at: http://profiles.nlm.nih.gov/NN/B/B/F/B/. Accessed November 17, 2005.

15. Centers for Disease Control and Prevention (CDC). Cigarette smoking attributable mortality: United States, 2000. MMWR Morb Mortal Wkly Rep 2005;52:842–844.

16. Katzel LI, Bleecker ER, Rogus EM, et al. Sequential effects of aerobic exercise training and weight loss in risk factors for coronary disease in healthy, obese middle-aged and older men. Metabolism 1997;46:1441–1447.

17. Hubert HB, Feinleb M, McNemara PM, et al. Obesity as an independent risk factor for cardiovascular disease: a 26-year follow-up of the participants in the Framingham Heart Study. Circulation 1983;67:968–977.

18. Grundy SM, Pasternak R, Greenland P, et al. Assessment of cardiovascular risk by use of multiple risk factor assessment equations: a statement for the healthcare professionals from the American Heart Association and the American College of Cardiology. Circulation 1999;100:1481–1492.

19. Eckel RH. Obesity and heart disease: a statement for healthcare professionals from the Nutrition Committee, American Heart Association. Circulation 1997;96:3248–3250.

20. Sowers JR. Obesity as a cardiovascular risk factor. Am J Med 2003;115(Suppl 8A):37S–41S.

21. Steinberger J, Daniels SR. Obesity, insulin resistance, diabetes, and cardiovascular risk for children; an American Heart Association scientific statement from the Atherosclerosis, Hypertension, and Obesity in the Young Committee (Council on Cardiovascular Disease in the Young) and the Diabetes Committee (Council on Nutrition, Physical Activity, and Metabolism). Circulation 2003;107:1448–1453.

22. Rodriguez BL, D'Agostino R, Abbott RD, et al. Risk for hospitalized stroke in men enrolled in Honolulu Heart Program and the Framingham Study: a comparison of incidence and risk factor effects. Stroke 2002;33:230–236.

23. Czernichow S, Mennen L, Bertrais S, et al. Relationship between changes in weight and changes in cardiovascular risk factors in middle aged French subjects: effect on dieting. Int J Obes Relat Metab Disord 2002;26: 1138–1143.

24. Pearson TA, Blair SN, Daniels SR, et al. AHA guidelines for primary prevention of cardiovascular disease and stroke: 2002 update: consensus panel guide to comprehensive risk reduction for adult patients without coronary or other atherosclerotic vascular diseases. Circulation 2002;106:388–391.

25. Wadden TA, Anderson DA, Foster GD. Two-year changes in lipids and lipoproteins associated with the maintenance of a 5% to 10% reduction in initial weight: some findings and some questions. Obes Res 1999;7:170–178.

26. National Institutes of Health; National Heart, Lung and Blood Institute; North American Association for the Study of Obesity. The Practical Guide to the Identification, Evaluation, and Treatment of Overweight and Obesity in Adults. National Institutes of Health, 2000. NIH publication No. 00-4084 October 2000.

27. Oster G, Thompson D, Edelsberg J, et al. Lifetime health and economic benefits of weight loss among obese persons. Am J Public Health 1999;89:1536–1542.

28. HHS Publication number: HHS-ODPHP-2005-01-DGA-A, Dietary Guidelines for Americans 2005, United States Department of Health and Human Services, United States Department of Agriculture. Available at: http://healthierus.gov/dietaryguidelines. Accessed February 8, 2007.

29. Clinical Guidelines on the Identification, Evaluation, and Treatment of Overweight and Obesity in Adults. Bethesda, MD: National Institutes of Health, U.S. Department of Health and Human Services, 1998. NIH Publication No. 98-4083.

30. Lee IM, Paffenbarger RS, Hennekens CH, et al. Physical activity, physical fitness and longevity. Aging (Milano) 1997;9:2–11.

31. Blair SN, Jackson AS. Physical fitness and activity as separate heart disease risk factors: a meta-analysis. Med Sci Sports Exerc 2001;33:762–764.

32. Powell KE, Thompson PD, Casperson CJ, et al. Physical activity and the incidence of coronary heart disease. Annu Rev Public Health 1987;8:253–287.

33. Goldstein LB, Adams R, Becker K, et al. Primary prevention of ischemic stroke: a statement for healthcare professionals from Stroke Council of the American Heart Association. Circulation 1996;94:857–862.

34. Fletcher GF, Balady G, Blair SN, et al. Statement on exercise benefits and recommendations for physical activity programs for all Americans: a statement for health professionals by the Committee on Exercise and Rehabilitation of the Council of Clinical Cardiology, American Heart Association. Circulation 1996;94:857–862.

35. Antman EM, Anbe DT, Armstrong PW, et al. ACC/AHA guidelines for the management of patients with ST-segment myocardial infarction: a report of the American College of Cardiology/American Heart Association Task Force on Practice Guidelines (Committee to Revise the 1999 Guidelines for the Management of Patients With Acute Myocardial Infarction). Circulation 2004;110:e82–e293.

36. Rossouw JE, Lewis B, Rafkind BM. The value of lowering cholesterol after myocardial infarction. N Engl J Med 1990;323:1112–1119.

37. Smith SC, Blair SN, Bonow RO, et al. AHA/ACC Guidelines for preventing heart attack and death in patients with atherosclerotic cardiovascular disease: 2001 update. A statement for healthcare professionals from the American Heat Association and the American College of Cardiology. Circulation 2001;104:1577–1579.

38. Leon AS, Franklin BA, Costa F, et al. Cardiac rehabilitation and secondary prevention of coronary heart disease. Circulation 2005;111:369–376.

39. Taylor RS, Brown A, Ebrahim S, et al. Exercise-based rehabilitation for patients with coronary heart disease: systematic review and meta-analysis of randomized trials. Am J Med 2004;116:682–697.

40. American Diabetes Association. Aspirin therapy. Diabetes Care 2004;27(Suppl 1):S72–S73.

41. Vuori IM. Dose response of physical activity and low back pain, osteoarthritis, and osteoporosis. Med Sci Sports Exerc 2001;33(6 Suppl):S551–S586.

42. Oldridge NB, Guyatt GH, Fisher ME, et al. Cardiac rehabilitation after myocardial infarction: combined experience of randomized clinical trials. JAMA 1988;260:945–950.

43. Centers for Disease Control and Prevention. Increasing physical activity: a report on recommendations of the Task Force on Community Preventive Services. MMWR Morb Mortal Wkly Rep 2001;50(No. RR-18):1.

44. U.S. Department of Agriculture and U.S. Department of Health and Human Services. Nutrition and Your Health: Dietary Guidelines for Americans, 5th ed. Home and Garden Bulletin no. 232. Washington, D.C.: U.S. Department of Agriculture, 2000, 44 pages.

45. American Heart Association. Delicious Decisions. Available at: http://www.deliciousdecisions.org/. Accessed March 23, 2004.

46. Thompson PD, Buchner D, Pina IL, et al. Exercise and physical activity in the prevention and treatment of atherosclerotic cardiovascular disease. Circulation 2003;107:3109–3116.

47. Knowler WC, Barrett-Connor E, Flowler SE, et al., for the Diabetes Prevention Program Research Group. Reduction in the incidence of type 2 diabetes with lifestyle intervention or metformin. N Engl J Med 2002;346:393–403.

48. Wing RR, Hill JO. Successful weight loss maintenance. Annu Rev Nutr 2001;21:323–341.

49. Polluck KM. Exercise in treating depression: broadening the psychotherapist's role. J Clin Psychol 2001;57:1289–1300.

50. Breslow RA, Ballard-Barbash R, Munoz K, et al. Long-term recreational physical activity and breast cancer in the National Health and Nutrition Examination Survey I epidemiology follow-up study. Cancer Epidemiol Biomarkers Prev 2001;10:805–808.

51. Slattery ML, Potter JD. Physical activity and colon cancer: confounding or interaction? Med Sci Sports Exerc 2002;34:913–919.

52. Blair SN, Jackson AS. Physical fitness and activity as separate heart disease risk factors: a meta-analysis. Med Sci Sports Exerc 2001;33:762–764.

53. U.S. Department of Health, Education, and Welfare. Smoking and Heath: Report of the Advisory Committee to the Surgeon General of the Public Health Services. Washington, D.C.: U.S. Department of Health, Education, and Welfare, Public Health Service, 1964. PHS Publication No. 1103. Available at: http://www.cdc.gov/tobacco/sgr/sgr_1964/sgr64.htm. Accessed November 17, 2005.

54. Pate RR, Pratt M, Blair SN, et al. Physical activity and public health: a recommendation from the Centers for Disease Control and Prevention and the American College of Sports Medicine. JAMA 1995;273:402–407.

55. U.S. Department of Health and Human Services. Physical activity and health: a report of the Surgeon General. Atlanta: U.S. Department of Health and Human Services, Centers for Disease Control and Prevention, National Center for Chronic Disease Prevention and Health Promotion, 1996.

56. Centers for Disease Control and Prevention. Available at: www.cdc.gov/nccdphp/dnpa/physical/recommendations/adults.htm. Accessed July 26, 2005.

57. National Institutes of Health: Consensus Development Panel on Physical Activity and Cardiovascular Health. Physical activity and cardiovascular health. JAMA 1996;276:214–246.

58. O'Connor GT, Buring JE, Yucef S, et al. An overview of randomized trials of rehabilitation and exercise after myocardial infarction. Circulation 1989;80:234–244.

59. Jolliffe JA, Rees K, Taylor RS, et al. Exercise based rehabilitation for coronary heart disease. Cochrane Database Syst Rev 2001;(1):CD001800.

60. Franklin BA, Bonzheim K, Gordon S, et al. Safety of medically supervised outpatient cardiac rehabilitation exercise therapy: a 16 year follow-up. Chest 1998;114:902–906.

61. Bluml BM, McKenney JM, Cziraky MJ. Pharmaceutical care services and results in project ImPACT: hyperlipidemia. J Am Pharm Assoc 2000;40:157–165.

CHAPTER 9

Stroke

OBJECTIVES

At the end of this chapter the reader should be able to:

1. Explain the risk associated with ischemic stroke.
2. Summarize the prevention and treatment options for stroke.
3. Describe appropriate nutritional strategies for patients at risk for stroke.
4. Suggest appropriate exercises for patients at risk for stroke.
5. Formulate a basic nutrition, exercise, and smoking-cessation program for a patient at risk for developing a stroke.

OVERVIEW OF STROKE

The incidence of **stroke** ranks as one of the most prevalent killers in the world and as the third leading cause of death in the United States behind diseases of the heart and cancer.[1,2] Stroke can be either ischemic or hemorrhagic in origin.[2] The majority of strokes (88%) are caused by **ischemia,** which has essentially the same pathophysiology as a **myocardial infarction.**[1,2] Many **ischemic strokes** result from an atherosclerotic buildup in the cerebral arteries, similar to the atherosclerotic buildup in the coronary arteries that results in myocardial infarctions.[2] **Hemorrhagic strokes,** which make up 12% of all strokes, result from bleeding in the brain.[1] Hemorrhagic strokes are not as prevalent as ischemic strokes but result in higher mortality rates.[1,2]

PREVALENCE, ECONOMIC COSTS, AND HEALTH RISKS ASSOCIATED WITH STROKE

Each year about 700,000 Americans are diagnosed with either their first stroke or a recurrent stroke.[1] Of this, about 500,000 are a first attack with the remainder being a recurring event. Blacks have almost twice the risk of a first stroke compared with whites, and women experience about 40,000 more strokes each year than men.[1] Stroke accounted for more than 1 of every 15 deaths in the United States in 2002, and because women live longer than men, women accounted for 61.5% of the deaths associated with stroke in 2002.[1]

The economic burden associated with stroke is great. It was estimated in 2005 that the direct and indirect costs of stroke were $6.8 billion.[1] Within 30 days of the onset of an acute stroke, the average cost of a mild ischemic stroke was $13,019 and for a severe ischemic stroke was $20,346.[1] In the United States, the mean lifetime cost associated with ischemic stroke is estimated to be $140,048.[1]

PATHOPHYSIOLOGY OF STROKE

A stroke is defined as a sudden onset of focal neurologic deficit that lasts for 24 hours or longer and is thought to be caused by the vascular system.[2] A **transient ischemic attack (TIA)** is the same definition as a stroke, but lasts for less than 24 hours and usually less than 30 minutes.[2] As stated above, a majority of strokes are ischemic in origin. The pathophysiology of an ischemic stroke is related to either vessel occlusion from atherosclerosis or a thrombus that occludes the vessel.[2,3] The atherosclerotic process that causes a stroke is the same as that which causes myocardial infarctions, as described in Chapter 8. Excess lipids and inflammatory cells that accumulate in the blood can result in plaque formation in the arteries. For a stroke, this occurs in cerebral arteries including the carotid arteries.[2] If the plaque formation ruptures, a thrombus can form and occlude the vessel at the site of the eruption or can break off and travel distally through smaller diameter vessels until it becomes lodged and does not allow blood flow past the clot.[2]

A thrombus can also develop as a result of blood stasis in the atria or ventricles, usually occurring from arrhythmias such as atrial fibrillation.[2,3] These are called cardiogenic emboli, and once they become dislodged from the atria or ventricle and mobilize, they pass through the aorta and move to the cerebral arteries.[2] Once in the cerebral arteries, the clot will travel downstream until it too becomes lodged because of the narrowing of vessel diameter. This then causes a stroke because little or no blood and oxygen can get behind the clot, causing an infarction. Ischemic strokes are sometimes called cerebral infarction, much like the term myocardial infarction.

The second and less prevalent type of stroke is a hemorrhagic stroke. These types of strokes occur as a result of the presence of blood in the brain parenchyma, which causes damage to the surrounding tissue.[2] As reported above, 12% of all strokes are hemorrhagic in origin.[1] Most hemorrhagic strokes occur as a result of intracerebral hemorrhage (9%), whereas the remaining (3%) are subarachnoid in origin.[2] The pooling of the blood in the brain parenchyma not only directly damages the brain tissue but also can compress the surrounding tissue and vessels, causing secondary ischemia.[2] Approximately 30% of strokes caused by intracerebral hemorrhages continue to grow larger during the first 24 hours.[2,4]

Hemorrhagic strokes can be caused by certain medications, trauma, and other factors. Ischemic strokes can be caused by several factors, many of which are modifiable.

TABLE 9–1	Environmental Factors Increasing the Risk of Ischemic Stroke

Hypertension
Cigarette smoking
Diabetes
Hyperlipidemia
Obesity
Physical inactivity
Alcohol abuse
Drug abuse
Asymptomatic carotid stenosis
Sickle cell disease
Atrial fibrillation
Hyperhomocysteinemia
Hypercoagulability
Hormone replacement therapy
Oral contraceptive use
History of transient ischemic attacks
Mitral valve stenosis
Dilated cardiomyopathy
Recent myocardial infarction
Coronary heart disease

Source: Welty TE. Cerebrovascular disorders. In: Koda-Kimble MA, ed. Applied Therapeutics: The Clinical Use of Drugs, 8th ed. Philadelphia: Lippincott Williams & Wilkins, 2005:55.1–55.20.

Because ischemic strokes are more prevalent and some of the risks can be modified through lifestyle changes, this chapter will focus on the primary and secondary prevention of ischemic stroke for patients who are at risk.

Several risk factors have been identified that can cause stroke. Some of these risk factors are modifiable and some are non-modifiable. The non-modifiable risk factors include age, race, gender, and family history.[5] For instance, the risk of stroke doubles for each successive decade of life after the age of 55 years.[5–7] The risk of ischemic stroke can decrease through the adoption of lifestyle changes as many risk factors for stroke are modifiable. A list of the modifiable risks factors for ischemic stroke is provided in Table 9-1.

STROKE DISEASE PREVENTION AND TREATMENT

Like **coronary heart disease,** the prevention and treatment of ischemic stroke can be separated into primary and secondary prevention strategies. Primary prevention strategies begin by recognizing the risk factors that can lead to an ischemic stroke and then treating or preventing the underlying causes.[5] As listed in Table 9-1, there are several risk factors that can lead to an ischemic stroke. Among the most documented modifiable risk factors for both ischemic and hemorrhagic stroke is **hypertension.**[5] Elevated **systolic blood pressure** with or without an elevation in **diastolic blood pressure** can increase the risk of stroke. High blood pressure that is defined as isolated systolic hypertension (systolic blood pressure >160 mm Hg and diastolic blood pressure <90 mm Hg), which is common in the elderly, is especially important to control to decrease stroke risk.[5,8] The relative risk for stroke in a 50-year-old patient with hypertension is four times that of a 50-year-old without hypertension.[5] However, the risk of stroke can be decreased 38% by adequately controlling blood pressure.[5]

Other major modifiable risk factors for stroke include smoking, **diabetes mellitus,** and hyperlipidemia. Individuals who smoke have approximately double the relative risk for an ischemic stroke compared with those who do not smoke.[5,9] The stroke risk reduction on cessation of smoking is approximately 50% at 1 year and is the same as nonsmokers 5 years after quitting.[5,10]

Patients with diabetes have an increased susceptibility for **atherosclerosis** and other atherogenic risk factors such as hypertension, **obesity,** and **dyslipidemia.**[5] Diabetes alone has been shown to be an independent risk for ischemic stroke and has an increased relative risk for stroke that ranges from nearly two times to six times that of individuals without diabetes.[5] Interestingly, controlling blood glucose does not reduce the risk of stroke in persons with diabetes, but controlling blood pressure in persons with diabetes significantly reduces stroke incidence.[5,11]

Dyslipidemia is an established risk factor for the development of coronary heart disease (CHD). Less is known about its effects on the risk of stroke. Some studies have found that an increased amount of blood **cholesterol** increases the rate of both CHD and thromboembolic stroke as well as the incidence of death associated with cerebral hemorrhage.[5,12–15] Other studies have shown that the use of 3-hydroxy-3-methylglutaryl coenzyme A (HMG-CoA) reductase inhibitors (statins) can reduce the progression of asymptomatic carotid atherosclerosis.[5,16–20] It appears that controlling blood lipids with statins may reduce the risk of stroke.

Obesity and **physical inactivity** have been established as potential modifiable risk factors for stroke but are less well documented. Increases in abdominal obesity in men and weight gain and **body mass index (BMI)** increases in women have been shown to be independent risk factors for stroke.[5,21,22] On the basis of this, weight loss and weight control are recommended. However, the reduction in stroke risk with weight loss has yet to be established.[5]

Much data exist regarding the risk for stroke as it relates to physical inactivity. It is stated that individuals who are sedentary have a risk of stroke that is 2.7 times greater than those who are physically active.[5] It is unknown, however, whether the benefits of **physical activity** in relation to stroke are related to reductions in blood pressure and controlling other risk factors such as diabetes and obesity.[5] The benefits for primary risk reduction of stroke are apparent even with light to moderate levels of activity as well as with increased amounts of recreational activity.[5]

The primary prevention of ischemic stroke can be approached through many lifestyle modification strategies. Clearly, controlling blood pressure and dyslipidemia and smoking cessation when appropriate can significantly decrease the risk of stroke. In addition, weight loss, physical activity, and proper nutrition that includes limiting alcohol intake may also decrease stroke risk independently as well as help control the risk factors that lead to stroke.[5]

Secondary stroke prevention is aimed at trying to prevent a recurring stroke or TIA in patients who have already experienced one or more strokes or TIAs. The lifestyle modification strategies that are involved in the secondary prevention of stroke or TIA are the same as those for primary stroke prevention. Therefore, emphasis is placed on controlling blood pressure, blood lipids, and tobacco use as well as weight control, physical activity, and proper nutrition. In addition, it is indicated that patients who have experienced a stroke or TIA be placed on medication(s) in addition to lifestyle modifications to further decrease stroke risk. A list of the medications used for secondary prevention of stroke is provided in Table 9-2.

TABLE 9–2   Medications Used to Treat and Prevent Stroke or Transient Ischemic Attack

Antiplatelets
Anticoagulants
Drugs to control blood pressure (see Chapter 6)
Drugs used to control blood lipids (see Chapter 7)

Several barriers to rehabilitation adherence and secondary prevention may exist for poststroke patients, their families, and caregivers. An evaluation of the physical, psychological, and emotional barriers to participation in physical rehabilitation and secondary prevention strategies should be assessed by a trained professional.[23] The primary factors that may act as barriers to stroke rehabilitation and secondary prevention include stroke severity, comorbidities, and clinical deficits.[23] Secondary factors include familial support, depression, poststroke fatigue, social integration, and cultural issues.[23]

Physical barriers are common in poststroke patients, and therefore a medical history and physical examination are important before recommending a physical activity program for both rehabilitation and to prevent subsequent strokes.[23] Such an evaluation may be beyond the scope of a pharmacist's capabilities and will most often need to be completed by a healthcare professional trained in this area. In addition, assessing the communication deficit will have a significant impact on the success of the rehabilitation program.[23] Alternative methods of communication may need to be established with the patient. Working with family members and caregivers on mutually derived goals and safety issues is also important to ensuring program adherence.[23]

Pharmacists can help with program adherence for patients at risk for stroke as well as patients who are poststroke through education. Many individuals who have not experienced a stroke may not understand the importance of implementing strategies such as blood pressure control, smoking cessation, and other lifestyle modifications. Many feel that there is nothing to treat as long as they do not feel bad or are not sick. Spreading the word about primary disease prevention can be a part of every healthcare provider's responsibilities. Pharmacists can support both primary and secondary stroke prevention by educating patients and family members about their importance. The more education patients have regarding their health, even when they are not sick, the more informed their decision making can be. Table 9-3 lists program adherence strategies for the prevention of stroke.

NUTRITION AND STROKE

Proper nutrition is an important component for reducing the risk of stroke as it is for reducing the risk of CHD.[5,24] Although the data regarding the general effects of nutrition on stroke risk are limited, there is evidence that increases in fruits and vegetables are advantageous toward reducing stroke risk. One study reported that individuals who consumed green leafy vegetables and citrus fruit and juice experienced a lower relative risk of stroke compared with a control group.[5,25] An increment of one serving per day was associated with a 6% lower risk of stroke.[5,25] Therefore, the American Heart Association (AHA) recommends that at least five servings of fruits and vegetables be consumed daily to reduce the risk of stroke.[5]

TABLE 9–3 Program Adherence Recommendations for Patients With or at Risk for Stroke

Professional patient evaluation for physical, psychological, and emotional barriers

Effective communication with patient and the patient's family and caregivers

Patient education about prevention and treatment

Ensure the patient has a clear understanding of the disease-prevention components and the importance of each

Multiple adherence strategies work better than a single approach

Weekly contact with patients for the first 4 weeks of the program, then monthly thereafter, to continually assess the patient's progress and troubleshoot problems

Set achievable goals

Obtain baseline assessment of dietary intake

Institute a self-monitoring program such as keeping a log of food intake and exercise participation

Identify patient-specific barriers to the lifestyle changes

Design a program that is reasonable, gradual, and easily implemented

Source: National Institutes of Health, National Heart, Lung, and Blood Institute. Third report of the National Cholesterol Education Program (NCEP) Expert Panel on Detection, Evaluation, and Treatment of High Blood Cholesterol in Adults (Adult Treatment Panel III). NIH Publication No. 02-5215, September 2002.

This recommendation from the AHA is consistent with the dietary recommendations discussed in the National Cholesterol Education Program, Adult Treatment Panel III Guidelines (NCEP ATP III) (http://www.nhlbi.nih.gov/guidelines/) and those discussed in the Seventh Report of the Joint National Committee of Prevention, Detection, Evaluation, and Treatment of High Blood Pressure (JNC 7) (http://www.nhlbi.nih.gov/guidelines/) as well as the Dietary Guidelines for Americans 2005 (http://www.healthierus.gov/dietaryguidelines/).[24,26–29] The recommendations stated in each of these guidelines are similar and primarily focus on promoting health and reducing the risk for CHD and other chronic diseases by lowering **low-density lipoprotein** cholesterol (LDL) and blood pressure. The overarching themes are to eat fewer calories, be more physically active, and make wiser food choices.[27] Because the pathophysiology of ischemic stroke and CHD are so similar, this information can and should also be applied to individuals who are implementing primary and secondary strategies of stroke prevention.

Chapters 1, 6, and 7 discuss in further detail specific information regarding dietary modifications for patients at risk for developing CHD and stroke. Refer to these chapters for further detail. Table 9-4 lists dietary recommendations for the treatment and prevention of stroke.

PHYSICAL ACTIVITY AND STROKE

Similar to patients with or at risk for CHD, physical activity can be addressed either as primary prevention for stroke or as rehabilitation and secondary prevention of stroke. It is well established that a major component of primary **cardiovascular disease** prevention is physical activity.[5,24] Some studies have also shown beneficial effects of physical activity in the primary prevention of stroke.[5,30–38] Because CHD and ischemic stroke

TABLE 9–4	Dietary Recommendations to Treat and Prevent Stroke

Nutrient	Recommendation
Total calories	Balance calorie intake with expenditure to obtain appropriate body weight
Carbohydrate[a]	50–60% of total calorie intake
Fruits and vegetables	At least 5 servings per day of each
Fiber	20–30 g/day
Protein	Around 15% of total calorie intake
Monounsaturated fat	Up to 20% of total calorie intake
Polyunsaturated fat	Up to 10% of total calorie intake
Saturated fat	Less than 7% of total calorie intake
Total fat	25–35% to total calorie intake
Dietary cholesterol	Less than 200 mg/day

[a]Most carbohydrate intake should come from whole grains, fruits, and vegetables.
Source: HHS Publication No. HHS-ODPHP-2005-01-DGA-A. Dietary Guidelines for Americans 2005, U.S. Department of Health and Human Services, U.S. Department of Agriculture. Available at: http://healthierus.gov/dietaryguidelines.
Source: National Institutes of Health, National Heart, Lung, and Blood Institute. Third report of the National Cholesterol Education Program (NCEP) Expert Panel on Detection, Evaluation, and Treatment of High Blood Cholesterol in Adults (Adult Treatment Panel III). NIH Publication No. 02-5215, September 2002.

share similar underlying pathophysiology, it seems logical that physical activity would decrease the risk for ischemic stroke as it does with CHD.[39] This, however, is not as well studied in stroke as it is with CHD. It is clear that physical activity provides protection against stroke.[39] But it is unclear whether a dose–response relationship exists. One study showed that men with low fitness levels had a 2.7 times greater risk for a stroke compared with men with moderate fitness levels and a 3.13 times greater risk for a stroke compared with men with a high fitness level.[39,40] Other studies that were less well designed, however, showed positive but less strong results in preventing stroke with physical activity. The recommendation for physical activity in primary stroke prevention is to participate in at least 30 minutes of moderate-intensity **exercise** on most if not all days of the week.[5] The physical activity should be aerobic in nature, with examples being walking, jogging, and cycling.[41–44] It is recommended that medical supervision accompany those patients who are at high risk for cardiac disease as discussed in Chapter 8.[5] Table 9-5 provides recommendations for the primary prevention of stroke.

Leisure Time, Commuting, and Occupational Physical Activity and Stroke Risk

Several studies have been conducted in an attempt to establish whether regular amounts of exercise decrease the risk for stroke. Some studies have shown that regular amounts of physical activity decrease stroke risk, although others are controversial. What about activity that is not necessarily planned or scheduled such as exercise?

Will increased physical activity in normal daily life decrease stroke risk? A Finnish study of more than 47,000 individuals between the ages of 25 and 64 attempted to answer these questions.[45]

A prospective study of individuals without a history of coronary heart disease, stroke, or cancer was completed between 1972 and 1997 (every 5 years) in which six independent self-administered questionnaires were completed by the participants.[45] The surveys asked the participants about smoking, alcohol consumption, socioeconomic factors, medical history, and physical activity, which included leisure time, occupational, and commuting to work physical activity. The self-reported leisure time activity was classified into three categories: (1) low (defined as almost completely inactive); (2) moderate (defined as some physical activity greater than 4 hours per week such as walking, cycling, or light gardening, but excluding travel to work); and (3) high (defined as vigorous physical activity for greater than 3 hours per week such as running, jogging, swimming, or regular exercise or competitive sports several times per week). Occupational physical activity was also classified as (1) low (defined as physically very easy such as sitting); (2) moderate (defined as standing or walking); and (3) active (defined as walking or lifting, or heavy manual labor such as industrial or farm work). Daily commuting was categorized as (1) using motorized transportation, (2) walking or bicycling 1 to 29 minutes, and (3) walking or bicycling 30 minutes or more. Study participants were followed until the end of 2003, and the mean follow-up time was 19 years.[45]

The main follow-up end point was the incidence of stroke, fatal or non-fatal, and ischemic or hemorrhagic. There were a total of 2,863 recorded stroke events, with 2,264 of them being ischemic in nature. After adjusting for age, area, study year, and other risk factors, the results showed that high leisure activity reduced all types of stroke including hemorrhagic. Moderate levels of activity reduced intracerebral hemorrhage and ischemic strokes but not subarachnoid stroke. In addition, those participants who commuted to work on foot or via bicycle less than 30 minutes per day had an 8% lower risk of total stroke compared with those who reported no activity. Those whose commute was 30 minutes or longer experienced an 11% lower risk of total stroke compared with physically inactive commuters. Also, occupations that are considered active were shown to be protective against stroke, but the results were not statistically significant after adjusting for leisure time and commuting physical activity.[45]

The results of this study further emphasize that healthcare professionals should be stressing the importance of overall physical activity. Disease risk reduction can occur by becoming more active in all aspects of life. Pharmacists can encourage individuals to participate in more leisure time physical activity and to take walks during work breaks and before and after work.

The secondary prevention and rehabilitation of stroke survivors with participation in physical activity has shown much potential value.[23] Many studies have demonstrated that patients who have experienced a stroke benefit from physical activity through physiologic, psychological, sensorimotor, strength, endurance, and functional effects of many different types of physical activity.[23,46–59] In addition to these rehabilitation effects, increased physical activity in patients who have survived a stroke has demonstrated a decreased cardiovascular disease risk and decreased risk for mortality from stroke and cardiac events.[23,60–63]

Three major goals exist with regard to physical activity in a poststroke patient. These goals are (1) preventing complications with prolonged inactivity because many

TABLE 9–5	Physical Activity Recommendations for the Primary Prevention of Stroke

Exercise Variable	Recommendation
Goals	Decrease risk for stroke and CVD Decrease risk factors for stroke and CVD such as elevated blood pressure, insulin resistance and glucose intolerance, elevated triglycerides concentrations, low HDL-C concentrations, obesity, CHD, and myocardial function
Type	Aerobic exercises (large muscle activities) such as walking, jogging, running, cycling, or individual aerobic exercise preference Resistance training can be adjunctive to aerobic exercises
Intensity	Moderate-intensity endurance activity
Duration	30 minutes or more continuous or intermittent exercise per day
Frequency	Most, preferably all, days of the week
Lifestyle activity	Increase overall daily activities through increasing the duration of activities of daily living (e.g., walking the dog, taking stairs, yard work, household duties)

Source: U.S. Department of Health and Human Services. Physical activity and health: a report of the Surgeon General. Atlanta: U.S. Department of Health and Human Services, Centers for Disease Control and Prevention, National Center for Chronic Disease Prevention and Health Promotion, 1996. CHD, coronary heart disease; CVD, cardiovascular disease; HDL-C, high-density lipoprotein cholesterol.

patients have physical disabilities, (2) reducing the risk for another stroke or a CHD event, and (3) increasing aerobic fitness levels. Other goals include improvements in quality of life, functional capacity and mobility, neurologic impairments, and motor function.[23]

Each patient who has experienced a stroke will have unique circumstances and needs with regard to physical activity. Therefore, healthcare professionals with experience in exercise programming with poststroke patients must evaluate and recommend specific exercises unique to the patient's needs. In general, stroke survivors are recommended to participate in aerobic, strength, **flexibility,** and neuromuscular exercises with goals such as those listed above.[23]

Aerobic exercises should focus on large muscle activities that can be performed and tolerated by the individual patient. These may include walking and stationary bicycling as well as arm ergometry and seated stepper.[23] Aerobic activities should be performed at 50 to 80% of the maximum heart rate, three to seven times per week for 20 to 60 minutes per session (or multiple 10-minute sessions).[23] Strength-building activities such as using weight machines, free weights, or resistance bands can be done to improve activities of daily living. It is recommended that one to three sets of 10 to 15 repetitions be performed for large muscle groups on 2 to 3 days per week.[23] Stretching exercises can help patients increase range of motion and prevent contractures and should be performed before and after aerobic and strength training. Neuromuscular exercises involve coordination and balance activities to improve the level of safety during activities of daily living. These activities can be performed on the same day as strength activities or 2 to 3 days per week.[23]

PHARMACY PRACTICE APPLICATION

A pharmacist can encounter many patients each day who have risk factors, such as those listed in Table 9-1, which can lead to a stroke. As discussed in other chapters, pharmacists are in an excellent position to discuss and design lifestyle interventions for patients who are at risk for having a first stroke. Encouraging, supporting, and designing physical activity, nutrition, weight loss, and smoking-cessation programs as well as helping patients control and monitor blood pressure and blood cholesterol are just some of the primary prevention strategies pharmacists can use with patients who are at risk.

Pharmacists can also help patients who have already experienced a stroke by helping them quit smoking, and controlling and monitoring their blood pressure, blood cholesterol, diabetes, and other risk factors for stroke and cardiovascular disease. In addition, educating patients about the benefits of proper nutrition and physical activity is important as well as encouraging and supporting their participation in rehabilitation programs. Lastly, pharmacists can help stroke survivors overcome barriers they may have to participating in such programs as well as other barriers they may have to participating in secondary prevention activities.

CASE STUDY

A.P. is a 57-year-old Hispanic female with a past medical history of hypertension for 5 years. She has been taking amlodipine 5 mg daily since her initial diagnosis. She has no other significant medical history, but her brother died of a myocardial infarction at age 47 years and her father died of a stroke at age 55 years. Her mother has diabetes mellitus but is otherwise in good health at age 82 years. In addition, A.P. smokes one and a half packs of cigarettes per day and has done so for the past 33 years. She states that she is very active with her job as a daycare provider and gets additional exercise by walking on a treadmill three times per week. She states that she tries to maintain a healthy diet with low sodium and little fast food. A.P. is 4′ 10″ tall and weighs 125 lb. Her average blood pressure in the pharmacy was measured at 164/88 mm Hg with a heart rate of 58 beats/min.

A.P. requests your assistance in analyzing her blood pressure. After educating A.P. about her blood pressure measurements in relation to optimal blood pressure and the risks of hypertension, she inquires about your wellness program. She decides to join your program. Results from her 4-day dietary analysis were as follows:

> *Average total caloric intake per day = 2,000 calories*
> *Carbohydrates = 58% of total calories*
> *Monounsaturated fats = 12% of total calories*
> *Polyunsaturated fats = 7% of total calories*
> *Saturated fats = 5% of total calories*
> *Total fats = 24% of total calories*
> *Protein = 18% of total calories*
> *Total dietary cholesterol = 150 mg*
> *Fiber = 21 g*
> *Calcium = 875 mg/day*
> *Potassium = 4,500 mg/day*
> *Magnesium = 526 mg/day*
> *Sodium = 2,025 mg/day*

Case Activities

1. *Write an SOAP note for A.P.*
2. *List A.P.'s risk factors for stroke and determine whether intervention is needed.*
3. *If needed, design a program that includes nutrition, exercise, and smoking-cessation counseling for A.P. that will decrease her risk for stroke.*

REFERENCES

1. American Heart Association. Heart Disease and Stroke Statistics—2005 Update. Dallas: American Heart Association, 2005.
2. Fagan SC, Hess DC. Stroke. In: Dipiro JT, ed. Pharmacotherapy: A Pathophysiologic Approach, 6th ed. New York: McGraw-Hill, 2005:415–427.
3. Welty TE. Cerebrovascular disorders. In: Koda-Kimble MA, ed. Applied Therapeutics: The Clinical Use of Drugs, 8th ed. Philadelphia: Lippincott Williams & Wilkins, 2005:55.1–55.20.
4. Fayad PB, Awad IA. Surgery for intracerebral hemorrhage. Neurology 1998;51(Suppl 3):S69–S73.
5. Goldstein LB, Adams R, Becker K, et al. AHA Scientific statement. Primary prevention of ischemic stroke: a statement for healthcare professionals from the Stroke Council of the American Heart Association. Circulation 2001;103:163–182.
6. Brown RD, Whisnant JP, Sicks JD, et al. Stroke incidence, prevalence and survival: secular trends in Rochester, Minnesota, through 1989. Stroke 1996;27:373–380.
7. Wolf PA, D'Agostino RB, O'Neal MA, et al. Secular trends in stroke incidence and mortality: the Framingham Study. Stroke 1992;23:1551–1555.
8. Staessen JA, Fagard R, Thijs L, et al. Randomized double-blind comparison of placebo and active treatment in older patients with isolated systolic hypertension: the Systolic Hypertension in Europe (Syst-Eur) Trial Investigators. Lancet 1997;350:757–764.
9. Shinton R, Beevers G. Meta-analysis of relation between cigarette smoking and stroke. BMJ 1989;298:789–794.
10. Wolf PA, D'Agostino RB, Kannel WB, et al. Cigarette smoking as a risk factor for stroke: the Framingham Study. JAMA 1988;259:1025–1029.
11. Tuomilehto J, Rastenyte D. Diabetes and glucose intolerance as risk factors for stroke. J Cardiovasc Risk 1999;6:241–249.
12. Qizilbash N, Jones L, Warlow C, et al. Fibrinogen and lipid concentrations as risk factors for transient ischemic attacks and minor ischemic strokes. BMJ 1991;303:605–609.
13. Kargman DE, Tuck C, Berglund LF, et al. High density lipoprotein: a potentially modifiable stroke risk factor: the Northern Manhattan Stroke Study [Abstract]. Neuroepidemiology 1996;15:20S.
14. Kargman DE, Tuck C, Berglund LF, et al. Elevated high density lipoprotein levels are more important in atherosclerotic ischemic stroke subtypes: the Northern Manhattan Stroke Study. Ann Neurol 1998; 44:442–443.
15. Qizilbash N, Lewington S, Duffy S, et al. Cholesterol, diastolic blood pressure and stroke: 13,000 strokes in 450,000 people in 45 prospective cohorts: Prospective Studies Collaboration. Lancet 1995;346:1647–1653.
16. Fine-Edelstein JS, Wolf PA, O'Leary DH, et al. Precursors of extracranial carotid atherosclerosis in the Framingham Study. Neurology 1994;44:1046–1050.
17. Blankenhorn DH, Selzer RH, Crawford DW, et al. Beneficial effects of Colestipol-niacin therapy on the common carotid artery: two- and four-year reduction of intima-media thickness measured by ultrasound. Circulation 1993;88:20–28.
18. Furgerg CD, Adams HP Jr, Applegate WB, et al. Effect of lovastatin on early carotid atherosclerosis and cardiovascular events: Asymptomatic Carotid Artery Progression Study (ACAPS) research group. Circulation 1994;90:1679–1687.
19. Crouse JR III, Byington RP, Bond MG, et al. Pravastatin, lipids and atherosclerosis in the carotid arteries (PLAC-II). Am J Cardiol 1995;75:455–459.
20. Hodis HN, Mack WJ, LaBree L, et al. Reduction in carotid arterial wall thickness using lovastatin and dietary therapy: a randomized controlled clinical trial. Ann Intern Med 1996;124:548–556.
21. Walker SP, Rimm EB, Ascherio A, et al. Body size and fat distribution as predictors of stroke among US men. Am J Epidemiol 1996;144:1143–1150.
22. Rexrode KM, Hennekens CH, Willett WC, et al. A prospective study of body mass index, weight change, and risk of stroke in women. JAMA 1997;277:1539–1545.
23. Gordon NF, Gulanick M, Costa F, et al. AHA Scientific Statement. Physical activity and exercise recommendations for stroke survivors. Circulation 2004;109:2031–2041.

24. National Institutes of Health, National Heart, Lung, and Blood Institute. Third report of the National Cholesterol Education Program (NCEP) Expert Panel on Detection, Evaluation, and Treatment of High Blood Cholesterol in Adults (Adult Treatment Panel III). NIH Publication No. 02-5215, September 2002.

25. Joshipura KJ, Acherio A, Manson JE, et al. Fruit and vegetable intake in relation to risk of ischemic stroke. JAMA 1999;282:1233–1239.

26. Chobanian AV, Bakris GL, Black HR, et al. Seventh report of the Joint National Committee on Prevention, Detection, Evaluation, and Treatment of High Blood Pressure. Hypertension 2003;42:1206–1252.

27. HHS Publication No. HHS-ODPHP-2005-01-DGA-A. Dietary Guidelines for Americans 2005, United States Department of Health and Human Services, United States Department of Agriculture. Available at: http://www.healthierus.gov/dietaryguidelines. Accessed February 8, 2007.

28. Antman EM, Anbe DT, Armstrong PW, et al. ACC/AHA guidelines for the management of patients with ST-segment myocardial infarction: a report of the American College of Cardiology/American Heart Association Task Force on Practice Guidelines (Committee to Revise the 1999 Guidelines for the Management of Patients With Acute Myocardial Infarction). Circulation 2004;110:e82–e293.

29. Smith SC, Blair SN, Bonow RO, et al. AHA/ACC guidelines for preventing heart attack and death in patients with atherosclerotic cardiovascular disease: 2001 update. A statement for healthcare professionals from the American Heart Association and the American College of Cardiology. Circulation 2001;104:1577–1579.

30. Fletcher GF. Exercise in the prevention of stroke. Health Rep 1994;6:106–110.

31. Abbott RD, Rodriguez BL, Burchfiel CM, et al. Physical activity in older, middle aged men and reduced risk of stroke: the Honolulu Heart Program. Am J Epidemiol 1994;139:881–893.

32. Kiely DK, Wolf PA, Cupples LA, et al. Physical activity and stroke risk: the Framingham Study. Am J Epidemiol 1994;140:608–620.

33. Haheim LL, Holme I, Hjermann I, et al. Risk factors of stroke incidence and mortality: a 12 year follow-up of the Oslo Study. Stroke 1993;24:1484–1489.

34. Manson JE, Stampfer MJ, Willett WC, et al. Physical activity and the incidence of coronary heart disease and stroke in women [Abstract]. Circulation 1995;91(Suppl):5.

35. Lindenstrom E, Boysen G, Nyboe J. Lifestyle factors and risk of cerebrovascular disease in women: the Copenhagen City Heart Study. Stroke 1993;24:1468–1472.

36. Gillum RF, Mussolino ME, Ingram DD. Physical activity and stroke incidence in women and men: the NHANES I Epidemiologic Follow-up Study. Am J Epidemiol 1996;143:860–869.

37. Sacco RL, Gan R, Boden-Albala B, et al. Leisure time physical activity and ischemic stroke risk: the Northern Manhattan Stroke Study. Stroke 1998;29:380–387.

38. Wannamethee G, Shaper AG. Physical activity and stroke in British middle aged men. BMJ 1992;304:597–601.

39. Katzmarzyk PT. Physical activity status and chronic diseases. In: Kaminsky LA, ed. ACSM's Resource Manual for Guidelines for Exercise Testing and Prescription, 5th ed. Philadelphia: Lippincott Williams & Wilkins, 2006:122–135.

40. Kohl HW III. Physical activity and cardiovascular disease: evidence for a dose response. Med Sci Sports Exerc 2001;33(Suppl):S472–S483.

41. Pate RR, Pratt M, Blair SN, et al. Physical activity and public health: a recommendation from the Centers for Disease Control and Prevention and the American College of Sports Medicine. JAMA 1995;273:402–407.

42. U.S. Department of Health and Human Services. Physical activity and health: a report of the Surgeon General. Atlanta: U.S. Department of Health and Human Services, Centers for Disease Control and Prevention, National Center for Chronic Disease Prevention and Health Promotion, 1996.

43. Centers for Disease Control and Prevention. Available at: http://www.cdc.gov/nccdphp/dnpa/physical/recommendations/adults.htm. Accessed July 26, 2005.

44. National Institutes of Health: Consensus Development Panel on Physical Activity and Cardiovascular Health. Physical activity and cardiovascular health. JAMA 1996;276:214–246.

45. Hu G, Sarti C, Jousilahti P, et al. Leisure time, occupational, and commuting physical activity and the risk of stroke. Stroke 2005;36:1994–1999.

46. Brinkman JR, Hoskins TA. Physical conditioning and altered self concept in rehabilitated hemiplegic patients. Phys Ther 1979;7:859–865.

47. Duncan P, Richards L, Wallace D, et al. A randomized controlled pilot study of a home based exercise program for individuals with mild and moderate stroke. Stroke 1998;29:2055–2060.

48. Engardt M, Knutsson E, Jonsson M, et al. Dynamic muscle strength training in stroke patients: effects of knee extension torque, electromyographic activity, and motor function. Arch Phys Med Rehabil 1995;76:419–425.

49. Gordon NF, Contractor A, Leighton RF. Resistance training for hypertension and stroke patients. In: Graves JE, Franklin BA, eds. Resistance Training for Health and Rehabilitation. Champaign, IL: Human Kinetics, 2001:237–251.

50. Hesse S, Bertlet C, Jahnke MT, et al. Treadmill training with partial body weight support compared with physiotherapy in nonambulatory hemiparetic patients. Stroke 1995;26:976–981.

51. Macko RF, DeSouza CA, Tretter LD, et al. Treadmill aerobic exercise training reduces the energy expenditure and cardiovascular demands of hemiparetic gait in chronic stroke patients: a preliminary report. Stroke 1997;28:326–330.

52. Macco RF, Smith GV, Dobrovolny CL, et al. Treadmill training improves fitness reserve in chronic stroke patients. Arch Phys Med Rehabil 2001;82:879–884.

53. Potempa K, Lopez M, Braun LT, et al. Physiological outcomes of aerobic exercise training in hemiparetic stroke patients. Stroke 1995;26:101–105.

54. Rimmer JH, Riley B, Creviston T, et al. Exercise training in a predominately African-American group of stroke survivors. Med Sci Sports Exerc 2000;32:1990–1996.

55. Sharp SA, Brouwer BJ. Isokinetic strength training of a hemiparetic knee: effects on function and spasticity. Arch Phys Med Rehabil 1997;78:1231–1236.

56. Shepherd RB. Exercise and training to optimize functional motor performance in stroke: driving neural reorganization? Neural Plast 2001;8:121–129.

57. Silver KH, Macko RF, Forrester LW, et al. Effects of aerobic treadmill training on gait velocity, cadence and gait symmetry in chronic hemiparetic stroke: a preliminary report. Neurorehabil Neural Repair 2000;14:65–71.

58. Weiss A, Suzuki T, Bean J, et al. High intensity strength training improves strength and functional performance after stroke. Am J Phys Med Rehabil 2000;79:369–376.

59. Whitall J, McCombe Waller S, Silver KH, et al. Repetitive bilateral arm training with rhythmic auditory cueing improves motor function in chronic hemiparetic stroke. Stroke 2000;31:2390–2395.

60. Thompson PD, Buchner D, Pina IL, et al. Exercise and physical activity in the prevention and treatment of atherosclerotic cardiovascular disease. Circulation 2003;107:3109–3116.

61. Lee CD, Blair SN. Cardiorespiratory fitness and stroke mortality in men. Med Sci Sports Exerc 2002;34:592–595.

62. Paffenbarger RS Jr, Hyde RT, Wing AL, et al. Physical activity, all cause mortality, and longevity in college alumni. N Engl J Med 1986;314:605–613.

63. Pate RR, Pratt M, Blair SN, et al. Physical activity and public health: a recommendation from the Centers for Disease Control and Prevention and the American College of Sports Medicine. JAMA 1995;273:402–407.

Peripheral Arterial Disease

At the end of this chapter the reader should be able to:

1. Explain the risks associated with peripheral arterial disease.
2. Summarize the prevention and treatment options for peripheral arterial disease.
3. Describe appropriate nutritional strategies for patients with peripheral arterial disease.
4. Suggest appropriate exercises for patients with risk factors for peripheral arterial disease.
5. Formulate a basic nutrition, exercise, and smoking-cessation program for a patient at risk for developing peripheral arterial disease.

OVERVIEW OF PERIPHERAL ARTERIAL DISEASE

Atherosclerosis, or a narrowing of the arteries as a result of plaque formation, is one of the most common causes of death.[1] Throughout the past several decades, the focus of atherosclerosis has been on the coronary arteries in the heart. It is well known, however, that atherosclerosis is a systemic disease, and if signs and symptoms of atherosclerosis are found in one region of the body, they are also likely to exist in other areas.[1] Other regions of the body where atherosclerosis is likely to exist besides the heart include the cerebrovascular, aortic, renal, and peripheral or lower extremity arteries.[1] This chapter will focus on the prevention and treatment of atherosclerosis of the lower extremity arteries.

A great deal of confusion exists concerning the terminology of atherosclerosis of the lower extremity arteries. The most common term used is **peripheral arterial disease (PAD).**[2] Others use the term peripheral vascular disease (PVD) to refer to both venous and arterial vascular disease. A new term that is being used is simply lower-extremity arterial disease. This term is not yet used widely; therefore, we will use the term PAD throughout the remainder of this chapter on the primary and secondary prevention of atherosclerosis in the lower extremity arteries.[2]

Prevalence and Health Risks Associated With Peripheral Arterial Disease

Peripheral arterial disease has traditionally been diagnosed and defined by the presence of lower-extremity pain with exertion, often called **claudication,** or absent or markedly diminished pulses on physical examination.[1] Of those individuals with PAD, only 10 to 30% have classic claudication symptoms.[1] It is currently more common and effective to use ankle–brachial index (ABI) to diagnose PAD because an ABI of 0.90 or less is 90% sensitive and 95% specific for PAD.[2] Current data from the Framingham Heart Study show that PAD prevalence is manifested in 3.9% of men and 3.3% of women between the ages of 55 to 64 years and 65 to 74 years, respectively.[2,3] Claudication occurs in 1.9% of men and 0.8% of women during these same age ranges.[2,3] Using ABI to define PAD, it has been found that 2 to 3% of men and women have PAD by the age of 50 years and approximately 20% have PAD at 75 years of age or older.[2] In addition, PAD seems to occur more frequently in Hispanic and African American individuals.[2]

Patients with PAD are at an increased risk for other diseases associated with **cardiovascular disease** (CVD). Patients with PAD have a risk for **myocardial infarction** that is four times greater than those without PAD and a two to three times increased risk for **stroke.**[1] Other data show that in patients with PAD, 85% have **coronary heart disease** and 60% have cerebrovascular disease with greater than 30% carotid artery stenosis.[1]

Pathophysiology of Peripheral Arterial Disease

Because atherosclerosis is a systemic phenomenon, the pathophysiology of PAD atherosclerosis is the same process as that described for coronary heart disease and stroke in Chapters 8 and 9, respectively, except that it occurs in the peripheral vasculature. The process is complex and involves the interrelated occurrences of lipid abnormalities, inflammation, platelet activation, **endothelial dysfunction,** thrombosis, and other factors.[4] Because the vascular structure and endothelial cells become damaged in the atherosclerotic process, the vasodilatory action of the arteries does not function properly and with the addition of plaque build-up, blood flow is impeded to the lower extremities.[5] Patients who have at least 50% atherosclerotic stenosis in their lower extremity arteries can begin to experience intermittent claudication symptoms during **exercise.**[5] Those with greater than 80% stenosis can experience symptoms during rest.[5] Similar to a myocardial infarction or unstable angina of the heart, if the atherosclerotic plaque becomes unstable, it can rupture, creating a thrombus, and occlude blood flow to the lower extremities.[5] The lower extremity arteries that are most commonly involved in PAD are the femoropopliteal-tibial and aortoiliac, along with carotid, vertebral, splenic, renal, and brachiocephalic.[6]

The risk factors that contribute to the development and progression of PAD are similar to other forms of atherosclerotic disease. The traditional non-modifiable risks of age, gender, family history, and race exist. In addition, the modifiable risks of smoking, **diabetes mellitus, dyslipidemia,** and **hypertension** remain as traditional risk factors for PAD.[5–8] Within these traditional, modifiable risks, smoking and diabetes have been shown to be the strongest risk factors for atherosclerotic vascular disease, including PAD.[7] Diabetes appears to be a greater risk factor for PAD in women than in men and is associated with peroneal and tibial atherosclerosis.[7] Cigarette smoking is associated with aortoiliac atherosclerosis, and young women who are heavy smokers have a distinct

TABLE 10–1	Environmental Risk Factors for Peripheral Arterial Disease

Age
Gender
Race
Family history
Cigarette smoking
Diabetes
Dyslipidemia
Hypertension
Physical inactivity
Homocysteinemia
Elevated lipoprotein (a)
Elevated apolipoprotein (apo) A-1
Elevated vascular cell adhesion molecule 1 (VCAM-1)
Elevated fibrinogen
Elevated intercellular adhesion molecule 1 (ICAM-1)
Elevated high-sensitivity C-reactive protein (hs-CRP)

Source: Smith SC, Milani RV, Arnett DK, et al. Atherosclerotic vascular disease conference. Writing group II: risk factors. Circulation 2004;109:2613–2616.

risk for hypoplastic aortoiliac syndrome.[7] Other, more novel risk factors have also been listed for atherosclerotic disease, including PAD. Among them are included lipoprotein(a), apolipoprotein (apo) A-1, high-sensitivity C-reactive protein (hs-CRP), and homocysteine.[7,8] A list of the risk factors for PAD is provided in Table 10-1.

PERIPHERAL ARTERIAL DISEASE PREVENTION AND TREATMENT

From a pharmacist's perspective, prevention of PAD can be approached with two different strategies. Because PAD is an atherosclerotic process that is similar to, and most often occurs in conjunction with, coronary heart disease (CHD) and ischemic cerebrovascular disease, the general primary prevention strategies for CHD, stroke, and PAD are the same. As discussed in Chapters 8 and 9, pharmacists are in an ideal position to offer primary prevention strategies to patients who may be at risk for PAD. The second strategy involves pharmacists' participation in the secondary prevention of PAD by controlling risk factors to prevent the further progression of cardiovascular disease.

For primary prevention, many of the modifiable risk factors listed in Table 10-1 can be monitored by pharmacists. As stated earlier, smoking and diabetes may be the most significant contributing risk factors to PAD.[7] Chapter 4 discusses smoking-cessation programs and strategies that pharmacists can use within their practice setting. Pharmacists can also assist patients with diabetes management to decrease PAD risk. In addition, hypertension and dyslipidemia programs can be offered as a service by pharmacists to not only manage those particular diseases but also decrease the overall risk for cardiovascular disease.

The American College of Cardiology/American Heart Association (ACC/AHA) Guidelines for the Management of Patients With Peripheral Arterial Disease discusses in great detail the treatment for lower extremity PAD (http://www.americanheart.org/presenter.jhtml?identifier=3004542).[8] The treatment for PAD outlined in these guidelines

TABLE 10–2	**Medications Used to Treat and Prevent Peripheral Arterial Disease**

Antihypertensive drugs (i.e., β-blockers and ACE inhibitors; see Chapter 6)
Antidyslipidemic drugs (i.e., HMG CoA reductase inhibitors; see Chapter 7)
Diabetes mellitus medications (see Chapter 12)
Nicotine replacement or bupropion (see Chapter 4)
Antiplatelet drugs

ACE, angiotensin-converting enzyme; HMG-CoA, 3-hydroxy-3-methylglutaryl coenzyme A.

is primarily focused on improving patient symptoms and cardiovascular risk reduction. As stated earlier in this chapter, patients with PAD are also at increased risk for heart attack and stroke. Therefore, secondary prevention of atherosclerotic vascular disease is an important aspect of treatment for patients with PAD.

Reducing the overall risk for cardiovascular disease in patients with PAD can be done through the use of lipid-lowering drugs, antihypertensive drugs, diabetes therapies, smoking cessation, and antiplatelet drugs.[8] Smoking-cessation programs can be used in the pharmacy practice setting as discussed in Chapter 4. However, it is beyond the scope of this chapter to discuss in detail each of the medications used to treat PAD. Controlling blood lipids, blood pressure, and diabetes for patients with PAD should be done by following the practice guidelines for each of the respective diseases. A list of the drugs used in the treatment of PAD is provided in Table 10-2.

Exercise is an important aspect of PAD treatment. As discussed earlier, claudication is a primary symptom of PAD and is characterized by walking-induced pain in one or both legs that does not subside until rest.[9] Claudication pain occurs because of insufficient blood flow to the muscles in the legs.[10] To avoid this leg discomfort, patients with PAD and claudication often decrease their walking pace and distance and, ultimately, **physical activity** in general.[9] This results in a decreased physical conditioning by as much as 50% in PAD patients compared with individuals of similar age without PAD.[9] This can then lead to a deconditioned state that results in patients becoming homebound and dependent on others, which often results in decreased quality of life.[9,11]

Lower Extremity Disease

As individuals age, the ability to maintain independence becomes a major quality-of-life factor. Persons who are able to transport themselves from place to place, such as the grocery store or shopping center, and who can perform simple household chores independently have been shown to exhibit a higher standard of quality of life. Mobility limitations can significantly decrease this independence. The term lower extremity disease, or LED, has been used to describe the condition of patients who experience either peripheral arterial disease (PAD) or peripheral neuropathy (PN).[12] Persons with LED are at increased risk for mobility limitations.[13,14]

A study conducted of more than 6,000 participants showed that during 1999 to 2002, approximately 20% of adults older than 40 years of age had LED.[12] Individuals with diabetes experienced nearly twice the prevalence of LED compared with those without diabetes. Among persons with limited mobility, the most frequently reported limitations were walking a quarter mile and walking up 10 steps without resting. Among patients who had the diagnosis of both LED and diabetes, 33% had difficulty walking a quarter mile and walking up 10 steps, and 6% reported difficulty walking from one room to another on the same level.[12]

Mobility limitations can have a spiral effect on patients. As the symptoms of LED become more prevalent, mobility declines over time and the overall amount of physical activity performed also declines. Attempts to perform physical activity can lead to further worsening of the symptoms, which can then cause many patients to stop activity. The sedentary lifestyle that ensues with mobility limitations then leads to physical deconditioning that can result in the inability to perform even simple tasks such as household cleaning and walking to get the mail and increased risks for cardiovascular disease. Therefore, maintaining or regaining mobility is an important issue for patients with PAD and LED to maintain independence and quality of life and decrease the risk for other diseases.

Pharmacists can become involved by identifying patients who may be at risk for LED, such as those with PAD and diabetes. Referring patients with LED to other healthcare professionals who offer treatment and rehabilitation is an excellent service that pharmacists can provide to their patients. Preventing the worsening of LED before it leads to severe mobility limitations can help patients maintain independence and a high-standard quality of life.

Exercise is recommended to patients with PAD to relieve their exertional symptoms, improve walking capacity, improve quality of life, and decrease atherosclerotic disease risk.[9] The improved exercise tolerance is thought to occur in part as a result of increased blood flow to the legs, more favorable redistribution of blood flow, reduced viscosity of the blood, greater reliance on aerobic metabolism and less on anaerobic metabolism, and improved walking efficiency.[10] Patients with PAD and intermittent claudication are recommended by the ACC/AHA guidelines to participate in supervised exercise training as an initial treatment modality along with medication and atherosclerotic disease risk reduction.[8] This exercise training should be performed for a minimum of 30 to 45 minutes at least three times per week for a minimum of 12 weeks.[8] It is important to note that the usefulness of an unsupervised exercise program is not well established as an effective initial treatment modality for patients with intermittent claudication.[8] The enrollment in a supervised program with electrocardiographic (ECG), heart rate, and blood pressure monitoring is recommended by the American College of Cardiology, the American Heart Association, and the American College of Sports Medicine.[8,9]

Walking is generally the preferred mode of activity and should be preceded by 5 to 10 minutes of warm-up activity, which usually consists of non–weight-bearing activity such as bicycling.[9] The initial walking workload should be set at a level that will cause claudication symptoms within 3 to 5 minutes after beginning the activity.[9] Patients should walk at this level until they reach a claudication pain of moderate severity (3 of 4 on the claudication pain scale), and then they should follow this by a brief period of standing or sitting until symptoms resolve.[8–10] This exercise-rest-exercise pattern should continue initially for a total of 35 minutes and be increased by 5 minutes each session until 50 minutes of continuous walking is accomplished.[8] Each exercise session should be followed by 5 to 10 minutes of cool-down activity similar to that performed during the warm-up.[8]

Similar to patients with CHD, stroke, and **heart failure,** supervising patients with PAD who are beginning an exercise program is in most cases beyond the scope of expertise of

TABLE 10–3 Program Adherence Recommendations for Patients With or at Risk for Peripheral Arterial Disease

Patient education about prevention and treatment

Ensure the patient has a clear understanding of the disease treatment and prevention components and the importance of each

Discuss the risk and benefit of each treatment alternative

Multiple adherence strategies work better than a single approach

Weekly contact with patients for the first 4 weeks of the program, then monthly thereafter, to continually assess the patient's progress and troubleshoot problems

Set achievable goals

Refer to a claudication exercise rehabilitation program

Exercise testing should be conducted before beginning an exercise program to ensure a safe and patient-specific exercise prescription

Obtain baseline assessment of dietary intake

Institute a self-monitoring program such as keeping a log of food intake and exercise participation

Identify patient-specific barriers to the lifestyle changes

Design a program that is reasonable, gradual, and easily implemented

Source: Hirsch AT, Haskal ZJ, Hertzer NR, et al. ACC/AHA guidelines for the management of patients with peripheral arterial disease (lower extremity, renal, mesenteric, and abdominal aortic): executive summary: a report of the American College of Cardiology/American Heart Association Task Force on Practice Guidelines (Writing Committee to Develop Guidelines for the Management of Patients With Peripheral Arterial Disease [Lower Extremity, Renal, Mesenteric, and Abdominal Aortic]). J Am Coll Cardiol 2006;47:1239–1312.

most pharmacists. The role of a pharmacist in the treatment of PAD with exercise is one of support and encouragement. Pharmacists can assist by helping patients maintain compliance with their treatment modalities. Table 10-3 lists suggestions that may help patients adhere to their treatment and prevention strategies. Managing the exercise prescriptions for patients who are at risk for but do not yet have PAD and other cardiovascular diseases can be done by pharmacists within their practice setting. This will be discussed in the physical activity section of this chapter.

NUTRITION AND PERIPHERAL ARTERIAL DISEASE

Proper nutrition is an important component in reducing the general risk for cardiovascular disease. There are no specific recommendations with regard to nutrition for the treatment and prevention of PAD. Therefore, the general recommendations set out in the National Cholesterol Education Program, Adult Treatment Panel III Guidelines (NCEP ATP III) (http://www.nhlbi.nih.gov/guidelines/) and those discussed in the Seventh Report of the Joint National Committee of Prevention, Detection, Evaluation, and Treatment of High Blood Pressure (JNC 7) (http://www.nhlbi.nih.gov/guidelines/) as well as the Dietary Guidelines for Americans 2005 (http://www.healthierus.gov/dietaryguidelines/) would apply for the primary and secondary prevention of PAD.[15–19] The recommendations stated in each of these guidelines are similar and primarily focus

TABLE 10–4   Dietary Recommendations for Patients With Peripheral Arterial Disease

Nutrient	Recommendation
Total calories	Balance calorie intake with expenditure to obtain appropriate body weight
Carbohydrate[a]	50–60% of total calorie intake
Fiber	20–30 g/day
Protein	Around 15% of total calorie intake
Monounsaturated fat	Up to 20% of total calorie intake
Polyunsaturated fat	Up to 10% of total calorie intake
Saturated fat	Less than 7% of total calorie intake
Total fat	25–35% of total calorie intake
Dietary cholesterol	Less than 200 mg/day

[a]Most carbohydrate intake should come from whole grains, fruits, and vegetables.
Source: HHS Publication o. HHS-ODPHP-2005-01-DGA-A. Dietary Guidelines for Americans 2005, U.S. Department of Health and Human Services, U.S. Department of Agriculture. Available at: http://healthierus.gov/dietaryguidelines. Accessed February 9, 2007.

on promoting health and reducing the risk for CHD and other chronic diseases by lowering **low-density lipoprotein** cholesterol (LDL) and blood pressure. The overarching themes are to eat fewer calories, be more physically active, and make wiser food choices.[17] Because the pathophysiology of PAD, **ischemic stroke,** and CHD are so similar, this information can and should also be applied to individuals who are implementing primary and secondary strategies of PAD prevention. Chapter 1 discusses specific information regarding dietary modifications for patients at risk for developing cardiovascular diseases. Table 10-4 lists dietary recommendations for the prevention of PAD.

PHYSICAL ACTIVITY AND PERIPHERAL ARTERIAL DISEASE

As discussed in Chapter 2, physical activity is an important component for overall health and decreased mortality rates. **Physical inactivity** is well established as a major modifiable risk factor for patients who are sedentary and at risk for developing cardiovascular disease.[20] Although the ACC/AHA Guidelines for the Management of Patients With Peripheral Arterial Disease do not specifically address the topic of exercise and primary disease prevention, general exercise guidelines apply to all Americans and especially to those who may be at risk for cardiovascular diseases such as PAD.[8] The American Heart Association has released a scientific statement that suggests all healthcare professionals promote increased physical activity among their patients.[20] Regular amounts of aerobic physical activity produce cardiovascular changes that increase exercise capacity, endurance, and **muscular strength** and prevent the incidence of heart disease in addition to decreasing the symptoms associated with cardiovascular disease.[20] Exercise can decrease the risk for and aid in controlling chronic diseases that can lead to atherosclerosis and heart disease such as **obesity, type 2 diabetes,** hypertension, and dyslipidemia as well as other diseases such as **osteoporosis,** depression, breast cancer, and colon cancer.[20–31]

The evidence supporting the incorporation of increased physical activity among all individuals in an effort to decrease the risk of atherosclerotic disease is very strong. Several prospective epidemiologic studies have supported the causal relationship between exercise and lower rates of CHD.[20,32–36] These studies show that individuals who participate in physical activity generally experience a CHD rate that is half that of sedentary individuals. Therefore, it is clear that primary CHD prevention strategies must incorporate increased physical activity as part of a disease prevention plan. The current recommendations by the AHA (http://www.americanheart.org/presenter.jhtml?identifier=1200013), Centers for Disease Control (CDC) (http://www.cdc.gov/nccdphp/dnpa/physical/recommendations/index.htm), American College of Sports Medicine (ACSM) (http://www.acsm.org/), and the Surgeon General (http://www.surgeongeneral.gov/) state that individuals should engage in 30 minutes or more of moderate-intensity physical activity on most (preferably all) days of the week.[20,21] Table 10-5 lists exercise recommendations for the prevention of CHD.

The role of the pharmacist with regard to physical activity and PAD is for the most part in the area of primary prevention. Pharmacists can identify patients who may be at greater risk for cardiovascular disease and recommend and monitor a physical activity program with the primary goal of decreasing that cardiovascular risk. In addition, patients who currently have PAD should participate in a supervised exercise program to decrease PAD symptoms as well as decrease overall cardiovascular risk. Pharmacists can encourage these patients to participate in such a program and assist them with strategies that can maintain and enhance adherence. All healthcare providers, including

TABLE 10–5 **Physical Activity Recommendations for Patients With Peripheral Arterial Disease**

Exercise Variable	Recommendation
Goals	Decrease risk for PAD and CVD
	Decrease risk factors for PAD and CVD such as diabetes, elevated blood pressure, elevated triglyceride concentrations, low HDL-C concentrations, obesity, stroke, myocardial function
	Increase exercise peak workload and endurance
Type	Aerobic exercises (large muscle activities) such as walking, jogging, running, cycling, or individual aerobic exercise preference
	Resistance training can be adjunctive to aerobic exercises
Intensity	Moderate intensity endurance activity
Duration	30 minutes or more continuous or intermittent exercise per day
Frequency	Most, preferably all days of the week
Lifestyle activity	Increase overall daily activities through increasing the duration of activities of daily living (e.g., walking the dog, taking stairs, yard work, household duties)

Source: U.S. Department of Health and Human Services. Physical activity and health: a report of the Surgeon General. Atlanta: U.S. Department of Health and Human Services, Centers for Disease Control and Prevention, National Center for Chronic Disease Prevention and Health Promotion, 1996.
CVD, cardiovascular disease; HDL-C, high-density lipoprotein cholesterol; PAD, peripheral arterial disease.

pharmacists, should educate their patients on the importance of physical activity for both primary and secondary disease prevention.

PHARMACY PRACTICE APPLICATION

Applying prevention strategies for PAD and other diseases to the regular work duties of a pharmacist is well within the scope of pharmacy practice. The primary goal of pharmacists and all healthcare professionals should be to prevent and treat disease. Cardiovascular disease is the most common cause of death in the United States, and as a result many of the patients who pharmacists come in contact with throughout the day have cardiovascular disease risk factors or the disease itself. Regardless of pharmacy practice setting, incorporating disease prevention strategies into the drug counseling of these patients should become a standard of practice for pharmacists as the profession is well positioned within the community to act as a reliable and easily accessible resource for patients.

CASE STUDY

B.N. is a 32-year-old white female with a medical history of **type 1 diabetes mellitus.** *She has been getting her insulin prescriptions filled at your pharmacy for the past 8 years. She is currently managing her blood glucose with split mixed injections of NPH and regular insulin before breakfast and again before the evening meal. After a conversation with you about disease prevention, she decides to enroll in your pharmacist-managed disease prevention program.*

On further analysis you discover that B.N. is not married, has no children, is 5′ 7″ tall, weighs 135 lb, and has a resting blood pressure of 138/88 mm Hg and a heart rate of 88 beats/min. She has a distant family history of CHD (uncle) but reports no participation in physical activity, and she frequently eats fast food and smokes one pack of cigarettes per day for the past 15 years. A blood lipid panel and hemoglobin A_{1c} level were unavailable. Her 4-day dietary analysis revealed the following:

> *Total caloric intake per day = 2,054 calories*
> *Carbohydrates = 45% of total calories*
> *Monounsaturated fats = 14% of total calories*
> *Polyunsaturated fats = 11% of total calories*
> *Saturated fats = 15% of total calories*
> *Total fats = 40% of total calories*
> *Protein = 15% of total calories*
> *Total dietary cholesterol = 425 mg*
> *Fiber = 12 g*
> *Calcium = 750 mg/day*
> *Potassium = 3,260 mg/day*
> *Magnesium = 328 mg/day*
> *Sodium = 4,562 mg/day*

Case Activities

1. *Write an SOAP note for B.N.*
2. *List B.N.'s risk factors for PAD and cardiovascular disease and determine whether intervention is needed.*
3. *If needed, design a program that includes nutrition, exercise, and smoking-cessation counseling for B.N. that will decrease her risk for PAD and atherosclerosis.*

REFERENCES

1. Faxon DP, Creager MA, Smith SC, et al. Atherosclerotic vascular disease conference. Executive summary. Circulation 2004;109:2595–2604.

2. Pasternak RC, Criqui MH, Benjamin EJ, et al. Atherosclerotic vascular disease conference. Writing group I: epidemiology. Circulation 2004;109:2605–2612.

3. Murabito JM, Evans JC, Nieto K, et al. Prevalence of clinical correlates of peripheral arterial disease in the Framingham Offspring Study. Am Heart J 2002;143:961–965.

4. Faxon DP, Fuster V, Libby P, et al. Atherosclerotic vascular disease conference. Writing group III: pathophysiology. Circulation 2004;109:2617–2625.

5. Spencer AP, Weart CW. Peripheral vascular disorders. In: Koda-Kimble MA, ed. Applied Therapeutics: The Clinical Use of Drugs, 8th ed. Philadelphia: Lippincott Williams & Wilkins, 2005:15.1–15.16.

6. Hoeben BJ, Talbert RL. Peripheral arterial disease. In: Dipiro JT, ed. Pharmacotherapy: A Pathophysiologic Approach, 6th ed. New York: McGraw-Hill, 2005:453–460.

7. Smith SC, Milani RV, Arnett DK, et al. Atherosclerotic vascular disease conference. Writing group II: risk factors. Circulation 2004;109:2613–2616.

8. Hirsch AT, Haskal ZJ, Hertzer NR, et al. ACC/AHA guidelines for the management of patients with peripheral arterial disease (lower extremity, renal, mesenteric, and abdominal aortic): executive summary: a report of the American College of Cardiology/American Heart Association Task Force on Practice Guidelines (Writing Committee to Develop Guidelines for the Management of Patients With Peripheral Arterial Disease [Lower Extremity, Renal, Mesenteric, and Abdominal Aortic]). J Am Coll Cardiol 2006;47:1239–1312.

9. Whaley MH, ed. ACSM's Guidelines for Exercise Testing and Prescription/American College of Sports Medicine. Philadelphia: Lippincott Williams & Wilkins, 2006:225–227.

10. Womack CJ, Gardner AW. Peripheral arterial disease. In: Durstine JL, Moore GE, eds. ACSM's Exercise Management for Persons With Chronic Diseases and Disabilities, 2nd ed. Champaign, IL: Human Kinetics, 2003:81–85.

11. Treat-Jacobson D, Halverson SL, Ratchford A, et al. A patient derived perspective of health related quality of life with peripheral arterial disease. J Nurs Scholarship 2002;34:55–60.

12. Eberhardt MS, Saydah S, Paulose-Ram R, Tao M. Mobility limitation among persons aged >40 years with and without diagnosed diabetes and lower extremity disease—United States, 1999–2002. MMWR Morb Mortal Wkly Rep 2005;54:1183–1186.

13. McDermott MM, Liu K, Greenland P, et al. Functional decline in peripheral arterial disease: associations with the ankle brachial index and leg syndrome. JAMA 2004;292:453–461.

14. Resnick HE, Vinik AI, Schwartz AV, et al. Independent effects of peripheral nerve dysfunction on lower-extremity physical function in old age: the Women's Health and Aging Study. Diabetes Care 2000;23:1642–1647.

15. National Institutes of Health, National Heart, Lung, and Blood Institute. Third report of the National Cholesterol Education Program (NCEP) Expert Panel on Detection, Evaluation, and Treatment of High Blood Cholesterol in Adults (Adult Treatment Panel III). NIH Publication No. 02-5215, September 2002.

16. Chobanian AV, Bakris GL, Black HR, et al. Seventh report of the Joint National Committee on Prevention, Detection, Evaluation, and Treatment of High Blood Pressure. Hypertension 2003;42:1206–1252.

17. HHS Publication No. HHS-ODPHP-2005-01-DGA-A. Dietary Guidelines for Americans 2005, U.S. Department of Health and Human Services, U.S. Department of Agriculture. Available at: http://healthierus.gov/dietaryguidelines. Accessed February 9, 2007.

18. Antman EM, Anbe DT, Armstrong PW, et al. ACC/AHA guidelines for the management of patients with ST-segment myocardial infarction: a report of the American College of Cardiology/American Heart Association Task Force on Practice Guidelines (Committee to Revise the 1999 Guidelines for the Management of Patients With Acute Myocardial Infarction). Circulation 2004;110:e82–e293.

19. Smith SC, Blair SN, Bonow RO, et al. AHA/ACC guidelines for preventing heart attack and death in patients with atherosclerotic cardiovascular disease: 2001 update. A statement for healthcare professionals from the American Heart Association and the American College of Cardiology. Circulation 2001;104:1577–1579.

20. Thompson PD, Buchner D, Pina IL, et al. Exercise and physical activity in the prevention and treatment of atherosclerotic cardiovascular disease. Circulation 2003;107:3109–3116.

21. Pate RR, Pratt M, Blair SN, et al. Physical activity and public health: a recommendation from the Centers for Disease Control and Prevention and the American College of Sports Medicine. JAMA 1995;273:402–407.

22. U.S. Department of Health and Human Services. Physical activity and health: a report of the Surgeon General. Atlanta: U.S. Department of Health and Human Services, Centers for Disease Control and Prevention, National Center for Chronic Disease Prevention and Health Promotion, 1996.

23. Centers for Disease Control and Prevention. Available at: www.cdc.gov/nccdphp/dnpa/physical/recommendations/adults.htm. Accessed July 26, 2005.

24. National Institutes of Health: Consensus Development Panel on Physical Activity and Cardiovascular Health. Physical activity and cardiovascular health. JAMA 1996;276:214–246.

25. Katzmarzyk PT. Physical activity status and chronic disease. In: Kaminsky LA, ed. ACSM's Resource Manual for Guidelines for Exercise Testing and Prescription. Philadelphia: Lippincott Williams & Wilkins, 2006: 122–135.

26. Knowler WC, Barrett-Connor E, Flowler SE, et al., for the Diabetes Prevention Program Research Group. Reduction in the incidence of type 2 diabetes with lifestyle intervention or metformin. N Engl J Med 2002;346: 393–403.

27. Vuori IM. Dose response of physical activity and low back pain, osteoarthritis, and osteoporosis. Med Sci Sports Exerc 2001;33(6 Suppl):S551–S586.

28. Wing RR, Hill JO. Successful weight loss maintenance. Annu Rev Nutr 2001;21:323–341.

29. Polluck KM. Exercise in treating depression: broadening the psychotherapist's role. J Clin Psychol 2001;57: 1289–1300.

30. Breslow RA, Ballard-Barbash R, Munoz K, et al. Long-term recreational physical activity and breast cancer in the National Health and Nutrition Examination Survey I epidemiology follow-up study. Cancer Epidemiol Biomarkers Prev 2001;10:805–808.

31. Slattery ML, Potter JD. Physical activity and colon cancer: confounding or interaction? Med Sci Sports Exerc 2002;34:913–919.

32. Lee IM, Paffenbarger RS, Hennekens CH, et al. Physical activity, physical fitness and longevity. Aging (Milano) 1997;9:2–11.

33. Powell KE, Thompson PD, Casperson CJ, et al. Physical activity and the incidence of coronary heart disease. Annu Rev Public Health 1987;8:253–287.

34. Blair SN, Jackson AS. Physical fitness and activity as separate heart disease risk factors: a meta-analysis. Med Sci Sports Exerc 2001;33:762–764.

35. U.S. Department of Health, Education, and Welfare. Smoking and Heath: Report of the Advisory Committee to the Surgeon General of the Public Health Services. Washington, D.C.: U.S. Department of Health, Education, and Welfare, Public Health Service, 1964. PHS Publication No. 1103. Available at: http://www.cdc.gov/tobacco/sgr/sgr_1964/sgr64.htm. Accessed December 15, 2005.

36. Sowers JR. Obesity as a cardiovascular risk factor. Am J Med 2003;115(Suppl 8A):37S–41S.

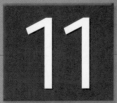
Heart Failure

OBJECTIVES

At the end of this chapter the reader should be able to:

1. Explain the risks associated with heart failure.
2. Summarize the treatment options available for heart failure.
3. Formulate a basic nutrition and physical activity program for patients at risk for heart failure.

OVERVIEW OF HEART FAILURE

Heart failure is a complex and often confusing disorder. As the prevalence of heart failure continues to rise, it is increasingly important for all healthcare providers to have not only a good understanding about the current treatments, but also knowledge about the effective strategies to prevent heart failure. Pharmacists can make a significant impact on the lives of patients who have heart failure by helping them manage the many medications that they may be taking. Additionally, pharmacists are ideally positioned to help reduce the risks associated with heart failure in selected patients. This chapter will discuss patients who are at risk for the development of heart failure and present strategies for pharmacists to help patients decrease those risks.

PREVALENCE, ECONOMIC COSTS, AND HEALTH RISKS ASSOCIATED WITH HEART FAILURE

Heart failure (HF) is characterized by the inability of the heart to adequately deliver oxygen to the body and has become a significant public health concern in the United States in recent decades.[1] Approximately 550,000 new cases of HF are diagnosed for the first time each year, and estimates predict that around 5 million Americans currently live with HF.[1,2] Heart failure accounts for 12 to 15 million physician office visits each year, with an incidence level that is approaching 10 per 1,000 people older than 65 years of age.[1,2] As a result of the increased prevalence of HF, it has become the most common Medicare diagnosis, costing more Medicare dollars than any other diagnosis. It is estimated that in 2005 the direct and indirect costs of HF were approximately $28 billion.[1,3] In addition, drug costs associated with HF in 2005 were almost $3 billion.[1,2]

The incidence of HF as well as the deaths associated with HF has continued to increase during the years despite improvements in both medication and non-medication treatments.[1] It is speculated that reasons associated with this include both the aging of the population and the recovery of patients after they have experienced a heart attack. Heart failure is primarily a condition of the elderly, and therefore, as patients get older, they are more likely to have HF. As will be explained later in the pathophysiology of HF, many patients obtain the diagnosis of HF after they have had a heart attack. The advances in the treatment of patients who are having a heart attack have improved a great deal in recent decades, resulting in more patients surviving such an event. Unfortunately, this has most likely resulted in an increased incidence of heart failure.[1]

PATHOPHYSIOLOGY OF HEART FAILURE

As stated above, HF is the inability of the heart to adequately deliver oxygen to the appropriate tissues of the body.[1] This is caused by an inability of the ventricles of the heart to fill with or eject blood.[1] HF is defined as a clinical syndrome because the diagnosis and classification are made on the basis of the symptoms that the patient is experiencing and the signs obtained from physical examination.[1] There is no single diagnostic test for HF because it is mostly a clinical diagnosis. Heart failure results in an impaired functional capacity, or the ability to perform physical tasks, as well as a decrease in the quality of life of the patients with this diagnosis.[1]

The clinical syndrome of HF can be caused by several different structural disorders of the heart. The most common cause of HF symptoms, however, is related to an impairment of the left ventricle of the heart.[1] Recall from anatomy class that the left ventricle is one of the four chambers in the heart. The left ventricle is the chamber that is primarily responsible for pumping blood out of the heart and to the body tissues. The volume of blood ejected from the heart during a particular unit of time (i.e., per minute) is called **cardiac output.** Structural impairment of the left ventricle will most often result in a decreased cardiac output. A decreased cardiac output will not allow for adequate amounts of blood to be circulated throughout the body, resulting in an insufficient amount of oxygen being delivered to the metabolizing tissues.[1]

Classic signs and symptoms resulting from HF include shortness of breath, fatigue, and fluid build-up in the lungs and extremities.[1] These findings commonly lead to a limited ability to perform physical tasks, such as **exercise,** as well as a decrease in the patient's quality of life. Not all symptoms are present at all times in patients with HF. Because of this, the older term "congestive heart failure or CHF" (which refers to having extra fluid in the body) has been replaced with the preferred term "heart failure."[1]

Heart failure is a disorder that progresses as a function of time and usually begins with myocardial injury.[4] In an attempt to compensate for this injury, the body responds in a number of ways to maintain adequate cardiac output.[1,4] Ironically, these compensatory mechanisms lead to HF symptoms and contribute to the further progression of HF. The current understanding of HF pathophysiology describes the activation of several endogenous neurohormones.[1,4] These neurohormonal changes play an important

TABLE 11–1	Environmental Risk Factors Leading to Heart Failure

Coronary heart disease
Myocardial infarction
Hypertension
Pulmonary hypertension
Dilated cardiomyopathy
Genetic causes
Valvular heart disease

role in causing the heart to change in shape and structure, often referred to as remodeling. These remodeling changes lead to HF symptoms.[1,4]

Several diseases have been identified that cause the initial myocardial injury that eventually leads to HF. Coronary artery disease, **hypertension,** and dilated cardiomyopathy have been identified as the cause of a majority of heart failure symptoms in the Western world.[1] As stated earlier, patients who experience a heart attack or multiple heart attacks can eventually experience HF symptoms. A common example is when a patient has a blocked coronary artery on the left side of the heart causing a lack of oxygen and myocardial tissue death to a part of the left ventricle. This can then lead to neurohormonal changes that cause myocardial remodeling, resulting in decreased cardiac output and heart failure symptoms. In fact, the HF guidelines written by the American College of Cardiology (ACC) and the American Heart Association (AHA) (http://www.americanheart.org/presenter.jhtml?identifier=3004542) state that any form of heart disease may ultimately lead to the HF syndrome.[1] A list of causes of HF is provided in Table 11-1.

HEART FAILURE PREVENTION AND TREATMENT

Because HF is a compilation of symptoms resulting in specific signs and symptoms rather than a disease that can be definitively diagnosed with specific tests, disease prevention is approached in a different manner. The primary goal in the prevention of HF is to adequately control the causes of myocardial injury.[1] This can then decrease the risks for obtaining HF symptoms.

Several diseases and lifestyle habits can lead to myocardial injury. Following the recommended guidelines of these diseases is an important first step in HF disease prevention. Patients with **atherosclerotic disease** (e.g., coronary, cerebral, and peripheral blood vessels) are likely to develop HF and, therefore, controlling the risk factors that lead to atherosclerotic disease can ultimately decrease the risk for HF.[1,5] Hyperlipidemia has been shown to significantly increase the risk for atherosclerotic disease and, therefore, adequately controlling blood lipid levels according to the **cholesterol** treatment guidelines can decrease the risk for HF.[1,6] In fact, treating high blood cholesterol according to the published guidelines has been shown to decrease the likelihood of death and of HF in patients who have previously had a heart attack.[7-10]

Elevated levels of systolic and, to a lesser extent, **diastolic blood pressure** are a major risk factor for the development of HF.[1] In one study, hypertension accounted for 39% of HF cases in men and 59% in women.[11] The lifetime risk of hypertension for those living in the United States is about 75%, with approximately one fourth of the American population currently having high blood pressure. Therefore, strategies to control hypertension are an important part in the prevention of HF. Long-term treatment of both systolic and diastolic blood pressure has been shown to decrease the risk of HF by as much as 50%.[12–15] Treating hypertension in patients who have previously had a heart attack can result in an 81% reduction in the incidence of HF.[13] Pharmacists and other healthcare providers should closely follow the current practice guidelines for treating hypertension to prevent the incidence of HF.[1,16]

Diabetes mellitus, insulin resistance, and **obesity** have all been shown to be important risk factors for the development of **coronary heart disease** and HF.[1,17–19] In addition, patients with the **metabolic syndrome** are also at increased risk for **cardiovascular disease** and therefore may have an increased risk for HF.[1,20] Adequately controlling blood glucose levels and body weight, as well as blood pressure and cholesterol levels, are important disease-prevention strategies for HF.

Several lifestyle modifications have also been identified to help decrease the risks associated with HF. Patients should strongly be advised about the hazards of smoking and alcohol use as well as the cardiotoxic effects of illicit drug use that can lead to HF.[1] Interestingly there is no direct evidence that controlling dietary sodium or participating in regular exercise can prevent the development of HF.[1] It is well known, however, that specific dietary changes and regular exercise control and decrease the risk for developing many diseases leading to heart disease as well as heart disease itself. This will be discussed in more detail later.

The ACC/AHA Heart Failure Guidelines classify HF into four stages.[1] Stage A consists of patients who are at risk for HF because they possess risk factors for HF such as those previously discussed (e.g., hypertension, atherosclerotic disease, diabetes, obesity, metabolic syndrome) but do not have structural heart disease or HF symptoms. Stage B consists of patients who do have structural heart disease (e.g., postmyocardial infarction) but are without HF symptoms. Stage C consists of patients with structural heart disease with prior or current symptoms of HF, and stage D consists of patients who are refractory to HF treatments and require specialized interventions.[1] The focus of this chapter is in the prevention of HF for patients who are at stage A or B and, to a lesser extent, treatment of HF for patients classified as stage C. Specific dietary and **physical activity** recommendations for patients at risk for HF as well as those with HF will be discussed in the following sections.

Beyond controlling the risk factors that can lead to HF, current treatment of HF is primarily focused on drug therapy. The major focus of drug therapy research and treatment in the past several years has been on decreasing the neurohormonal changes that take place during the progression of HF. Decreasing neurohormonal activation through the use of certain drugs has been shown to decrease myocardial remodeling and HF symptoms as well as improve survival.[1] It is beyond the scope of this chapter to discuss the effects of each of the drugs used to treat HF, but a list of the drug classes used in HF treatment is provided in Table 11-2.

TABLE 11–2   Medications Used to Treat Heart Failure

Angiotensin-converting enzyme (ACE) inhibitors
Angiotensin receptor blockers (ARB)
Aldosterone blockers
β-Blockers
Digoxin
Diuretics

Digoxin Pharmacokinetic and Exercise Interaction

Certain physiologic changes that occur during exercise may have an effect on the absorption, distribution, metabolism, and elimination of some drugs.[21] Exercise may affect the distribution of drugs by altering certain physiologic parameters that are key to drug distribution. The distribution of drugs is dependent on the delivery of the drug to the tissues, the ability of the drug to pass through tissue membranes, and the binding of the drug to plasma proteins.[21] During exercise drug distribution can theoretically be altered in several ways. Exercise decreases blood flow to inactive tissues, which may affect the delivery of the drug as well as the washout of drug from tissues in which drug is already present.[21] Plasma volume decreases during exercise, which causes an increase in plasma protein concentration resulting in increased drug–plasma protein binding. In addition, exercise causes blood pH to decrease, leading to decreased binding of acidic drugs to plasma albumin. An increase in body temperature during exercise can also have an effect on protein binding as this is temperature dependent.[21]

Digoxin, commonly used in patients with heart failure, has been shown to bind to skeletal muscle, altering its distribution.[21] The question is, "Does exercise significantly increase the binding of digoxin to skeletal muscles and do digoxin blood concentration levels decrease as a result of this binding?" Several studies relating exercise and digoxin **pharmacokinetics** have been published.[22–27] In one study, 10 healthy men received digoxin 0.5 mg/day for 2 weeks and then performed cycling exercises for 1 hour at a heart rate of 140 beats/min on two separate occasions. The objective of the study was to see whether skeletal muscle digoxin binding increased as a result of the exercise.[22] Muscle biopsies performed before and at several intervals after the exercises revealed that serum digoxin levels were significantly decreased ($P < 0.001$), whereas skeletal muscle concentration of digoxin was significantly increased ($P < 0.01$) when compared with levels measured during rest periods. This indicates that digoxin binds to actively working muscles, decreasing blood concentrations during single sessions of physical activity. Digoxin levels returned to normal within 1 hour after the exercise session. Several other studies have reported similar findings.[23–26]

Another study attempted to see whether similar digoxin binding occurs as a result of an exercise-training program rather than a single session of exercise.[27] Eighteen healthy men and women, both young and old, participated in a 16-week training program to discover whether such digoxin binding changes would occur. The results showed that no significant differences were found in pharmacokinetic variables of digoxin of participants who completed the exercise-training program versus those in a control group ($P > 0.05$).[27] In addition, no differences were found in younger versus older participants.

Therefore, pharmacists and other healthcare professionals should be aware that a digoxin concentration shift during exercise may occur. This shift in digoxin concentration may result in a lack of digoxin effectiveness. It is important to note that these studies were in healthy individuals rather than patients with heart failure. In addition, the clinical significance of this concentration shift has not been studied, and further research is needed to show how much, if any, this digoxin concentration shift will affect a heart failure patient's clinical outcomes.

TABLE 11–3 Program Adherence Recommendations for Patients With Heart Failure

Provide empathetic reinforcement

Provide consistent monitoring

Organize care delivery system by scheduling appointment and sending reminders

Provide proper patient education on both lifestyle modifications and medications

Collaborate with other healthcare professionals, especially the patient's physician

Individualize the lifestyle modification regimen

Promote a social support system

Organize the medications, possibly through the use of pillboxes, to decrease medication administration confusion

---

Program adherence to lifestyle change recommendations for patients with HF stage A or B is similar to that of other diseases. However, patients with HF may be unique from other patients in that many times they are required to take several medications not only to treat HF but to treat other coexisting diseases. Therefore, medication compliance can also become an issue. Several strategies can be used to improve patient motivation and compliance to adhere to both medication regimen and lifestyle modifications. Table 11-3 lists several strategies healthcare providers can use while treating patients with risk factors for HF as well as HF itself.

NUTRITION AND HEART FAILURE

The ACC/AHA heart failure guidelines offer no specific recommendations by way of nutrition for patients with HF. The only recommendation that is somewhat related is with regard to dietary sodium intake. Patients with stage C or D HF are recommended to partake in "moderate sodium restriction" because it may help to decrease the likelihood of fluid retention.[1] It is not stated, however, how much sodium is recommended per day. The other nutrition-related recommendation states that the use of nutritional supplements as treatment for HF is not indicated in patients with current or prior symptoms of HF.[1]

Because a great many of the HF recommendations focus on the prevention of HF symptoms (stages A and B), it would behoove pharmacists and other healthcare professionals to be familiar with dietary recommendations that decrease the incidence of coronary heart disease and hypertension.[16,28] Chapters 1, 6, and 7 discuss the 2005 Dietary Guidelines (http://www.healthierus.gov/dietaryguidelines/), the Dietary Approaches to Stop Hypertension (DASH) eating plan, and dietary recommendations to lower blood cholesterol, respectively. Please refer to these chapters for details regarding proper nutrition for preventing coronary heart disease and hypertension.

A particularly helpful eating plan for patients who are attempting to prevent HF as well as those who currently are experiencing symptoms of HF may be the DASH eating plan with low sodium intake.[29,30] The DASH eating plan emphasizes increased consumption of fiber, potassium, magnesium, and calcium and a decreased consumption of saturated fat and cholesterol. In addition, the DASH low-sodium eating plan recommends a sodium intake of 1,500 mg/day.[29,30] It has been shown that patients with hypertension who adopt the DASH eating plan with a 1,500-mg/day sodium intake can decrease their

TABLE 11–4   Dietary Recommendations for Patients With Heart Failure

Nutrients	Nutrient Target
Fat (% of total kcal)	27%
Saturated	6%
Monounsaturated	13%
Polyunsaturated	8%
Carbohydrates (% of total kcal)	55%
Protein (% of total kcal)	18%
Cholesterol	150 mg/day
Fiber	31 g/day
Potassium	4,700 mg/day
Magnesium	500 mg/day
Calcium	1,240 mg/day
Sodium	1,500 mg/day

Source: U.S. Department of Health and Human Services, National Institutes of Health. Facts about the DASH eating plan. Publication No. 03-4082, May 2003.

systolic blood pressure by an average of 11.5 mm Hg. Adopting this type of eating plan may be particularly beneficial for those patients who are stage A or B HF to prevent HF symptoms as well as those with stage C or D to prevent fluid retention. Table 11-4 highlights the DASH dietary recommendations.

PHYSICAL ACTIVITY AND HEART FAILURE

Before the mid 1980s it was generally accepted that patients with HF should avoid physical activity in hopes that bed rest might decrease the symptoms associated with HF and in the belief that physical activity would contribute to the further decline of the ability of the left ventricle to pump blood.[1,31–35] The current belief is completely opposite of these past views. It is now believed that patients who cannot participate in physical activity because of HF symptoms suffer from physical deconditioning, which can further exacerbate HF symptoms and produce further exercise intolerance and decreased quality of life.[1,36,37] In addition, lack of physical activity in patients with HF has been shown to produce adverse psychological effects as well as inhibit the ability of the peripheral blood vessels to function properly.[1,38,39] As a result, it is now believed that physical activity might improve the clinical status of patients with HF and may even attenuate the rate of HF progression.[1,36,40–42]

Unfortunately, there is currently very little long-term research to show the effects of physical conditioning in patients with HF. In fact only one such study has been published, which reports that exercise training was associated with a reduction in the risk of hospitalization and death.[43] It is currently unknown, however, which specific patients with HF are likely to respond favorably to exercise training or optimal exercise protocols for patients with HF.[1] Therefore, the current recommendation regarding exercise from the ACC/AHA is that it should be considered for all stable outpatients with chronic HF who are able to participate and should be used in conjunction with the recommended drug therapy.[1]

Although shortness of breath with physical exertion is a hallmark symptom of HF, approximately two thirds of exercising HF patients are limited by leg fatigue while exercising.[31] This premature leg fatigue is related to the inability of the heart to supply adequate blood and oxygen to the working muscles, creating an excess of lactic acid build-up in the muscles.[31] This causes a hyperventilation response during exercise and early fatigue. With time, exercise training can improve peripheral adaptations and cardiac function so that participation in physical activity can be easier, which may in turn decrease the risks for coronary heart disease and improve the patient's functional capacity, independence, and quality of life.

It is important to note that most of the data that have been obtained from patients with HF who participate in a physical conditioning program have been from a structured and supervised setting. Stage C and particularly stage D HF patients should exercise in a controlled and supervised environment such as a cardiac rehabilitation center or other setting with appropriately trained personnel. Some stage B patients should also exercise in a supervised setting depending on the extent of their individual structural heart damage. Formal exercise training programs have been shown to be effective at decreasing the symptoms associated with HF and improving the capacity to perform physical work.[31] Improving a patient's ability to sustain a low level of physical work can improve independence and quality of life.[1,31]

Unfortunately, the ACC/AHA heart failure guidelines offer little information by way of specific exercise recommendations for patients with HF. This is most likely because of the individual program that each patient requires. However, several items should be noted when working with exercising patients who have HF: (1) clinical status can change quickly for HF patients so proper personnel should be present to assess signs and symptoms; (2) warm-up and cool-down should be prolonged; (3) emphasis should be placed on longer exercise duration and frequency rather than on increased exercise intensity; (4) using heart rate to measure exercise intensity should be avoided and rate of perceived exertion (RPE) tables should be chosen in its place; (5) an electrocardiogram (ECG) is required for patients with a history of irregular heart rhythms; and (6) a work rate that may produce a drop in the ability of the left ventricle and heart muscle to function properly or that creates excess burden on the lungs should not be exceeded.[31,44] Specific physical activity suggestions for patients with HF are listed in Table 11-5.

TABLE 11–5 Physical Activity Recommendations for Patients With Heart Failure

Exercise Variable	Recommendation
Goals	Improve functional capacity, improve quality of life and maintain independence, decrease risk for coronary heart disease, monitor symptoms of worsening heart failure
Type	Aerobic exercises (large muscle activities) such as walking or bicycling Resistance training with light weight avoiding static muscle contractions
Intensity	Light to moderate RPE 11–16
Duration	20–40 minutes continuous or intermittent per day
Frequency	Progressively move to most days of the week
Lifestyle activity	Increase overall daily activities as tolerated through increasing the duration of activities of daily living (e.g., walking around the house, walking to get the mail, going to the grocery store)

RPE, rating of perceived exertion.

PHARMACY PRACTICE APPLICATION

This chapter illustrates that HF syndrome is a complex and debilitating disorder for those with the diagnosis. Recommendations for the treatment of HF primarily focus on proper drug therapy management and, to a much lesser extent, the use of exercise and proper nutrition. In addition, patients with HF pose unique challenges for healthcare providers as health status and signs and symptoms of HF can frequently change. Applying aggressive intervention strategies for nutrition and physical activity programming should not be the focus for patients with HF from the pharmacist's perspective. Pharmacists have been shown to be a valuable healthcare provider to patients with HF in previous studies by recommending appropriate medications and dosing.[45] It is likely to be beyond the scope of pharmacy practice to solely monitor exercise regimens and eating plans for patients who have the diagnosis of HF and are currently or have recently experienced symptoms of HF. As discussed above, patients with these characteristics should only perform exercise in supervised settings such as cardiac rehabilitation centers. Pharmacists, however, can still play a key role with these patients by encouraging them to participate and adhere to such programs in addition to monitoring their HF drug therapy regimen. Also, pharmacists can communicate with cardiac rehabilitation facilities to provide current medication therapy with the patient's permission.

With regard to HF and lifestyle modifications, pharmacists can be most effective at preventing HF in patients with risk factors for the syndrome by counseling them on lifestyle preventive strategies such as exercise, proper nutrition, weight loss, and smoking cessation. As stated earlier in this chapter, the most common causes of HF are coronary artery disease, particularly from **myocardial infarction,** and hypertension. Recall from their respective chapters in this book that the lifestyle modification strategies of physical activity, proper nutrition, weight loss, and tobacco cessation are key interventions in preventing coronary artery disease and myocardial infarction and in treating and preventing hypertension. Pharmacists can be effective at preventing HF by identifying their patients who are at risk and should encourage, implement, and monitor lifestyle modification strategies in such patients.

Because the role of a pharmacist in incorporating lifestyle modifications with regard to HF is most applicable for patients who pose risk factors for the syndrome, the following case study will be from the perspective of preventing HF rather than treating a patient who currently has HF symptoms.

CASE STUDY

*B.J. is a 45-year-old female who has been a patron of your pharmacy for 3 months. She has a past medical history of hypertension for 1 year and **dyslipidemia** for 4 years. She is sedentary with a BMI of 34 kg/m² (5′4″ tall and 199 lb), follows no specific eating plan, and does not drink alcohol or smoke tobacco. She does admit to eating "on the go" frequently owing to the busy schedules of her five children. Her current medications include hydrochlorothiazide 12.5 mg daily and rosuvastatin 10 mg daily. Her most recent cholesterol panel was taken 6 months ago and revealed total cholesterol 167, LDL 115, HDL 56, and triglycerides 145. Her current blood pressure, which you measured in the pharmacy, averaged 128/82 mm Hg with a resting heart rate of 82 beats/min.*

You notice B.J. has been reading some of the literature you have displayed in the pharmacy about disease-prevention pharmacy services. On asking her whether she has any questions about the material, she states that she wishes she were healthier. After you visit with B.J. she states that she is interested in adopting lifestyle modifications such as exercise and weight loss. She completes a 3-day dietary analysis that reveals the following results:

> *Average total caloric intake per day = 2,687 calories*
> *Carbohydrates = 43% of total calories*
> *Monounsaturated fats = 12% of total calories*
> *Polyunsaturated fats = 10% of total calories*
> *Saturated fats = 18% of total calories*
> *Total fats = 40% of total calories*
> *Protein = 20% of total calories*
> *Total dietary cholesterol = 320 mg*
> *Fiber = 10 g*
> *Calcium = 605 mg/day*
> *Potassium = 3,015 mg/day*
> *Magnesium = 327 mg/day*
> *Sodium = 3,375 mg/day*

Case Activities

1. *Write an SOAP note for B.J.*
2. *Write short- and long-term dietary and exercise goals for B.J.*
3. *Write an exercise prescription and dietary suggestions for B.J.*
4. *Design a weight-loss program for B.J.*

REFERENCES

1. Hunt SA, Abraham WT, Chin MH, et al. ACC/AHA 2005 guideline update for the diagnosis and management of chronic heart failure in the adult: a report of the American College of Cardiology/American Heart Association Task Force on Practice Guidelines (Writing Committee to Update the 2001 Guidelines for the Evaluation and Management of Heart Failure). American College of Cardiology Web Site. Available at: http://www.acc.org/clinical/guidelines/failure//index.pdf. Accessed November 4, 2005.
2. American Heart Association. Heart Disease and Stroke Statistics: 2005 Update. Dallas: American Heart Association, 2005.
3. Massie BM, Shah NB. Evolving trends in the epidemiologic factors of heart failure: rationale for preventive strategies and comprehensive disease management. Am Heart J 1997;133:703–712.
4. Parker RB, Patterson JH, Johnson JA. Heart failure. In: Dipiro JT, et al., eds. Pharmacotherapy: A Pathophysiologic Approach, 6th ed. New York: McGraw-Hill, 2005:219–260.
5. Smith SC Jr, Blair SN, Bonow RO, et al. AHA/ACC Scientific Statement: AHA/ACC guidelines for preventing heart attack and death in patients with atherosclerotic cardiovascular disease: 2001 update: a statement for healthcare professionals from the American Heart Association and the American College of Cardiology. Circulation 2001;104:1577–1579.
6. National Institutes of Health, National Heart, Lung, and Blood Institute. Third report of the National Cholesterol Education Program (NCEP) Expert Panel on Detection, Evaluation, and Treatment of High Blood Cholesterol in Adults (Adult Treatment Panel III). NIH Publication No. 02–5215, September 2002.
7. Grundy SM, Cleeman JI, Merz CN, et al. Implications for recent clinical trials for the National Cholesterol Education Program Adult Treatment Panel III guidelines. J Am Coll Cardiol 2004;44:720–732.
8. Kjekshus J, Pedersen TR, Olsson AG, Faergeman O, Pyorala K. The effects of simvastatin on the incidence of heart failure in patients with coronary artery heart disease. J Card Fail 1997;3:249–254.
9. Lewis SJ, Moye LA, Sacks FM, et al. Effect of pravastatin on cardiovascular events in older patients with myocardial infarction and cholesterol levels in the average range: results of the Cholesterol and Recurrent Events (CARE) trial. Ann Intern Med 1998;129:681–689.
10. Prevention of cardiovascular events and death with pravastatin in patients with coronary heart disease and broad range of initial cholesterol levels. The Long-Term Intervention with Pravastatin in Ischemic Disease (LIPID) Study Group. N Engl J Med 1998;339:1349–1357.
11. Vakili BA, Okin PM, Devereux RB. Prognostic implications of left ventricular hypertrophy. Am Heart J 2001;141:334–341.

12. Effects of treatment on morbidity in hypertension, II: results in patients with diastolic blood pressure averaging 90 through 114 mm Hg. JAMA 1970;213:1143–1152.

13. Kostis JB, Davis BR, Cutler J, et al., for the SHEP Cooperative Research Group. Prevention of heart failure by antihypertensive drug treatment in older persons with isolated systolic hypertension. JAMA 1997;278: 212–216.

14. Izzo JL Jr, Gradman AH. Mechanisms and management of hypertensive heart disease: from left ventricular hypertrophy to heart failure. Med Clin North Am 2004;88:1257–1271.

15. Baker DW. Prevention of heart failure. J Card Fail 2002;8:333–346.

16. Chobanian AV, Bakris GL, Black HR, et al. Seventh report of the Joint National Committee on Prevention, Detection, Evaluation, and Treatment of High Blood Pressure. Hypertension 2003;42:1206–1252.

17. Taegtmeyer H, McNulty P, Young ME. Adaptation and maladaptation of the heart in diabetes: part I: general concepts. Circulation 2002;105:1727–1733.

18. Kenchaniah S, Evans JC, Levy D, et al. Obesity and the risk of heart failure. N Engl J Med 2002;347:305–313.

19. He J, Ogden LG, Bazzano LA, Vupputuri S, Loria C, Whelton PK. Risk factors for congestive heart failure in US men and women: NHANES I epidemiologic follow-up study. Arch Intern Med 2001;161:996–1002.

20. Wilson PW, Grundy SM. The metabolic syndrome: practical guide to organs and treatment: part I. Circulation 2003;108:1422–1424.

21. Lenz TL, Lenz NJ, Faulkner MA. Potential interactions between exercise and drug therapy. Sports Med 2004;34:293–306.

22. Joreteg T, Jorestrand T. Physical exercise and binding of digoxin to skeletal muscle—effect of muscle activation frequency. Eur J Clin Pharmacol 1984;27:567–570.

23. Jogestrand T, Anderson K. Effect of physical exercise on the pharmacokinetics of digoxin during maintenance treatment. J Cardiovasc Pharmacol 1989:14:73–76.

24. Pederson KE, Madsen J, Kjaer K, et al. Effects of physical activity and immobilization on plasma digoxin concentration and renal digoxin clearance. Clin Pharmacol Ther 1983;34:303–308.

25. Grille W, Welter U, Johnson K, et al. Effects of physical activity on serum concentrations of digoxin and digitoxin. Eur J Clin Pharmacol 1996;50:237–239.

26. Laursen SO, Pedersen KE, Klitgaard NA. Influence of physical activity on plasma digoxin in hospitalised patients. Dan Med Bull 1987;34:115–117.

27. Jessup JV, Lowenthal DT, Pollock ML, et al. The effects of exercise training on the pharmacokinetics of digoxin. J Cardiopulmonary Rehabil 2000;20:89–95.

28. HHS Publication No. HHS-ODPHP-2005-01-DGA-A. Dietary Guidelines for Americans 2005, U.S. Department of Health and Human Services, U.S. Department of Agriculture. Available at: http://healthierus.gov/dietaryguidelines. Accessed February 9, 2007.

29. Appel LJ, Moore TJ, Obarzanek E, et al. A clinical trial of the effects of dietary patterns on blood pressure. N Engl J Med 1997;336:1117–1124.

30. Sacks FM, Svetkey LP, Vollmer WM, et al. Effects on blood pressure of reduced dietary sodium and the dietary approaches to stop hypertension (DASH) diet. N Engl J Med 2001;344:3–10.

31. Myers JN, Brubaker PH. Chronic heart failure. In: Durstine JL, ed. ACSM's Exercise Management for Persons With Chronic Diseases and Disabilities, 2nd ed. Champaign, IL: Human Kinetics, 2003:64–69.

32. McDonald CD, Burch GE, Walsh JJ. Prolonged bed rest in the treatment of idiopathic cardiomyopathy. Am J Med 1972;52:41–50.

33. Hochman JS, Healy B. Effect of exercise on acute myocardial infarction in rats. J Am Coll Cardiol 1986;7: 126–132.

34. Oh BH, Ono S, Rockman HA, Ross J Jr. Myocardial hypertrophy in the ischemic zone induced by exercise in rats after coronary reperfusion. Circulation 1993;87:598–607.

35. Jugdutt BI, Michorwski BL, Kappagoda CT. Exercise training after anterior Q wave myocardial infarction: importance of regional left ventricular function and topography. J Am Coll Cardiol 1988;12:362–372.

36. McKelvie RS, Teo KK, McCartney N, Humen D, Montague T, Yusuf S. Effects of exercise training in patients with congestive heart failure: a critical review. J Am Coll Cardiol 1995;25:789–796.

37. Mancini DM, Walter G, Reichek N, et al. Contribution of skeletal muscle atrophy to exercise intolerance and altered muscle metabolism in heart failure. Circulation 1992;85:1364–1373.

38. Sinoway LI. Effect of conditioning and deconditioning stimuli on metabolically determined blood flow in humans and implications for congestive heart failure. Am J Coll Cardiol 1988;62:45E–48E.

39. North TC, McCullagh R, Tran ZV. Effect of exercise on depression. Exerc Sport Sci Rev 1990;18:379–415.

40. Piepoli MF, Flather M, Coats AJ. Overview of studies of exercise training in chronic heart failure: the need for a prospective randomized multicentre European trial. Eur Heart J 1998;19:830–841.

41. Orenstein TL, Parker TG, Butany JW, et al. Favorable left ventricular remodeling following large myocardial infarction by exercise training: effect on ventricular morphology and gene expression. J Clin Invest 1995; 96:858–866.

42. Wang J, Yi GH, Knecht M, et al. Physical training alters the pathogenesis of pacing induced heart failure through endothelium-mediated mechanisms in awake dogs. Circulation 1997;96:2683–2692.

43. Belardinelli R, Georgiou D, Cianci G, Purcaro A. Randomized, controlled trial of long-term moderate exercise training in chronic heart failure: effects on functional capacity, quality of life, and clinical outcome. Circulation 1999;99:1173–1182.

44. U.S. Department of Health and Human Services. Physical activity and health: a report of the Surgeon General. Atlanta: U.S. Department of Health and Human Services, Centers for Disease Control and Prevention, National Center for Chronic Disease Prevention and Health Promotion, 1996.

45. Gattis WA, Hasselblad V, Whellan DJ, O'Connor CM. Reduction in heart failure events by the addition of a clinical pharmacist to the heart failure management team. Arch Intern Med 1999;159:1939–1945.

Diabetes Mellitus

At the end of this chapter the reader should be able to:

1. Explain the risks associated with diabetes mellitus.
2. Summarize the prevention and treatment options for diabetes mellitus.
3. Describe appropriate nutritional strategies for patients with diabetes mellitus.
4. Suggest appropriate exercises for patients with diabetes mellitus.
5. Formulate a basic nutrition and exercise program for a patient with diabetes mellitus.

OVERVIEW OF DIABETES MELLITUS

Diabetes mellitus is one of the most prevalent and debilitating chronic health conditions in the United States. In 2000, diabetes was listed as the sixth leading cause of death in the United States, accounting for more than 69,000 total deaths.[1] Individuals with diabetes can be afflicted with either type 1 or type 2 diabetes mellitus. Most patients with diabetes (about 90 to 95%) have type 2 diabetes, which is also sometimes referred to as non–insulin-dependent diabetes mellitus (NIDDM) or adult-onset diabetes mellitus.[2,3] Lifestyle modifications can have a significant impact on the prevention and control of type 2 diabetes. Pharmacists are well positioned to assist patients at risk for type 2 diabetes in prevention and treatment of this disease. Patients with type 1 diabetes can also benefit greatly from lifestyle modifications such as **exercise** to reduce the risk for cardiovascular disease.

PREVALENCE, ECONOMIC COSTS, AND HEALTH RISKS ASSOCIATED WITH DIABETES MELLITUS

In 2003, the prevalence of physician-diagnosed diabetes was more than 14 million new cases with an estimated additional 6 million undiagnosed diabetes patients in the United States.[3] From 1990 to 2006, the prevalence of those diagnosed with diabetes had increased 61%.[3] In 2002, 7.3% of the overall U.S. adult population was diagnosed with diabetes mellitus. The prevalence of diabetes more than doubles, however, when looking at the American Indian and the Alaska Native adult populations. In these populations, the prevalence of diabetes in 2002 was 15.3%.[3] American Indians or Alaska Natives are 2.6 times more likely to be diagnosed with diabetes compared with the non-Hispanic population. In addition, there is a disproportionately high prevalence of diabetes diagnosed in non-Hispanic blacks (11.7%) and Mexican Americans (9.6%) when compared with non-Hispanic whites (4.8%).[3] The worldwide prevalence of diabetes mellitus in 2000 was 2.8% but is projected to be 4.4% by the year 2030.[3] In 2004, the U.S. Department of Health and Human Services announced that approximately 40% of U.S. adults between the ages of 40 and 74 years (about 41 million people) had pre-diabetes.[3] Individuals with pre-diabetes are known to be at risk for diabetes mellitus, heart disease, and **stroke,** and many people with pre-diabetes do not know they have pre-diabetes or such risks.[3]

Preliminary 2003 statistical reports estimate that diabetes mellitus caused approximately 74,000 deaths in the United States and was an underlying or contributing cause of death in approximately 224,000 individuals.[3] Persons with diabetes mellitus are most likely to die of diseases related to the cardiovascular system. Heart disease death rates among adult patients with diabetes are two to four times higher than in adults without diabetes, and at least 65% of individuals with diabetes die of causes related to the heart or blood vessels.[3] In addition, the risk of stroke is about two to four times higher in patients with diabetes, and about 73% of patients with diabetes have a blood pressure of 130/80 mm Hg or greater or use prescription medications for **hypertension.**[3]

The economic burden of diabetes is substantial. In 2002 the total direct and indirect cost associated with diabetes was approximately $132 billion in the United States with direct costs making up $92 billion of this amount.[3,4] The average annual healthcare costs for a person with diabetes in 2002 was $13,243.[4] The average annual healthcare costs in 2002 for a person without diabetes was $2,560, representing a difference of $10,683.[4]

PATHOPHYSIOLOGY OF DIABETES MELLITUS

Diabetes is a syndrome that results from an absolute or relative lack of insulin to the cells of the body.[2] It is called a syndrome because diabetes is a group of metabolic disorders that are usually clinically characterized by high blood glucose levels or hyperglycemia.[5] Normal fasting blood glucose levels should be less than 100 mg/dL.[2] Impaired glucose tolerance is diagnosed when fasting blood glucose levels are less than 126 mg/dL, and impaired fasting glucose is defined as a glucose level between 100 and 125 mg/dL.[2] Diabetes in a non-pregnant adult is defined as a fasting glucose of 126 mg/dL or greater.[2]

The two most common types of diabetes are classified as type 1 and type 2. Women who develop diabetes as a result of the stress of pregnancy are classified as having gestational diabetes.[5] Other less common types of diabetes can be caused by infections, drugs, genetic defects, pancreatic destruction, and endocrinopathies.[5] This chapter will primarily focus on the prevention and treatment of type 1 and type 2 diabetes mellitus.

Type 1 Diabetes Mellitus

Type 1 diabetes mellitus occurs in 5 to 10% of the diabetic population and is character-ized by an absolute lack of insulin or the inability of the pancreas to make and secrete insulin.[5] This inability to produce insulin results from an autoimmune destruction of the beta cells of the pancreas.[5] At the time of diagnosis in 90% of patients with type 1 diabetes, immune destruction antibodies can be found.[5] These antibodies include islet cell antibodies, antibodies to glutamic acid decarboxylase, and antibodies to insulin.[5]

Most patients with type 1 diabetes are diagnosed before age 30, with peak diagno-sis between the ages of 12 and 14.[2] Clinical presentation consists of moderate to severe symptoms that generally progress rapidly.[2] Symptoms can include polyuria, polydipsia, fatigue, weight loss, and ketoacidosis.[2] Family history of type 1 diabetes is usually not strong, and treatment includes insulin, exercise, and proper eating habits.[2]

Type 2 Diabetes Mellitus

Type 2 diabetes mellitus accounts for 90 to 95% of all diabetics and is characterized by a relative lack of insulin.[2] This means that the tissue may be resistant to the insulin, there may be a defect in insulin secretion, or there may be an increase in hepatic glucose out-put. As type 2 diabetes progresses, all three of these pathogenetic occurrences may be hap-pening at the same time.[2] Most patients with type 2 diabetes present with **obesity,** which itself can cause insulin resistance.[5] These patients also often have high blood pressure, high triglyceride levels, low **high-density lipoprotein (HDL)** cholesterol levels, and high inhibitor plasminogen activator-1 (PAI-1) levels.[5] The compilation of these factors puts patients at high risk for macrovascular complications such as cardiovascular disease.[5]

Patients with type 2 diabetes usually present with the disease at ages older than 40 years.[2] There are, however, a disturbing number of adolescents now presenting with type 2 diabetes. Most adolescents who are diagnosed with diabetes are type 1, but some clinics are now reporting that one third to one half of all new cases of childhood dia-betes are type 2.[3] Symptoms at clinical presentation include mild polyuria and fatigue.[2] This type of diabetes has a strong genetic predisposition; therefore specific strategies to help control the risk factors for type 2 diabetes can be very helpful. Treatment of type 2 diabetes includes weight loss, a proper eating plan, exercise, oral antidiabetic agents, and possibly insulin.[2]

As stated earlier, patients with diabetes are at an increased risk for several compli-cations. Among the most prevalent of these complications are diseases related to the cardiovascular system. Heart disease and stroke account for about 65% of deaths in people with diabetes, and about 73% of adults with diabetes have a blood pressure of 130/80 mm Hg or greater or use prescription medications to treat hypertension.[6] Other complications related to diabetes in the United States include blindness, kidney disease, nervous system disease, amputations, dental disease, complications with pregnancy, bio-chemical imbalances (diabetic ketoacidosis, hyperosmolar coma), and higher inci-dences of pneumonia and influenza.[6]

Several risk factors have been identified that can lead to diabetes.[7] Some of these risk factors are non-modifiable and some are modifiable. Regardless of whether the risk is modifiable or not, patients who possess certain risk factors should be tested for dia-betes even if they are asymptomatic. Pharmacists can screen for these risk factors in their daily practice and either test the patient's blood glucose themselves or refer them to their physician for further evaluation. A list of the risk factors for diabetes is provided in Table 12-1.

TABLE 12–1	Environmental Risk Factors Leading to Diabetes Mellitus

Age > 45 years

Body mass index > 25 kg/m²

Physical inactivity

First-degree relative with diabetes

Members of the following ethnic populations:
   African American
   Latino
   Native American
   Asian American
   Pacific Islander

Hypertension

HDL cholesterol < 35 mg/dL or triglyceride level > 250 mg/dL

Women who have delivered a baby weighing >9 pounds or have been diagnosed with gestational diabetes mellitus

Women with polycystic ovary syndrome (PCOS)

Other clinical conditions associated with insulin resistance (PCOS, acanthosis nigricans)

History of vascular disease

Rapid progression (days to weeks) of:
   Polyuria
   Polydipsia
   Fatigue
   Weight loss
   Ketoacidosis

Source: Carlisle BA, Kroon LA, Koda-Kimble MA. Diabetes mellitus. In: Koda-Kimble MA, ed. Applied Therapeutics: The Clinical Use of Drugs, 8th ed. Philadelphia: Lippincott Williams & Wilkins, 2005:50.1–50.86. HDL, high-density lipoprotein.

DIABETES MELLITUS DISEASE PREVENTION AND TREATMENT

Because type 1 diabetes is an autoimmune disorder, it is difficult to implement strategies to prevent the absolute lack of insulin that occurs. It is well known, however, that patients with diabetes are at a greater risk for cardiovascular complications. As a result, patients with type 1 diabetes can benefit from lifestyle prevention strategies that decrease the risks for cardiovascular disease. These strategies include **physical activity,** proper eating habits, and smoking cessation. Obesity is usually not a problem with type 1 diabetes patients, but if patients are overweight or obese, a weight-loss program should also be included in the prevention strategies.

Lifestyle modification prevention strategies for patients with type 2 diabetes are also very important. Although a strong genetic component to type 2 diabetes exists, prevention strategies can help not only to prevent cardiovascular complications as in type 1 patients, but also to decrease the risk for type 2 diabetes altogether.[7] As 90 to 95% of patients with diabetes are type 2 diabetics, lifestyle modification prevention strategies are integral when learning about diabetes care. In addition, these same prevention strategies can be used to help treat type 2 diabetics and improve the overall health of these patients.[7]

Lifestyle intervention strategies for type 2 diabetes patients are usually centered on weight loss, as 60 to 90% of type 2 diabetics are obese.[2] Accomplishing weight loss is preferred by using physical activity in combination with proper eating habits. As stated earlier, diabetes is characterized as a compilation of metabolic disorders. Because of this, proper food intake becomes a priority not only for disease prevention, but for disease treatment (blood glucose control) as well. In addition, many patients with diabetes also have hypertension and poor blood lipid profiles.[2,5] Therefore, assisting patients with diabetes in controlling blood pressure, blood lipids, and blood glucose through the use of lifestyle modifications becomes a priority.[7] Patients with type 2 diabetes who smoke are also strongly encouraged to engage in a smoking-cessation program to help decrease their overall risk for cardiovascular disease and other smoking-related diseases. Therefore, the lifestyle modification treatment and prevention strategies for patients with type 2 diabetes include weight loss, physical activity, proper nutrition, and tobacco cessation (if applicable).

Several studies in recent years have been published to show that lifestyle interventions are an important part of diabetes care.[7,12] In one particular study, the Diabetes Prevention Program showed that non-diabetic persons with elevated fasting and postload glucose concentrations could dramatically affect their insulin sensitivity and their conversion from impaired glucose tolerance to type 2 diabetes through the use of lifestyle modifications.[8] Patients in this study (n = 3,243) were randomly assigned to a regimen of either usual care, placebo, or intensive lifestyle intervention.[8] The lifestyle intervention arm of the study consisted of achieving and maintaining a 7% body weight reduction through a healthy low-**calorie,** low-fat diet and encouraging physical activity of moderate intensity, such as brisk walking, for at least 150 minutes per week.[8] The study was originally designed to be ongoing for 5 years but was stopped after 2.8 years because of the conclusive nature of the results. The results showed that participants who received usual care developed type 2 diabetes at a rate of 7.8% each year compared with a 4.8% rate in those receiving lifestyle intervention.[8] This represents a 58% reduction in the development of diabetes in the lifestyle group compared with only a 31% reduction in the usual care group.[8]

Interestingly, impressive results were achieved in the Diabetes Prevention Program Study with only modest adjustments in lifestyle modification. The average weight loss was only 8 pounds, and the exercise program was an average of 30 minutes of walking 5 days each week.[8] It should also be noted that the individuals randomized to the lifestyle intervention arm participated in a 16-lesson curriculum covering diet, exercise, and behavior modification that was taught on a one-to-one basis during the first 24 weeks of study enrollment with subsequent group sessions as needed.[8] This aspect of the study emphasizes the importance of adequate patient education, and counseling and behavioral modification strategies when implementing lifestyle modifications.

Although the Diabetes Prevention Program showed that lifestyle modifications can work better than usual care, it is important to also emphasize to patients the importance of taking their diabetes medications. Some patients will have difficulty adhering to the lifestyle modification regimen and may not be afforded intense one-on-one patient counseling. Therefore, most patients should take medications to help control their type 2 diabetes, and all patients with type 1 diabetes must take insulin. Table 12-2 contains a list of medications that are commonly prescribed for patients with diabetes.

As with any disease in which lifestyle modification strategies are implemented, program compliance and patient motivation become an important part of the success of the individual patient. This was certainly shown to be the case in the Diabetes Prevention

TABLE 12–2	Medications Used to Treat Diabetes Mellitus

Oral agents
  Alpha-glucosidase inhibitors
  Biguanides
  Non-sulfonylurea insulin secretagogues
  Sulfonylureas (first- and second-generation)
  Thiazolidinediones
  Combination oral products
Subcutaneous injection
  Insulin
  Others

Program in which participants who were receiving the lifestyle intervention treatment were given 16 one-on-one lessons that covered diet, exercise, and behavioral modification to help participants achieve their specific goals.[8] Each lesson was flexible to the patient's schedule, culturally sensitive, and individualized. Most healthcare providers would ideally like to spend as much time as possible with patients to maximize the patient's success in the program. Even if clinicians are on a tight time schedule and cannot afford to spend 16 one-on-one sessions with patients, it is important to note that the more time that is spent with patients about behavioral change, the more likely they will be to adhere to the program. This was proven to be the case when talking to smokers about smoking cessation where as little as 3 minutes of counseling on every clinic visit about not smoking yielded greater smoking cessation success rates. This strategy can also be applied to patients with diabetes. Each time patients with diabetes come into the pharmacy for a prescription refill, pharmacists can talk to them about treatment and adherence to their eating plan and exercise regimen.

One of the areas of diabetes management that has been shown to be an integral component of diabetes care is diabetes self-management education.[13] Self-management training sessions for patients with diabetes have been shown to help patients adjust to daily regimens of diabetes management and to improve glycemic control. Self-management education can be conducted in an inpatient or an outpatient setting and is especially effective if done by an interdisciplinary team. The goal of the self-management training is to ultimately achieve and maintain optimal glucose control. This can be accomplished by teaching patients with diabetes about the connection between important glucose control factors such as proper nutrition, physical activity, emotional or physical stress, and medications. Patients learn how to respond appropriately and continually to each of the factors to maintain optimal glucose control.[13]

It is well known that self-management education is a critical part of diabetes care, and medical treatment without such care is considered inadequate.[13] Many studies have shown that self-management education leads to reductions in costs that are related to all types of diabetes care. In addition, self-management education has also been shown to decrease lower-extremity amputation rates, medication costs, and emergency room visits and hospitalizations.[13]

Pharmacists can be a valuable component of an interdisciplinary team focused on diabetes care in the inpatient and outpatient setting. In addition, pharmacists working in the community setting without other healthcare professionals in close proximity can also be indispensable to patients with diabetes by helping them treat their disease, prevent complications, and adhere to their individual diabetes regimen. Several program

TABLE 12–3   Program Adherence Recommendations for Patients With Diabetes Mellitus

Individualize the treatment and prevention plan

Talk with patients about their treatment plan (including lifestyle modification strategies) each time they come to the pharmacy for a prescription refill

Solicit the help of other healthcare professionals to emphasize the importance of lifestyle modification and diabetes care

Educate patients about the factors that can influence blood glucose control and how these factors work together to achieve and maintain optimal blood glucose levels (e.g., proper nutrition, physical activity, emotional or physical stress, and medications)

Set achievable goals

Institute a self-monitoring program such as keeping a log of food and medication intake and exercise participation

Identify patient-specific barriers to the lifestyle changes

Design a program that is reasonable, gradual, and easily implemented

Provide effective communication with the patient and the patient's family and caregivers

Involve the patient in the decision-making process

Source: National Institutes of Health, National Heart, Lung, and Blood Institute. Third report of the National Cholesterol Education Program (NCEP) Expert Panel on Detection, Evaluation, and Treatment of High Blood Cholesterol in Adults (Adult Treatment Panel III). NIH Publication No. 02-5215, September 2002.

adherence strategies are listed in Table 12-3 that can be used by pharmacists when working with patients with diabetes.[14]

NUTRITION AND DIABETES MELLITUS

Proper nutrition for patients with diabetes is essential to the optimal management of blood glucose and to the prevention of diabetes complications. Nutritional concepts when treating patients with diabetes are often referred to as medical nutrition therapy (MNT) and have become a big part of diabetes self-management education. Because diabetes is considered a metabolic disorder that is associated with abnormalities in carbohydrate, fat, and protein metabolism, nutrition in patients with diabetes has been much studied. Nutritional recommendations for patients with diabetes, however, are much like those that are recommended for patients with a high risk for cardiovascular disease, as well as those for the general population.

The American Diabetes Association (ADA; http://www.diabetes.org/for-health-professionals-and-scientists/cpr.jsp) has established a set of nutrition principles and recommendations for patients with diabetes.[15] Within these recommendations are goals for medical nutrition therapy that can be applied to all patients with diabetes. The four goals that the ADA has established are to (1) attain and maintain optimal metabolic outcomes including blood glucose, blood lipid, and blood pressure levels; (2) prevent and treat chronic complications of diabetes by modifying nutrient intake to prevent and treat obesity, **dyslipidemia,** cardiovascular disease, hypertension, and nephropathy; (3) improve health through healthy food choices and physical activity; and (4) address individual nutritional needs, taking into consideration the patient's cultural and lifestyle needs while respecting the patient's wishes and willingness to change.[15] These four goals should be applied and individualized to all patients with diabetes when discussing their medical nutrition therapy.

Carbohydrates and Diabetes

The general recommendation by the ADA is that it is important for patients with diabetes to consume carbohydrates that are derived from whole grains, fruits, vegetables, and low-fat milk as part of a healthy diet. Many factors can influence the glycemic response of foods including the amount of carbohydrate and the type of sugar.[15] The ADA recommends that the total amount of carbohydrate in meals or snacks consumed each day is more important than the source or type of carbohydrate consumed.[15] This is true for both type 1 and type 2 diabetics.

Sucrose, a disaccharide containing glucose and fructose, and sucrose-containing foods have proven not to have a significant effect on glycemic levels of patients with diabetes and therefore do not need to be restricted in these patients.[15] In fact, the ADA recommends that sucrose be substituted for other carbohydrate sources. Additionally, the U.S. Food and Drug Administration (FDA)–approved non-nutritive sweeteners (saccharin, aspartame, acesulfame potassium, and sucralose) are safe for patients with diabetes when consumed within the acceptable daily intake levels established by the FDA.[15]

Patients with type 1 diabetes have been shown in studies to have a strong relationship between premeal insulin dose and the response to glucose levels after a meal to the total carbohydrate content of the meal. As a result, the ADA suggests that patients with type 1 diabetes adjust their premeal insulin dose based on the carbohydrate content of the meal. There is some evidence also to show that it is important for type 1 diabetics who receive fixed doses of insulin to maintain day-to-day consistency with carbohydrate intake.[15]

Monounsaturated fats may be able to be substituted for some carbohydrate intake in patients with diabetes. There is a concern, however, for the increased caloric content that this may bring to the patient. The consensus from the ADA is that carbohydrate and monounsaturated fat intake together should provide 60 to 70% of a diabetes patient's total calorie intake.[15] It is important to consider the metabolic profile and weight loss needs of the patient when recommending specific foods so as to prevent the intake of too many calories.

Protein and Diabetes

Most Americans (including those with diabetes) consume 15 to 20% of their calories as protein. It has been demonstrated in patients with type 2 diabetes that moderate hyperglycemia can contribute to an increased turnover in protein, which suggests the increased need for protein. It has also been shown in patients with type 1 diabetes that adequate protein intake is needed to maintain proper blood glucose levels.[15] Because most American adults consume at least 50% more protein than required, patients with diabetes appear to be protected against protein malnutrition when consuming a usual diet.[15] Therefore, the expert consensus of the ADA recommends that protein intake of 15 to 20% of total calories (usual protein intake) is adequate for patients with diabetes and normal renal function.[15]

Dietary Fats and Diabetes

The primary goals for fat intake for patients with diabetes are essentially the same as those for patients without diabetes: to limit saturated fat and **cholesterol** intake.[15]

Persons with diabetes appear to be more sensitive to dietary cholesterol than the general public. Because patients with diabetes are at increased risk for cardiovascular disease, particular attention to saturated fat and cholesterol intake should be made by the patient and healthcare providers.

The ADA recommends that less than 10% of the total calories should come from saturated fats. Individuals who have **a low-density lipoprotein (LDL)** cholesterol of greater than 100 mg/dL may receive additional benefit from a saturated fat intake of less than 7% of the total caloric intake.[15] Dietary cholesterol intake should be less than 300 mg/day or less than 200 mg/day for those with LDL cholesterol levels greater than 100 mg/dL. In addition, the intake of *trans* **fatty acids** should be limited as in patients without diabetes.[15] Table 12-4 lists dietary recommendations for patients with diabetes mellitus.

Vitamins and Minerals and Diabetes

The recommendations for vitamin and mineral intake for patients with diabetes are the same as those for the general public. Aside from calcium intake to prevent bone loss and folate supplements to prevent birth defects, patients with diabetes do not need to take additional vitamin and mineral supplementation. This is assuming that the patient does not have a specific underlying deficiency.[15] Patients who consume a healthy balanced diet can obtain all the vitamins and minerals necessary for normal physiologic function.

Alcohol and Diabetes

Alcohol can have both a hypoglycemic and hyperglycemic effect on patients with diabetes. Patients who consume alcohol in a short period of time, without food, and in excessive amounts can significantly affect their blood glucose levels. Patients with type 1

TABLE 12-4   Dietary Recommendations for Patients With Diabetes Mellitus

Nutrient	Recommendation
Balance calorie intake with expenditure to obtain appropriate body weight	
Carbohydrate[a]	50–60% of total calorie intake (carbohydrate plus monounsaturated fat together should make up 60–70% of total calorie intake)
Fiber	20–30 g/day
Protein	15–20% of total calorie intake
Monounsaturated fat	Up to 20% of total calorie intake (carbohydrate plus monounsaturated fat together should make up 60–70% of total calorie intake)
Polyunsaturated fat	Up to 10% of total calorie intake
Saturated fat	Less than 10% of total calorie intake (less than 7% for patients with LDL cholesterol levels >100 mg/dL)
Total fat	25–35% of total calorie intake
Dietary cholesterol	Less than 300 mg/day (less than 300 for patients with LDL cholesterol levels >100 mg/dL)

[a]Most carbohydrate intake should come from whole grains, fruits, vegetables, and low-fat dairy products.
Source: American Diabetes Association. Position Statement. Nutrition principles and recommendations in diabetes. Diabetes Care 2004;27(Suppl 1):S36–S46.
LDL, low-density lipoprotein.

or type 2 diabetes, however, who consume moderate amounts of alcohol with food have shown no acute effects on blood glucose or insulin levels.[15] Therefore, the ADA's recommendations concerning alcohol consumption are the same for patients with diabetes and for those without diabetes. That is, individuals who choose to drink alcohol should limit daily intake to one drink for adult women and two drinks for adult men. One drink is defined as 12 oz of beer, 5 oz of wine, or 1.5 oz of distilled spirits.[15]

Nutrition and Type 1 Diabetes

The nutritional recommendations to maintain a healthy lifestyle for the general public that are discussed in Chapter 1 can also be applied to patients with type 1 diabetes.[15] The unique aspect about patients with type 1 diabetes is that they must integrate an insulin regimen into their daily lifestyle that is in coordination with meals and snacks. Because of the vast number of insulin options available today and the uniqueness of each individual's eating habits, each patient with diabetes should have a personalized regimen that fits his or her lifestyle. Patients receiving intensive insulin therapy should dose premeal insulin based on the total carbohydrate content of the meal or snack to obtain optimal postprandial glucose levels.[15] Patients who receive fixed insulin doses and do not adjust premeal insulin doses should try to maintain a consistent carbohydrate intake throughout each meal or snack.[15] In addition to carbohydrates, it is also important for patients with type 1 diabetes to watch their intake of fats and proteins in relation to their total calorie intake. Excess calories lead to increased body weight, which can affect blood glucose levels as well as blood lipids, blood pressure, and general health.[15]

Nutrition and Type 2 Diabetes

Nutritional recommendations to maintain a healthy lifestyle for the general public that are discussed in Chapter 1 can also be applied to patients with type 2 diabetes.[15] The emphasis of nutrition therapy for patients with type 2 diabetes focuses on decreasing total caloric intake as well as decreasing saturated fat, cholesterol, and sodium intake.[15] Many people with type 2 diabetes are obese and hypertensive and have dyslipidemia. This places them at high risk for cardiovascular disease and other complications. Therefore, the goal of a proper eating plan for patients with diabetes is to decrease the risk for cardiovascular disease along with weight loss to improve insulin sensitivity. Physical activity, along with nutrition therapy, is an important aspect to the treatment of patients with type 2 diabetes because it can lead to improved blood glucose levels, improved insulin sensitivity, and reduced cardiovascular risk. Nutritional strategies that promote weight loss should be applied to these patients on an individualized basis to provide the best opportunity for weight loss. Patients with type 2 diabetes sometimes require insulin therapy as well. For these patients, the same strategies for insulin and carbohydrate intake should be applied as in patients with type 1 diabetes.

PHYSICAL ACTIVITY

Physical activity is one of the hallmarks of diabetes management. Physical activity has an insulin-like effect that enhances the uptake of glucose, allowing for better glycemic control, even in the presence of glucose deficiencies.[16] Physical activity also improves glucose tolerance, improves insulin sensitivity, decreases glycosylated hemoglobin (HbA_{1c}), decreases insulin requirements, improves lipid profile, reduces blood pressure, assists in weight management, increases physical work capacity, decreases cardio-vascular disease risk, and improves overall well-being.[16] The exercise recommendations for patients with type 1 diabetes without complications are similar to those that are recommended for healthy individuals without disease.[17] The recommendations for patients with type 2 diabetes are very similar to those recommended for patients who are obese and have dyslipidemia and hypertension (Table 12-5).[17]

The ADA recommends that persons with diabetes participate in at least 150 minutes per week of moderate-intensity aerobic physical activity or at least 90 minutes per week of vigorous aerobic exercise.[7] The ADA further recommends that physical activity be distributed over at least 3 days per week with no more than two consecutive days

TABLE 12–5	Physical Activity Recommendations for Patients With Diabetes Mellitus	
Exercise Variable	**Type 1 Diabetes**	**Type 2 Diabetes**
Goals	Prevent the onset of disease Increase work capacity Improve overall well-being	Improve insulin sensitivity Reduce risk for cardiovascular disease Reduce body weight while maintaining lean body tissue Improve functional performance including activities of daily living
Types	Large muscle activities (e.g., walking, bicycling, dancing, rowing, swimming, water aerobics, tennis, racquetball, gardening, lawn mowing)	Large muscle activities (e.g., walking, bicycling, dancing, rowing, swimming, water aerobics, tennis, racquetball, gardening, lawn mowing)
Intensity	Moderate to vigorous	Very low to moderate[a]
Duration	At least 30 minutes of accumulated activity	5 to 10 minutes (initially), 20 to 60 minutes (more advanced; or 2 to 3 sessions/day of 10 to 30 minutes each)
Frequency	Most days of the week	2 to 4 times per week (for initial 2 to 8 weeks) Most days of the week (after initial 8 weeks)
Resistance training	All major muscle groups 1 set 15–20 repetitions, 2 to 3 times per week (rest at least 48 hours between sessions)	All major muscle groups 1 set 15–20 repetitions, 2 to 3 times per week (rest at least 48 hours between sessions)
Lifestyle activities	Increase overall daily activities through increasing the duration of activities of daily living (e.g., walking the dog, taking stairs, yard work, household duties)	

[a]Emphasize increasing duration rather than intensity.
Sources: Whaley MH, ed. ACSM's Guidelines for Exercise Testing and Prescription, 7th ed. Philadelphia: Lippincott Williams & Wilkins, 2006:207–211; Verity LS. Diabetes mellitus and exercise. In: Kaminsky LA, ed. ACSM's Resource Manual for Guidelines for Exercise Testing and Prescription, 5th ed. Philadelphia: Lippincott Williams & Wilkins, 2006:470–479.

without participation.[7] The American College of Sports Medicine (ACSM) recommends aerobic physical activity for patients with diabetes three to four times per week for 20 to 60 minutes at a moderate intensity.[16] In addition, the ACSM further recommends that patients with type 2 diabetes accumulate a minimum of 1,000 kcal per week of physical activity or 2,000 kcal per week or more if weight loss is a goal.[16] It is important to note that the increased sensitivity of insulin that is important for type 2 diabetics occurs during the physical activity session and for up to 48 hours after exercise.[18] Therefore, physical activity is recommended to be repeated at least every 48 hours to maintain this effect and obtain optimal blood glucose control.[7,18]

In addition to aerobic exercise, resistance training in patients without complications has been shown to be beneficial to patients with diabetes by improving insulin sensitivity.[7,16] The ACSM recommends one set of exercises for each major muscle group.[16] The goal is to increase the repetitions to 15 to 20 per exercise for a minimum frequency of two times per week with a minimum of 48 hours of rest between sessions.[16]

Proper Footwear and Exercise

Diabetes mellitus can cause many complications, of which one is diabetic neuropathy. Two of the most common consequences of diabetic neuropathy are amputation and foot ulcerations.[7] Early recognition and management of the risk factors that lead to foot ulcerations and amputations can prevent or delay these outcomes.[7]

Several risks are associated with foot ulcerations or amputations that include having diabetes for longer than 10 years, poor glycemic control, and cardiovascular, retinal, or renal complications.[7] Specific risks associated with just amputation as a result of diabetic neuropathy include peripheral neuropathy with loss of protective sensation, altered biomechanics, evidence of increased pressure (erythema, hemorrhage under callus), bony deformity, peripheral vascular disease, history of ulcers or amputation, and severe nail pathology.[7] Because of these risks, the ADA recommends that all patients with diabetes have a comprehensive foot examination performed in the primary care setting along with education regarding self-examinations.[7]

Patients with diabetes are strongly encouraged to exercise because of the many added benefits of the prevention and management of diabetes complications. It is very important, however, when counseling diabetic patients about exercise to discuss proper footwear. Patients should be educated that sensory loss may occur with the progression of diabetes. This means that diabetics may lose the ability to feel whether a shoe or sock is not fitting correctly, a blister is developing, or other foot and ankle ailments are occurring as a result of exercising.

Therefore, the ADA recommends that persons with diabetes use footwear that cushions and distributes pressure evenly on the foot. People with body deformities (e.g., hammertoe, prominent metatarsal heads, or bunions) may need extra-wide shoes. Also, non–weight-bearing physical activity may be required for people who cannot tolerate weight-bearing activity.

Patients at high risk for foot ulcerations and amputation should understand the implications of the loss of the protective sensation in the foot, the importance of foot monitoring on a daily basis, proper foot care including nail and skin care, and the selection of appropriate footwear. The pharmacist can discuss each of these items when counseling patients with diabetes as part of the diabetes self-monitoring program and in discussions about proper physical activity.

Physical Activity and Type 1 Diabetes

During physical activity in a person without diabetes there is an increase in glucagon output and an increased glucose uptake by peripheral muscles to adequately perform the activity. As a result, more glucose is released from the liver to continually supply the blood with glucose, and insulin levels naturally decrease to prevent blood glucose levels from becoming too low during exercise.[18] Peripheral blood glucose supply is determined by the individual person's conditioning as well as hepatic glucose output. In other words, the body has naturally occurring counterregulatory mechanisms that keep the blood glucose levels from getting too high (hyperglycemia) or too low (hypoglycemia) during exercise.

In patients with type 1 diabetes, these counterregulatory mechanisms do not work as well, and glycemic control in response to exercise is more difficult. Glycemic control in patients with type 1 diabetes is determined by many factors that the patients must manage himself or herself. Among these are included the metabolic control of blood glucose, the physical conditioning of the patient, prior physical activity and food intake, the intensity and duration of the activity, the integrity of the autonomic nervous system, and the type and timing of the insulin the patient is using.[18]

Physical activity can be used by patients with type 1 diabetes to more effectively control their blood glucose. One of the most critical aspects of optimal blood glucose control is to teach the patients how to manage all the variables that can affect blood glucose as part of the self-management process. Anticipating the need for food before and after physical activity, monitoring the effect of physical activity on blood glucose measurements after participation in exercise, and appropriately adjusting insulin dose in response to physical activity are effective measures to control blood glucose levels. It is important that healthcare professionals work with diabetic patients to teach them how to manage their own blood glucose levels by adjusting insulin doses and food intake as needed. Making the patient a diabetes expert yields better glycemic control and fewer diabetic complications.[18]

Because glucose uptake is altered during exercise, patients with type 1 diabetes will need to either reduce insulin dosage before an exercise session or consume extra glucose depending on the patient, the patient's insulin regimen, and whether the exercise was planned or unplanned. For planned exercise, a reduction in insulin dosage may be the preferred choice to prevent hypoglycemia.[15] For unplanned exercise, additional glucose may be needed.[15]

Moderate-intensity exercise increases glucose uptake by 2 to 3 mg/kg per minute above usual requirements.[15] Therefore, a 70-kg patient would need 8.4 to 12.6 g of carbohydrate per hour of moderate-intensity physical activity.[15] If the exercise session is more intense, more carbohydrate would be needed.[15] Another, more general recommendation is to consume 15 g of carbohydrate before or after moderate-intensity physical activity depending on the blood glucose level.[18] If the activity is very strenuous, 30 g of carbohydrate may be needed.[18]

Blood glucose levels differ for each patient, and likewise each patient has a different blood glucose response to exercise. Therefore, it is extremely important for healthcare providers to stress the importance of monitoring blood glucose levels before and after an exercise session. Physical activity can be very beneficial to patients with type 1 diabetes and may actually decrease insulin dosages. It has been shown that improving physical conditioning through exercise training can decrease daily subcutaneous insulin requirement by 20 to 30%.[18,19]

Physical Activity and Type 2 Diabetes

A physical activity program for a patient with type 2 diabetes is much like that of a patient who is obese with dyslipidemia and hypertension. Weight loss and increases in physical activity level are the key factors to this type of program. Increased physical activity and weight loss improves insulin sensitivity, which results in better glycemic control. As stated earlier, improved insulin sensitivity resulting from physical activity continues to occur for up to 48 hours after the exercise session.[18] Therefore, physical activity should be repeated at least every 48 hours to maintain this effect.[18] In addition, physical activity improves lipid profiles and helps to control blood pressure, both of which are important to the treatment of type 2 diabetes.

Approximately 40% of all patients with type 2 diabetes will also require daily insulin injections.[17] Close monitoring of blood glucose levels before and after exercise is also important for type 2 diabetics, especially if taking insulin. The same principles of consuming extra glucose before or after exercise to prevent hypoglycemia should also apply to these patients. Again, vigilant monitoring of glucose levels by the patient is a key factor to obtaining optimal glycemic control.

Safety Considerations

Several safety issues must be discussed with the diabetic patient before beginning an exercise program. First, all patients must undergo an extensive medical evaluation particularly for the cardiovascular, nervous, renal, and visual systems before beginning a program to rule out any underlying diabetes complications that may compromise the patient's safety. Second, patients must be educated about the risks for hypoglycemia and hyperglycemia that may result from exercise. Hypoglycemia is defined as a blood glucose level of less than 80 mg/dL or a rapid drop in glucose and may last as long as 48 hours after exercise.[16] Hyperglycemia, defined as a blood glucose level of greater than 300 mg/dL, is a particular risk for patients with type 1 diabetes who have poor glycemic control. It is recommended to avoid exercise if fasting glucose is greater than 250 mg/dL and ketosis is present and to use caution if glucose is greater than 300 mg/dL and no ketosis is present.[16,20] Carbohydrate intake or insulin injections should be adjusted before exercise based on blood glucose and exercise intensity to prevent hypoglycemia associated with exercise.[16] If preexercise blood glucose is less than 100 mg/dL, 20 to 30 g of additional carbohydrate should be ingested before beginning the activity for patients on insulin or insulin-secretagogue therapy.[7] Supplementary carbohydrates, however, are generally not necessary for individuals treated with diet, metformin, alpha-glucosidase inhibitors, or thiazolidinediones without insulin or a secretagogue.[7] Signs and symptoms of hypoglycemia and hyperglycemia are listed in Table 12-6.

Additionally, it is important to counsel patients who exercise late in the evening that they may need to increase consumption of carbohydrates before going to bed so as to decrease the risk of becoming hypoglycemic while sleeping. Other practical recommendations for exercise include wearing good shoes, practicing good hygiene, exercising with a partner, wearing a diabetes identification tag, planning exercise sessions in advance, and keeping a daily log of blood glucose levels in relation to time of medication administration and exercising time and intensity.[17]

Another important factor for diabetics who take insulin before exercising is to consider the injection site with the type of activity that is to be performed. Studies have shown that injecting insulin directly into a limb that is about to be exercised can alter the absorption of the insulin and therefore alter the glycemic control. Injecting insulin

TABLE 12–6	Signs and Symptoms of Hypoglycemia and Hyperglycemia
Hypoglycemia	Fainting or feeling faint, hand tremors, sweat, dizziness, crying, drowsiness, excessive hunger, fatigue, irritability, unsteady gait, apathy, blurred vision, confusion, delusion, double vision, loss of consciousness, convulsions, headache, inability to concentrate, nervousness, slurred speech, somnolence, poor concentration
Hyperglycemia	Weakness, increased thirst, dry mouth, soft eyeballs, frequent and scant urination, decreased appetite, nausea, vomiting, abdominal tenderness, acetone breath, Kussmaul respirations

into the thigh just before cycling showed an increased rate of insulin absorption during the first 10 minutes of activity by 135% and by 50% over the entire exercising time (60 minutes) compared with rest.[21] This increased absorption resulted in a greater decrease in blood glucose during the recovery period after exercise compared with injecting insulin into the abdomen.[21] Therefore, the ACSM recommends avoiding insulin injections into exercising limbs to lower the risk of hypoglycemia associated with exercise.[16] The preferred injection site is in the abdomen.[16]

Patients with diabetes can have several disabilities that have resulted from the disease. Each of these disabilities may have its own set of precautions relating to exercise to ensure patient safety. A list of disabilities and their precautions relating to exercise is provided in Table 12-7.

PHARMACY PRACTICE APPLICATION

For years pharmacists have been an integral healthcare provider to patients with diabetes. Many pharmacists have earned the distinction of being a certified diabetes educator (CDE) by spending a significant amount of their career educating and treating patients with diabetes. Other non-certified pharmacists in almost every pharmacy practice setting have also made significant contributions to the lives of patients with diabetes. Many examples have been published that document the advantages of a pharmacist working with diabetic patients. In the mid 1970s pharmacists in an ambulatory care setting demonstrated that pharmacist-to-patient teaching was effective at improving the quality of both the process and outcomes of diabetes care.[22] Diabetic patients in this study experienced fewer medication errors, fewer changes in therapy, fewer hospital admissions, and greater compliance in keeping appointments compared with a control group.[22]

Other research has shown that pharmacists who were granted the authority to change drug therapy in diabetic patients were able to show that these patients experienced significantly improved blood glucose control compared with patients who were treated by pharmacists who could only recommend drug therapy changes.[23] In addition to improved clinical outcomes, pharmacists have been able to demonstrate a cost savings when they work with diabetes patients. The city of Asheville, NC, was able to save $14,000 during the first 6 months and $20,246 during a 12-month period when pharmacists were involved in the treatment of city employees with diabetes.[24] Other studies were able to show a cost per patient savings of $144 to $640 per year with pharmacy services.[25,26]

Implementing diabetes care services into the pharmacy practice setting can be done to any degree in almost any setting. The degree of care can range from simply

TABLE 12–7   Safety Precautions for Exercising With Diabetes Complications

Diabetes-Related Complication	Recommendations With Exercise
Peripheral neuropathy	Take proper care of feet to prevent foot ulcers
	Limit weight-bearing exercise for patients with significant peripheral neuropathy
Autonomic neuropathy	Monitor signs and symptoms of hypoglycemia because of the inability of the patient to recognize them
	Monitor signs and symptoms of silent ischemia because of the inability to perceive angina
	Monitor blood pressure after exercise to manage hypotension and hypertension associated with vigorous exercise
	Understand that the heart rate and blood pressure response to exercise may be blunted and that the use of perceived exertion may help guide exercise intensity
	Use precautions for poor thermoregulation in both hot and cold environments
Retinopathy	For moderate non-proliferative diabetic retinopathy, avoid activities that dramatically elevate blood pressure
	For severe non-proliferative diabetic retinopathy, avoid exercise that increases blood pressure >170 mm Hg
	For proliferative diabetic retinopathy avoid strenuous activities, Valsalva maneuvers, or activities of pounding or jarring
Nephropathy	Limit exercise to low to moderate intensities and discourage strenuous intensities when physical work capacity is low

Source: Whaley MH, editor. ACSM's Guidelines for Exercise Testing and Prescription, 7th ed. Philadelphia: Lippincott Williams & Wilkins, 2006:207–211.

questioning patients about their care to offering a diabetes clinic that monitors every aspect of diabetes self-management. Pharmacy settings can range from hospital, to community and ambulatory care, to long-term care. It is important for pharmacists to understand that they can play a significant role in the health of diabetes patients. It is also important to understand that pharmacists are a part of the healthcare team and that a team approach, which includes the patient, to treating the disease is optimal. Proper glucose control and the prevention and management of diabetic complications are the responsibility of both the healthcare provider and the patient. Pharmacists, along with other healthcare providers, can provide patients the skills and motivation they need to become diabetes experts. When diabetic patients becomes their own best primary care giver, optimal outcomes are achievable.

CASE STUDY

A.M. is a 21-year-old white female with a 6-year history of type 1 diabetes. She has no other medical history but does have a family history of cardiovascular disease as her father had a heart attack at age 42 years. A.M. does not smoke, is sedentary, and follows no specific diet to manage her diabetes. She has been getting her diabetes medication and supplies at your pharmacy since the onset of her disease, and you and the pharmacy staff have worked with her in the past to teach her how to measure her blood sugar with a blood glucose monitor. During A.M.'s last trip to the pharmacy to refill her insulin, she mentioned to you that she has been having trouble lately keeping her blood glucose level within the normal range, especially on the weekends. A.M. states that she knows that it is important to keep her blood sugar under control and requests your help. She is 5′6″ tall, weighs 130 lb, has a resting blood pressure of 116/72 mm Hg, heart rate of 78 beats/min, HbA₁C of 7.0%, and a fasting blood glucose of 105 mg/dL. She also admits to drinking five alcoholic beverages each night from Thursday through Saturday. A.M. decides to enroll in your diabetes management program. A.M. completes a 3-day dietary analysis as part of the diabetes management program and the results are as follows:

> *Total caloric intake per day = 1,910 calories*
> *Carbohydrates = 47% of total calories*
> *Monounsaturated fats = 8% of total calories*
> *Polyunsaturated fats = 17% of total calories*
> *Saturated fats = 20% of total calories*
> *Total fats = 45% of total calories*
> *Protein = 8% of total calories*
> *Total dietary cholesterol = 350 mg*
> *Fiber = 12 g*
> *Calcium = 1,050 mg/day*
> *Potassium = 4,500 mg/day*
> *Magnesium = 400 mg/day*
> *Sodium = 2,000 mg/day*

Case Activities

1. *Write an SOAP note for A.M.*
2. *List A.M.'s risk factors for diabetes complications and determine whether an intervention is needed.*
3. *Design a program that includes nutrition and exercise counseling for A.M. that will improve her glucose control and decrease her risk for diabetes complications.*

REFERENCES

1. Mokdad AH, Marks JS, Stroup DF, Gerberding JL. Actual causes of death in the United States, 2000. JAMA 2004;291:1238–1245.
2. Carlisle BA, Kroon LA, Koda-Kimble MA. Diabetes mellitus. In: Koda-Kimble MA, ed. Applied Therapeutics: The Clinical Use of Drugs, 8th ed. Philadelphia: Lippincott Williams & Wilkins, 2005:50.1–50.86.
3. American Heart Association. Heart Disease and Stroke Statistics—2006 Update. Available at: http://americanheart.org/downloadable/heart/113535864858055–1026_HS_Stats06book.pdf. Accessed January 28, 2006.
4. Centers for Disease Control and Prevention. At a glance: diabetes. Atlanta: U.S. Department of Health and Human Services, Centers for Disease Control and Prevention, Coordinating Center for Health Promotion, 2005.
5. Triplitt CL, Reasner CA, Isley WL. Diabetes mellitus. In: Dipiro JT, ed. Pharmacotherapy: A Pathophysiologic Approach, 6th ed. New York: McGraw-Hill, 2005:1333–1367.
6. Centers for Disease Control and Prevention. National diabetes fact sheet: general information and national estimates on diabetes in the United States, 2005. Atlanta: U.S. Department of Health and Human Services, Centers for Disease Control and Prevention, 2005.
7. American Diabetes Association. Position Statement. Standards of medical care in diabetes—2006. Diabetes Care 2006;29(Suppl 1):S4–S42.
8. Knowler WC, Barrett-Conner E, Fowler SE, et al. Reduction in the incidence of type 2 diabetes with lifestyle intervention or metformin. N Engl J Med 2002;346:393–403.
9. Pan XR, Li GW, Hu YH, et al. Effects of diet and exercise in preventing NIDDM in people with impaired glucose tolerance: the Da Quig IGT and Diabetes Study. Diabetes Care 1997;20:537–544.

10. Buchanan TA, Xiang AH, Peters RK, et al. Prevention of pancreatic beta-cell function and prevention of type 2 diabetes by pharmacological treatment of insulin resistance in high risk Hispanic women. Diabetes 2002;51:2796–2803.

11. Chiasson JL, Josse RG, Gomis R, Hanefeld M, Karasik A, Laakso M. Acarbose for prevention of type 2 diabetes mellitus: the STOP-NIDDM randomized trial. Lancet 2002;359:2072–2077.

12. Tuomilehto J, Lindstrom J, Eriksson JG, et al. Prevention of type 2 diabetes mellitus by changes in lifestyle among subjects with impaired glucose tolerance. N Engl J Med 2001;344:1343–1350.

13. American Diabetes Association. Position Statement. Third-party reimbursement for diabetes care, self-management education, and supplies. Diabetes Care 2006;29(Suppl 1):S68–S69.

14. National Institutes of Health, National Heart, Lung, and Blood Institute. Third report of the National Cholesterol Education Program (NCEP) Expert Panel on Detection, Evaluation, and Treatment of High Blood Cholesterol in Adults (Adult Treatment Panel III). NIH Publication No. 02-5215, September 2002.

15. American Diabetes Association. Position Statement. Nutrition principles and recommendations in diabetes. Diabetes Care 2004;27(Suppl 1):S36–S46.

16. Whaley MH, ed. ACSM's Guidelines for Exercise Testing and Prescription, 7th ed. Philadelphia: Lippincott Williams & Wilkins, 2006:207–211.

17. Verity LS. Diabetes mellitus and exercise. In: Kaminsky LA, ed. ACSM's Resource Manual for Guidelines for Exercise Testing and Prescription, 5th ed. Philadelphia: Lippincott Williams & Wilkins, 2006:470–479.

18. Feld S. The American association of clinical endocrinologists medical guidelines for the management of diabetes mellitus: the AACE system of intensive diabetes self-management—2002 update. Endocr Pract 2002;8(Suppl 1):40–82.

19. Devlin JT, Hirshman M, Horton ED, Horton ES. Enhanced peripheral and splanchnic insulin sensitivity in NIDDM men after single bout of exercise. Diabetes 1987;39:434–439.

20. American Diabetes Association. Physical activity/exercise in diabetes. Diabetes Care 2003;26(Suppl):S73–S77.

21. Koivisto VA, Felig P. Effects of leg exercise on insulin absorption in diabetic patients. N Engl J Med 1978;298:79–83.

22. Sczupak CA, Conrad WF. Relationship between patient-oriented pharmaceutical services and therapeutic outcomes of ambulatory patients with diabetes mellitus. Am J Hosp Pharm 1977;34:1238–1242.

23. Cooper JW. Consultant pharmacist contribution to diabetes mellitus patient outcomes in two nursing facilities. Cons Pharm 1995;10:40–45.

24. American Pharmacists Association. Available at: http://www.aphanet.org/AM/Template.cfm?Section=Pharmacy_Practice&CONTENTID=2907&TEMPLATE=/CM/HTMLDisplay.cfm. Accessed February 8, 2006.

25. Munroe WP, Kunz K, Dalmady-Israel C, Potter L, Schonfeld WH. Economic evaluation of pharmacist involvement in disease management in a community pharmacy setting. Clin Ther 1997;19:113–123.

26. Borgsdorf LR, Miano JS, Knapp KK. Pharmacist managed medication review in a managed care system. Am J Hosp Pharm 1994;51:772–777.

Obesity

At the end of this chapter the reader should be able to:

1. Explain the health risks associated with obesity.
2. List the treatment options available for obesity.
3. Describe the components of proper nutrition for patients who are obese.
4. Suggest appropriate exercises for patients who are obese.
5. Formulate a basic nutrition and exercise program for a patient who is obese.

OVERVIEW OF OBESITY

The incidence of obesity among American adults has risen significantly in the past 20 years. The problem is not only isolated to adults; the prevalence among children is also increasing. Pharmacists and other healthcare providers have daily contact with patients who are obese for weight-related and non–weight-related medical conditions. This frequent contact provides pharmacists and others the opportunity to provide patient interventions that may lead to weight loss, lower incidences of chronic disease, and improved overall health. This chapter, along with Chapter 3, discusses weight-loss and weight-maintenance strategies that pharmacists can use when treating obese patients.

PREVALENCE, ECONOMIC COSTS, AND HEALTH RISKS ASSOCIATED WITH OVERWEIGHT AND OBESITY

The number of Americans who are overweight or obese has become a significant public health problem in recent years. It is reported that approximately 65% of the U.S.

adult population is either obese or overweight, with more than 30% of the adult population being obese.[1] **Obesity** appears to be slightly more prevalent in females (33.2%) compared with males (27.6%).[1] The prevalence is especially high in black and Mexican American females (49.0% and 38.4%, respectively) compared with white, Hispanic or Latino, and Asian females (30.7%, 25.4%, and 7.0%, respectively). From 1999 to 2002 the prevalence of obesity increased 75%.[1] In addition, it is estimated that 300,000 U.S. adults die each year of causes related to obesity.[2]

The estimated annual cost attributed to obesity-related diseases in the United States is approximately $100 billion.[3] In addition, hospital costs related to obesity among children and adolescents were estimated at $127 million during 1997 to 1999.[4]

PATHOPHYSIOLOGY OF OBESITY

Obesity is defined as having excess body fat that often leads to additional and significant health problems. Overweight and obesity can be assessed using several different methods such as body mass index, height and weight tables, girth measurements, body fat distribution, and body fat percentage.[5] **Body mass index (BMI)** is one of the most common and easy to use methods to assess patients for overweight and obesity. Patient height and weight can be applied to a BMI table (such as in Appendix B) or hand calculated by using one of the following two formulas:[5,6]

$$[\text{weight (pounds)}/\text{height (inches}^2)] \times 703$$

OR

$$[\text{weight (kg)}/\text{height (m}^2)]$$

The *Clinical Guidelines on the Identification, Evaluation, and Treatment of Overweight and Obesity in Adults* (http://www.nhlbi.nih.gov/guidelines/) defines a normal BMI as 18.5 to 24.9 kg/m².[5] Overweight is defined as having a BMI of 25.0 to 29.9 kg/m², and obesity and extreme obesity are defined by a BMI of 30.0 to 39.9 and 40 kg/m² or greater, respectively.[5]

One caution to using BMI to assess a patient's health status is that it may not work to accurately assess the overweight or obese status with all individuals. Because the calculation uses height and weight measurements to calculate BMI, individuals with a high degree of muscle mass may appear to have a falsely high BMI. Therefore, using body fat percentage method for these individuals along with BMI may give a more accurate depiction of the patient's health status as it relates to body size.

There are several contributing factors that can lead an individual to become overweight or obese. These factors are listed in Table 13-1. Two of the most common causes of obesity in the United States and other developed countries are an excess in calorie intake combined with a lack of physical activity. To maintain current body weight, a balance between calories that are taken in through food consumption and calories that are expended through metabolism and physical activity is required. When the body takes in more calories than it is expending, a positive caloric balance is obtained and weight is gained. When the body expends more calories than it consumes through the diet, a **negative caloric balance** is obtained and weight is lost.[7]

Obesity is associated with several serious comorbid conditions as well as with increased mortality. Increases in body weight and body fat and the central distribution

TABLE 13–1   Environmental Risk Factors Leading to Obesity

Excess calorie intake
Physical inactivity
Environmental factors
Hypothalamic disorder
Endocrine disorder
Genetic disorder

Source: Clinical Guidelines on the Identification, Evaluation, and Treatment of Overweight and Obesity in Adults. Bethesda, MD: National Institutes of Health, U.S. Department of Health and Human Services, 1998. NIH Publication No. 98-4083.

of body fat are contributors to increasing the prevalence of comorbid conditions.[8] Many of the associated diseases that increase mortality are caused by increases in cardiovascular disease. A list of disease outcomes resulting from obesity is provided in Table 13-2.

Obesity can significantly shorten the lifespan of individuals. A 20-year-old white male with a BMI of greater than 45 kg/m² is estimated to have 13 years of life lost as a

TABLE 13–2   Disease Outcomes Resulting From Obesity

Category	Disease or Condition
Cardiovascular	Hypertension
	Hypercholesterolemia
	Hypertriglyceridemia
	Decreased high-density lipoprotein
	Stroke
	Coronary artery disease
	Left ventricular hypertrophy
	Heart failure
Metabolic	Insulin resistance
	Diabetes mellitus
Respiratory	Sleep apnea
	Obstructive pulmonary disease
Cancer	Endometrial cancer
	Breast cancer
	Prostate cancer
	Colon cancer
Musculoskeletal	Osteoarthritis
Psychological	Depression
Other	Gallbladder disease
	Pregnancy complications
	Menstrual irregularities
	Stress incontinence
	Hirsutism
	Hiatus hernia

Source: Clinical Guidelines on the Identification, Evaluation, and Treatment of Overweight and Obesity in Adults. Bethesda, MD: National Institutes of Health, U.S. Department of Health and Human Services, 1998. NIH Publication No. 98-4083.

result of obesity. A 20-year-old white female with the same BMI can expect to have 8 years of life lost as a result of obesity. These same estimates for black males and females are 20 and 5 years, respectively, of life lost as a result of obesity. An optimal BMI between 20 and 25 kg/m^2 is associated with the lowest risk of mortality. A BMI of less than 20kg/m^2 and greater than 30 kg/m^2 is associated with a moderate to very high risk of mortality.[5]

OBESITY DISEASE PREVENTION AND TREATMENT

The overarching goals in a weight-loss program that guide the more patient-specific goals are to (1) prevent further weight gain, (2) reduce body weight, and (3) maintain a lower body weight for a long period.[5] Before beginning a weight-loss program the healthcare practitioner and patient must first establish clear and measurable goals that are specifically designed for that patient. The *Clinical Guidelines on the Identification, Evaluation, and Treatment of Overweight and Obesity in Adults* recommend a starting weight-loss goal of 10% of the initial body weight.[5] Once the patient has had a successful initial 10% weight loss, an assessment of the program by the practitioner and patient should be done and further weight-loss goals defined. The Guidelines recommend that a reasonable time frame for the initial 10% weight loss is during a 6-month period. It is recommended that weight loss at a rate of 1 to 2 pounds per week is appropriate for patients to maintain adequate basal metabolism and to achieve their 10% weight reduction within 6 months.[5]

Obesity is now being thought of as a chronic disease rather than a temporary condition that can be resolved with weight loss. Therefore, after patients have successfully obtained their weight-loss goals, an aggressive maintenance strategy should be initiated. The weight-maintenance program should consist of dietary therapy, physical activity, and behavior therapy and should be continued indefinitely.[6] Included in this strategy is continued follow-up from their healthcare practitioner. The incidence of weight gain after successful participation in a weight-loss program is high and should be prevented with weight-maintenance goals and a follow-up plan. A follow-up plan with the pharmacist can be implemented and scheduled around regular medication refill times. The number of follow-up visits with each patient will be specific to the individual needs of that patient, but can range from monthly to once every 6 months.

Childhood Obesity

Like adults, the number of children who are overweight and obese has increased dramatically in the past several decades. Many factors have been suggested as contributing to the cause of the obesity epidemic in children. Many social and environmental factors such as reduced physical education in schools, increased homework loads, campus vending machines, larger portion sizes, television, fast food restaurants, video games, and others are blamed for the increasing number of obese children.[9] Even though it is recommended that childhood obesity be prevented and treated in the clinical setting, healthcare providers must have an understanding of the many social and environmental factors that contribute to obesity and work toward modifying these factors if obesity in children is expected to decline.[9]

Many of the suggested social and environmental factors that have been theorized as causes of childhood obesity have been shown not to be substantiated. Research looking back to the 1970s has shown that school homework has not significantly increased during the past three decades and is not likely to be a contributor to the obesity epidemic.[9] The amount of free time of children, however, has substantially declined in recent years. Since 1981, the total weekly free time of children has declined by 12% and the time spent away from home, particularly in school, daycare, and after-school activities has increased.[9] In addition, unstructured playtime has also decreased to make time for more organized activities. It was previously thought that children are not spending as much time playing organized sports as in previous years, but this is not the case. Children in 1997 reported participating in organized sports 73 minutes longer per week compared with children in 1981.[9] Other activities that occupy more of children's time than in previous decades are shopping and personal care time. The categories in which children are actually spending fewer minutes per week compared with the early 1980s are in general playing time and other passive leisure activities, and they on average watch less television (−246 min/week).[9] Therefore, children are participating in more structured activities today than they were in the early 1980s; however, playtime has decreased, and organized sports time has increased. In addition, some have contributed the increase in childhood obesity to a decrease in walking or biking as a form of transportation for children. Research, however, has shown that this has changed little during the past few decades.[10]

Many of the frequent and significant hypotheses on weight gain address changes in food and diet. It has been shown that eating as a primary activity has declined in recent decades. Although this may initially seem to be a positive aspect in the fight against obesity, it is quite the opposite. This information indicates that there is a shift away from family "sit-down" meals and toward snacking. As reported above, children are involved in more activities than in the past and are therefore eating quick, convenient meals. The food industry has accommodated this trend, but, unfortunately, these types of foods are often low in nutritional value and high in calories. The intake of chips, crackers, popcorn, and pretzels tripled from the mid 1970s to the mid 1990s.[10] The intake of soft drinks has doubled during this same period.[10] In addition, it is less expensive to purchase fast convenient foods versus fresh fruits and vegetables. Starting from a baseline of 100 during 1982 to 1984, the price index for soft drinks has only increased to 126 by 2002, representing an increase below that of the general inflation. By contrast, the price index of fresh fruits and vegetables increased to 258 by 2002, representing an increase that far exceeds that of general inflation.[10]

Pharmacists, as members of the healthcare community, can be advocates for better overall health in children. Pharmacists can educate and encourage parents and children about the importance of healthy eating and physical activity. Much work is needed both in the clinical setting with individual patients and in the social and environmental factors that contribute to obesity. Healthcare providers have a responsibility to promote overall good health in all factors that contribute to childhood obesity.

Weight-Loss and Weight-Maintenance Strategies

An effective weight-control program incorporates a combination of several treatment strategies. Available strategies include dietary therapy, **physical activity,** behavior therapy, pharmacotherapy, and surgery. The appropriate treatment strategy will depend on the patient's BMI and comorbidities. The Guidelines recommend that everyone participate in the lifestyle modification components of dietary therapy and physical activity unless they are contraindicated.[5] Incorporating these treatment strategies is important because they have not only been shown to improve the success of a weight-loss program, but have also been shown to decrease some of the comorbidities associated with obesity. Specific details regarding these therapies are discussed later in this chapter.

Behavior Therapy

Behavior therapy is a critical aspect of a weight-loss program because it incorporates techniques that can be used to overcome barriers that exist within the dietary therapy and physical activity programs.[6] As with other aspects of a weight-loss program, behavior therapy needs to be individualized to the patient. Before attempting to motivate the patient for change, the practitioner must first evaluate the patient's readiness for change and the patient's own self-motivation level. The behavior therapy plan should include important themes such as setting appropriate and achievable goals and focusing on the main outcomes of the program. The most important outcome of a weight-loss program should be to improve the patient's health.[6] Monitoring progress is a continuous and ongoing process and is the responsibility of both the patient and the healthcare practitioner. Behavior therapy is recommended along with dietary therapy and physical activity for all patients with a BMI of 25 kg/m² or greater.[6] Table 13-3 lists important aspects of the behavior therapy plan that can help improve patient adherence.

Pharmacotherapy

The use of medication to treat obesity is suggested to be appropriate if the patient has a BMI of 27 to 29.9 kg/m² with the existence of comorbidities.[6] Obesity medications are appropriate to use in patients with a BMI of 30 kg/m² or greater regardless of the presence of comorbidities.[6] There are currently six commonly used drugs that have U.S. Food and Drug Administration (FDA) approval to be used for weight loss.[11] Since 1973 only two of these six drugs have been approved, and these same two drugs are the only ones approved for long-term use. The two drugs are orlistat and sibutramine. As a result, these are the most commonly prescribed weight-loss medications used today.

TABLE 13–3   Program Adherence Recommendations in a Weight-Loss Program

Assess weight-loss history, attitudes, and beliefs before beginning a weight-loss program
Build a constructive partnership between the patient and the pharmacist
Set achievable goals
Maintain adequate follow-up with the patient (especially within first 6 months)
Have a long-term weight-maintenance plan that incorporates follow-up appointments
Have patient self-monitor progress by recording daily food intake and checking body weight weekly
Have patient identify external cues that stimulate undesired eating
Have patient eat breakfast daily
Have patient exercise regularly
Focus on the most important outcome—health improvement
Congratulate patient on successes
Do not criticize shortcomings

Source: The Practical Guide. Identification, Evaluation, and Treatment of Overweight and Obesity in Adults. Bethesda, MD: National Institutes of Health, U.S. Department of Health and Human Services, 2000. NIH Publication No. 00-4084.

TABLE 13-4 Drug Classes Used for Weight Loss

Noradrenergic agents
Noradrenergic and serotonergic agent
Lipase inhibitor

It is important to note that sibutramine has been shown to produce significant increases in both **systolic** and **diastolic blood pressure** as well as heart rate.[6] Therefore, sibutramine should not be used in patients with a history of coronary artery disease, **stroke,** heart failure, or arrhythmias and should be used with caution in patients with pulmonary hypertension.[12] Measuring blood pressure at baseline and throughout treatment is recommended regardless of whether comorbidities exist. Medications with FDA approval for weight loss are listed in Table 13-4.

Surgery

The use of surgery to promote weight loss is an option in patients with the existence of comorbidities and a BMI of 35 to 39 kg/m² or in patients without comorbidities and a BMI of 40 kg/m² or greater.[5] Weight-loss surgery should be reserved for patients in whom other weight-loss treatments have failed and who have clinically severe obesity.[6] Two types of surgical procedures have been shown to produce effective weight loss in patients. Banded gastroplasty limits gastric volume and therefore decreases food intake, and gastric bypass alters digestion in addition to limiting food intake. Both procedures have shown significant weight loss sustained for 5 years or greater, and both are recommended to integrate programs of dietary counseling, physical activity, and behavior therapy before and after surgery.[6]

NUTRITION AND OBESITY

Dietary therapy is a key component of weight-loss and weight-maintenance therapy as most overweight and obese persons will need adjustments in caloric intake to lose weight. The dietary therapy component of weight loss focuses on teaching patients how to modify their individual diet to decrease calorie intake. It is very important that calorie reduction recommendations are not too aggressive and are made with the goal of slow and progressive weight loss through moderate calorie reduction. In addition, the composition of the diet should be balanced and structured in a way that decreases other possible cardiovascular risk factors such as **hypertension, dyslipidemia,** and **diabetes mellitus.**

The focus of weight loss through dietary therapy is to create a **caloric deficit** by decreasing the caloric intake. To achieve this caloric deficit, a low-calorie diet is recommended that consists of at least 1,000 to 1,200 kcal/day for most women and 1,200 to 1,600 kcal/day for most men.[6] The specific caloric intake for each patient should be individualized and chosen with the patient's baseline caloric intake and body weight in mind. Healthcare practitioners should emphasize to patients that moderate dietary changes should be incorporated rather than drastic dietary changes. This will help maintain patient compliance to the weight-loss regimen and produce slow and progressive weight loss. A diet that is individually designed to create a deficit of 500 to 1,000 kcal/day should be adequate to produce a 1- to 2-pound weight loss per week.[6]

It should be noted that very low calorie diets (<800 kcal/day) require extra dietary supplementation and are only recommended in specific patients for short periods. The amount of weight loss is similar with low-calorie diets and very low calorie diets; however, the incidence of weight regain is greater with very low calorie diets.[5,6] Only specialized practitioners with experience in the use of very low calorie diets should recommend this type of therapy.

Successful dietary therapy is dependent on modifying the patient's diet to create a caloric deficit while allowing for all the necessary dietary allowances and also maintaining food preferences of the patient. This can be challenging but is achievable through detailed patient consultation. The patients must be involved in this process. It is oftentimes helpful to give the patient several appropriate choices and allow the patient to choose the diet. This allows them to self-monitor their intake and improves compliance as stated in the behavior therapy section. The keys to success for dietary therapy are to (1) educate patients regarding the calorie value of foods they are choosing as well as the composition (carbohydrate, fats, and protein) by reading the nutrition label, (2) avoid overconsumption of high-calorie foods, (3) reduce portion size, and (4) maintain adequate water intake. Specific dietary composition recommendations from the Guidelines are listed in Table 13-5.

PHYSICAL ACTIVITY AND OBESITY

Physical activity is an important component of a weight-loss program for several reasons. Increasing physical activity, along with decreasing calorie intake, will help promote a

TABLE 13–5   Dietary Recommendations for Patients Who Are Overweight or Obese

Nutrient	Recommendation
Total calories[a]	Approximately 500–1,000 kcal/day reduction from usual intake
Carbohydrate[b]	55% or more of total calories
Fiber	20–30 g/day
Protein	Approximately 15% of total calories
Monounsaturated fat	Up to 15% of total calories
Polyunsaturated fat	Up to 10% of total calories
Saturated fat	8–10% of total calories
Total fat	30% or less of total calories
Dietary cholesterol	<300 mg/day
Sodium chloride	No more than 100 mmol/day (approximately 2.4 g of sodium, or approximately 6 g of sodium chloride)
Calcium	1,000–1,500 mg/day

[a]It is recommended that alcohol not be consumed as part of the daily caloric intake as it will increase the total calories but has also been shown to be associated with obesity in epidemiologic studies.
[b]Most carbohydrate intake should come from whole grains, fruits, and vegetables.
Source: The Practical Guide. Identification, Evaluation, and Treatment of Overweight and Obesity in Adults. Bethesda, MD: National Institutes of Health, U.S. Department of Health and Human Services, 2000. NIH Publication No. 00-4084.

caloric deficit needed for weight loss. In addition, physical activity improves maintenance of weight loss, decreases the loss of fat-free mass–associated weight loss, and improves cardiovascular and metabolic health independent of weight loss.[6,7]

Physical activity may be one of the most important components involved in the maintenance of weight loss. Maintaining body weight can occur directly by increasing caloric expenditure through physical activity. It can also occur indirectly by promoting a positive behavior change in which the patient decreases food consumption. The influence of physical activity on food intake is not well known, but it is thought to have a possible impact on calorie intake in some individuals.[13]

Decreasing body weight by reducing body fat and maintaining lean body tissue (along with patient safety) is the main goal in the treatment of overweight and obese patients. Including physical activity into a weight-loss regimen along with dieting has been shown to significantly reduce the amount of lean tissue lost during weight loss ($P < 0.05$).[14] Individuals who will most likely be successful during a weight-loss program include those who are slightly or moderately obese, have upper body fat distribution, have no history of weight cycling, became overweight as an adult, and have a sincere desire to lose weight.[13]

Many overweight and obese patients have been sedentary for many years. As a result, these patients may lack the confidence, motivation, and skills needed to participate in physical activities. Therefore, some patients may need supervision when first beginning a physical activity program. Safety should always be the highest priority for patients beginning a physical activity program, especially if they have little experience being physically active. Physical injury may be one of the primary reasons for discontinuation of physical activity in obese patients.[13] A patient who becomes injured while exercising will be increasingly difficult to motivate to continue the program after the injury heals.[6] Overweight and obese patients must always obtain clearance from their physician before beginning an exercise program.[7] Some patients may require testing for cardiopulmonary disease before beginning, depending on their symptoms and comorbidities.[6]

Depending on the prior experiences and the length of time the patient has been sedentary, the physical activity program should begin very slowly and proceed gradually. For some patients, an initial program may begin with increasing the activities of daily living. Examples of this could include work around the house, such as vacuuming, ironing, cooking, gardening, or painting a room.[6] Other patients may begin at a level that includes a slow 10-minute walk around the neighborhood, riding a stationary bicycle, or swimming at a slow pace. Still others may be able to work at a greater intensity by walking more briskly, rowing or cycling at a greater intensity, or using other non-impact aerobic machines. Recreational sports such as tennis, racquetball, and basketball are also good activities that will increase caloric expenditure and improve the patient's cardiovascular profile. It is important to remember that overweight and obese patients are at increased risk for orthopedic injuries if they participate in high-impact activities such as running. These types of activities should be avoided until the patient has lost a sufficient amount of weight and has improved their aerobic capacity with other activities.

The activities that are appropriate for each patient should be individualized. Decisions on the type and amount of activity will depend on the patient's comorbidities, prior experiences, and specific preferences.[7] Many patients should begin with non–weight-bearing activities or very low intensity weight-bearing activities and progress to greater intensity activities. Many of the activities that are chosen, such as walking or cycling, can be performed for short amounts of time (e.g., 5 to 10 minutes) several times per day. It is important to begin a program with short-duration activities that are preferable to the patients. This will be more encouraging and enjoyable and lead to better compliance. The progression of the activities should begin with 2 to 3 days per week and progress to most days of the week. It is important also to emphasize an increase in duration over intensity for the initial several weeks of the program. This will decrease the risks for injury and improve compliance. The American College of Sports Medicine recommends that overweight and obese adults progress to a minimum of 150 minutes of moderate-intensity exercise per week and, when possible, progress to greater than 200 minutes of moderate-intensity exercise per week.[7] Greater and more effective results will be experienced with a longer duration of activity. Therefore, patients who have weight loss as their goal should attempt to increase physical activity duration up to 60 minutes per day.

Resistance and flexibility exercises are also important activities to include in a physical activity program for weight loss. Resistance training activities can be effective at helping maintain lean tissue as well as increasing strength to improve functional activities such as activities of daily living, vocational activities, and improved self-confidence. Resistance training can be performed using stretch bands or strength training equipment. Flexibility exercises should be performed as part of a proper warm-up and cool-down and can also help improve patients' functional capacities by improving activities of daily living.

Suggested exercise guidelines for patients who are overweight and obese are provided in Table 13-6.

PHARMACY PRACTICE APPLICATION

Because pharmacists regularly treat patients with a variety of medical conditions, they are well positioned to counsel overweight and obese patients regardless of whether they are taking medication for weight loss. Knowing the medical history of a patient and the medications being taken can allow the pharmacist to accurately assess the health risks of a patient based on his or her body weight and comorbidities. In a community pharmacy

TABLE 13–6 **Physical Activity Recommendations for Patients Who Are Overweight or Obese**

Goals	Reduce risk for cardiovascular disease
	Reduce body weight while maintaining lean body tissue
	Improve functional performance including activities of daily living
Type of activity	Large muscle activities (e.g., walking, bicycling, dancing, rowing, swimming, water aerobics, tennis, racquetball, gardening, lawn mowing)
Intensity[a]	Very low to moderate
Duration[a]	5–10 minutes (initially)
	20–60 minutes (more advanced; or 2–3 sessions/day of 10–30 minutes each)
Frequency	2–4 times per week (for initial 2–8 weeks)
	Most days of the week (after initial 8 weeks)
Lifestyle activity	Increase overall daily activities inside and outside of home

[a]Emphasize increasing duration rather than intensity.

Source: ACSM Position Stand on the Appropriate Intervention Strategies for Weight Loss and Prevention of Weight Regain for Adults. Med Sci Sports Exerc 2001;33:2145–2156.

setting, pharmacist interventions regarding weight loss can conveniently take place at the same time the patient comes to the pharmacy to pick up medications or at the time drug counseling occurs. Pharmacists practicing in a hospital setting can address weight-loss issues with patients and begin to assess their willingness to participate in a weight-loss program. This is also a good opportunity to educate patients about the benefits of weight loss and the important components involved in a weight-loss program. It is important for pharmacists to work in close contact with the patient's physician and other healthcare providers to keep the patient's safety the highest priority and to update the other healthcare providers on the status of the patient's progress with the weight-loss program.

CASE STUDY

J.M. is a 38-year-old female who comes into the pharmacy to fill a prescription for one of her three children. She notices the preventive health information display and handouts in the pharmacy. After obtaining counseling about the medication for her child, she inquires about a weight-loss program that the pharmacy offers and states that she currently does not participate in an exercise program of any kind. She is 5′ 3″ tall, weighs 180 lb, and has a resting heart rate of 90 beats/min and blood pressure of 117/66 mm Hg. J.M. agreed to participate in a weight-control program and proceeded to complete a 3-day dietary analysis, which revealed the following:

> *Ave caloric intake per day = 2,775 calories*
> *Carbohydrates = 45% of total calories*
> *Monounsaturated fats = 15% of total calories*
> *Polyunsaturated fats = 15% of total calories*
> *Saturated fats = 15% of total calories*
> *Total fats = 45% of total calories*
> *Protein = 10% of total calories*
> *Total dietary cholesterol = 250 mg*
> *Fiber = 15 g*
> *Calcium = 800 mg/day*

Case Activities

1. *Write an SOAP note for J.M.*
2. *Write short- and long-term dietary and exercise goals for J.M.*
3. *Write an exercise prescription and dietary suggestions for J.M.*
4. *Design a weight-loss program for J.M.*

REFERENCES

1. American Heart Association. Heart Disease and Stroke Statistics—2005 Update. Dallas: American Heart Association, 2005.
2. Allison DB, Fontaine KR, Manson JE, Stevens J, VanItallie TB. Annual deaths attributable to obesity in the United States. JAMA 1999;282:1530–1538.
3. Centers for Disease Control and Prevention. State-specific prevalence of obesity among adults with disabilities—eight states and the District of Colombia, 1998–1999. MMWR Morb Mortal Wkly Rep 2002;51:805.
4. Centers for Disease Control and Prevention. Available at: www.cdc.gov/nccdphp/pe_factsheets. Accessed October 13, 2006.
5. Clinical Guidelines on the Identification, Evaluation, and Treatment of Overweight and Obesity in Adults. Bethesda, MD: National Institutes of Health, U.S. Department of Health and Human Services, 1998. NIH Publication No. 98-4083.

6. The Practical Guide. Identification, Evaluation, and Treatment of Overweight and Obesity in Adults. Bethesda, MD: National Institutes of Health, U.S. Department of Health and Human Services, 2000. NIH Publication No. 00-4084.

7. ACSM position stand on the appropriate intervention strategies for weight loss and prevention of weight regain for adults. Med Sci Sports Exerc 2001;33:2145–2156.

8. Fletcher BJ, Grundy SM. Obesity: impact on cardiovascular disease. Circulation 1998;98:1472–1476.

9. Sturn R. Childhood obesity—what we can learn from existing data on societal trends, part 1. Prev Chronic Dis 2005. Available at: http://www.cdc.gov/pcd/issues/2005/jan/04_0038.htm. Accessed October 13, 2006.

10. Sturn R. Childhood obesity—what we can learn from existing data on societal trends, part 2. Prev Chronic Dis 2005. Available at: http://www.cdc.gov/pcd/issues/2005/apr/04_0039.htm. Accessed October 13, 2006.

11. North American Association for the Study of Obesity. Available at: http://www.obesityonline.org/slides/slide01.cfm?tk=37&dpg=2. Accessed January 27, 2005.

12. Package insert. Meridia (sibutramine hydrochloride monohydrate). North Chicago, IL: Abbott Laboratories, December 2004.

13. Wallace JP. Obesity. In: Durstine JL, Moore GE, eds. ACSM's Exercise Management for Persons With Chronic Diseases and Disabilities. Champaign, IL: Human Kinetics, 2003:149–156.

CHAPTER 14

Metabolic Syndrome

OBJECTIVES

At the end of this chapter the reader should be able to:

1. Explain the risks associated with the metabolic syndrome.
2. Summarize the prevention and treatment options for the metabolic syndrome.
3. Describe appropriate nutritional strategies for patients with the metabolic syndrome.
4. Suggest appropriate exercises for patients with the metabolic syndrome.
5. Formulate basic nutrition, exercise, weight-loss, and smoking-cessation programs for a patient with the metabolic syndrome.

OVERVIEW OF METABOLIC SYNDROME

Metabolic syndrome has been defined as a "constellation" of metabolic risk factors in one individual.[1,2] These interrelated risk factors are thought to directly promote the development of atherosclerotic **cardiovascular disease** and are strongly associated with **type 2 diabetes mellitus** or the risk for this condition.[2] The metabolic risk factors involved include atherogenic **dyslipidemia** (elevated **triglycerides** and apolipoprotein B, small **low-density lipoprotein (LDL)** particles, and low amounts of **high-density lipoprotein (HDL)** cholesterol concentrations), elevated blood pressure, elevated plasma glucose, a prothrombotic state, and a proinflammatory state.[2]

PREVALENCE, ECONOMIC COSTS, AND HEALTH RISKS ASSOCIATED WITH METABOLIC SYNDROME

Using the National Cholesterol Education Program (NCEP) Adult Treatment Panel III (ATP III), it was estimated in 2002 that approximately 47 million Americans have metabolic syndrome.[1,3,4] The age-adjusted prevalence for metabolic syndrome in 2002 was 23.7%, and as Americans get older the prevalence increases.[3] In 2004, a different study using the same criteria estimated the prevalence to be 30% of adult Americans. In 2002, Mexican Americans had the highest prevalence of any race at 31.9%, with whites at 23.8% and African Americans at 21.6%.[3] Also in 2002, the overall prevalence was similar between men (24.0%) and women (23.4%). Among African Americans, however, women had a 57% higher prevalence than men as was the case with Mexican Americans in which women had a 26% higher prevalence than men.[3] Additionally, the risk for **coronary heart disease (CHD)** in individuals with metabolic syndrome was 7.4% compared with 3.6% in individuals without metabolic syndrome ($P < 0.001$).[3] Therefore, persons with metabolic syndrome are about two times more likely to have prevalent CHD compared with persons without metabolic syndrome after adjusting for established risk factors.[3]

It is also estimated that the prevalence of metabolic syndrome among U.S. adolescents is high. In 2003, an estimated 1 million U.S. adolescents between the ages of 12 and 19 years met the criteria for the diagnosis of metabolic syndrome.[3] This represents 4.2% of adolescents in the United States with males accounting for 6.2% and females accounting for 2.1% of the adolescent population.[3] Of the adolescents with metabolic syndrome, almost 74% were overweight and more than 25% were at risk for becoming overweight.[3]

Because of the relative newness of the diagnosis metabolic syndrome, little cost analysis data currently exist. One study, however, showed that the combination of **physical inactivity,** overweight, and **obesity** were associated with 23% of health plan healthcare charges and 27% of national healthcare charges between 1996 and 1999.[5] Charges associated with these risk factors were highest for the group that was 65 years of age and older and for those with chronic conditions. However, nearly half of the charges came from the group between the ages of 40 and 64 years without chronic disease.[5]

PATHOPHYSIOLOGY OF METABOLIC SYNDROME

As stated in the introduction, metabolic syndrome is a compilation of metabolic risk factors. It is currently unknown whether metabolic syndrome has a single cause or whether each of the underlying risk factors has independent pathophysiology that combines to create elevated cardiovascular risk for the patient.[1,2] The most important of the underlying risk factors are abdominal obesity and insulin resistance. A list of the risk factors for metabolic syndrome is provided in Table 14-1.

The NCEP ATP III guidelines (http://www.nhlbi.nih.gov/guidelines/) were one of the first to set criteria for diagnosis of metabolic syndrome.[1] More recently the American Heart Association and National Heart, Lung, and Blood Institute (AHA/NHLBI) (http://www.americanheart.org/presenter.jhtml?identifier=3004542) published a scientific statement on the diagnosis and management of metabolic syndrome.[2] The AHA/NHLBI largely use the same criteria as the NCEP ATP III guidelines for diagnosis with slight modifications. The criteria essentially consist of five risk components with each having a measured range to confirm diagnosis. Diagnosis of the metabolic syndrome is confirmed when the patient has three of five of the following criteria: (1) elevated waist circumference ($\geq$102 cm in men, $\geq$88 cm in women); (2) elevated triglycerides ($\geq$150 mg/dL or treatment for elevated triglycerides); (3) reduced HDL cholesterol (<40 mg/dL in men, <50 mg/dL in women, or treatment for reduced HDL

TABLE 14-1   Environmental Risk Factors Leading to Metabolic Syndrome

Abdominal obesity
Insulin resistance
Physical inactivity
Aging
Hormonal imbalance
Genetic predisposition
Ethnic predisposition
Atherogenic dyslipidemia
Raised blood pressure
Prothrombotic state
Proinflammatory state

Source: National Institutes of Health, National Heart, Lung, and Blood Institute. Third report of the National Cholesterol Education Program (NCEP) Expert Panel on Detection, Evaluation, and Treatment of High Blood Cholesterol in Adults (Adult Treatment Panel III). NIH Publication No. 02-5215, September 2002.

cholesterol); (4) elevated blood pressure (≥130 mm Hg systolic or ≥85 mm Hg diastolic or drug treatment for hypertension); and (5) elevated fasting glucose (≥100 mg/dL or drug treatment for elevated glucose).[2]

Having the diagnosis of metabolic syndrome has been shown to increase the patient's risk for atherosclerotic cardiovascular disease by twofold.[2] The pathophysiology of the syndrome is not well understood. Therefore, to understand why a patient with metabolic syndrome has an increased risk for atherosclerotic cardiovascular disease the pathophysiology for each risk factor in relation to increased risk for cardiovascular disease can be studied separately. Please refer to the pathophysiology section of each risk factor's respective chapter (**hypertension,** dyslipidemia, **diabetes mellitus,** and obesity) for greater pathophysiology clarification.

Mental Stress and Metabolic Syndrome

Mental stress has traditionally been linked as a risk factor for coronary heart disease (CHD). Retrospective and prospective studies have both shown that stress at the workplace can increase the risk for CHD.[6–8] The biologic mechanisms that link stress and CHD, however, are currently unknown. Some studies in the past have found that social gradient and work stress increase the risks for both metabolic syndrome and CHD.[6,9,10] Other studies have shown that work stress increases the risk for components of metabolic syndrome, but conclusions are not consistent.[6,11,12]

One particular project set out to design a prospective study to investigate the association between stress at work and its influence on the metabolic syndrome by repeatedly measuring work stress during a person's career.[6] Repeatedly measuring stress over time is thought to give an accurate representation of the exposure to psychosocial stress and its cumulative effects on health.[6] This particular study followed 10,308 participants for an average of 14 years, and work stress was measured on four different occasions. The participants were between the ages of 35 and 55 years at the beginning of the study and worked for 1 of 20 civil service departments in London, England, between the years 1985 and 1999.[6] Data on the components of metabolic syndrome were collected toward the end of the study and used the definition from the National Cholesterol Education Program (NCEP) Adult Treatment Panel III (ATP III) guidelines.[1]

The results of the study showed that a dose-response relationship exists between the exposure to work stressors during a 14-year period and the risk for metabolic syndrome, regardless of other risk factors.[6] The participants in the study who reported stress on three or more occasions (defined as chronic stress) were more than twice as likely to have metabolic syndrome compared with those without stress ($P = 0.01$) After excluding the participants who were obese at baseline, the authors concluded that the participant's preexisting physiologic risk is unlikely to explain the observed association with the metabolic risk and, therefore, it is likely that stress caused the syndrome.[6]

It is unknown whether the increased risk for metabolic syndrome was caused by the effects of chronic stress on insulin resistance, resting blood pressure, and lipoprotein metabolism. The authors of the study state, however, that prolonged stress may affect the autonomic nervous system and neuroendocrine activity directly, contributing to the increased risk for the syndrome.[6] This, along with increased blood pressure and inflammation caused by increased stress, may be the cause for increased metabolic syndrome risk and may partially explain the relationship between stress and CHD.

Healthcare providers can easily get into the habit of solely focusing on traditional risk factors like blood pressure and lipid levels when assessing CHD risk. The effect of mental stress on physiologic changes, however, should not be overlooked. Pharmacists can counsel patients about the importance of chronic stress on CHD risk and use the opportunity to emphasize increased **physical activity** as a strategy to improve both physical and mental health.

METABOLIC SYNDROME PREVENTION AND TREATMENT

Disease-prevention strategies are very important for patients with metabolic syndrome. Some patients may have an elevated short-term (within 10 years) risk, but all patients will have an elevated long-term risk for atherosclerotic cardiovascular disease.[2] A Framingham score (see Appendix A) should be assessed on each patient with the syndrome to determine short-term risk. Patients who already have atherosclerotic cardiovascular disease and diabetes have the highest short-term risk and should be treated with the most intensive interventions. Other patients may also have elevated short-term risk without these conditions, which will depend on the severity of each risk scored in the Framingham assessment.[2] Therefore, even in patients with metabolic syndrome, the short-term risk assessment depends on the Framingham scoring. However, because of the risk factors involved, patients with metabolic syndrome are at long-term risk regardless of Framingham score. Therefore, disease-prevention strategies should be used for every patient with metabolic syndrome to decrease long-term cardiovascular risks.[2]

The clinical management of metabolic syndrome is focused not only primarily on the prevention of cardiovascular disease but also on prevention of type 2 diabetes.[2] First-line prevention and treatment efforts center around smoking cessation, reducing LDL cholesterol, reducing blood pressure, and reducing blood glucose levels.[2] The intensity of the therapy will depend on the risk of the individual. Lifestyle intervention therapies are considered first-line intervention to reduce both short- and long-term metabolic risk factors.[2] The major lifestyle interventions include weight loss, increased physical activity, and dietary modifications.

Obesity, especially abdominal obesity, appears to have a high degree of atherogenicity.[2] The goal for patients with metabolic syndrome is to reduce body weight by 7 to 10% during the first year of therapy.[2] Thereafter, weight loss should continue with the ultimate desired goal of a body mass index (BMI) of less than 25 kg/m^2.[2] In addition, male patients should aim for a waist circumference of less than 40 inches and female patients, a waist circumference of less than 35 inches. Weight reduction should be accomplished through a combination of increased physical activity, decreased caloric intake, and behavioral modifications.[2] It is important to remind patients that even small amounts of weight loss are associated with significant health benefits.[2]

Physical activity is recommended for 30 minutes per day, five days per week at a moderate intensity.[2] Because weight loss is usually one of the primary goals for a patient with metabolic syndrome, it is preferred that physical activity ultimately be performed for 60 minutes on almost every day of the week.[2] Accumulated greater amounts of physical activity throughout each day through lifestyle activities should be stressed. In addition, patients with existing cardiovascular disease or high-risk CVD should be advised to **exercise** under direct medical supervision.[2]

An atherogenic diet consists of high amounts of saturated fat, *trans* fat, and **cholesterol.** Therefore, for patients with metabolic syndrome to decrease their risk for CVD, saturated fats should comprise less than 7% of total daily calories with total fat intake representing 25 to 35% of the total calories.[2] In addition, cholesterol intake should be limited to less than 200 mg/day, and *trans* fat intake should be minimized.[2] It is also recommended that most of the dietary fat consumed should be unsaturated, and refined and simple sugar intake be limited.[2]

As stated in the list of risk factors, most patients with metabolic syndrome display a prothrombotic and proinflammatory state.[2] A prothrombotic state is characterized by elevations of plasminogen activator-1 and fibrinogen, and a proinflammatory state is characterized by elevations of C-reactive protein.[2] There are currently no specific drugs available to treat either of these two conditions. However, low-dose aspirin is often recommended for patients with the metabolic syndrome and a Framingham score of 10% or greater, those with diabetes or CVD, and other high-risk patients.[2] In addition, recommendations for drug therapy for persons with elevated blood pressure (http://www.nhlbi.nih.gov/guidelines/), dyslipidemia (http://www.nhlbi.nih.gov/guidelines/), and diabetes (http://www.diabetes.org/for-health-professionals-and-scientists/cpr.jsp) should follow the established guidelines of the AHA, NHLBI, and American Diabetes Association to treat each condition (Table 14-2).[2]

TABLE 14–2   **Medications Used to Treat Metabolic Syndrome[a]**

Antiplatelet agents (e.g., low-dose aspirin especially for Framingham score ≥10%, and those with CVD, DM, or other high-risk conditions)

Medications used to treat high blood pressure (see Chapter 6)

Medications used to treat dyslipidemia (see Chapter 7)

Medications used to treat type 2 diabetes (see Chapter 12)

---

[a]No specific medications currently recommended for metabolic syndrome.

CVD, cardiovascular disease; DM, diabetes mellitus.

TABLE 14-3   **Program Adherence Recommendations for Patients With Metabolic Syndrome**

Ensure the patient has a clear understanding of the TLC components and the importance of each

Recommend that multiple adherence strategies work better than a single approach

Establish weekly contact with patients for the first 4 weeks of the program, then monthly thereafter, to continually assess the patient's progress and troubleshoot problems

Set achievable goals

Obtain baseline assessment of dietary intake

Institute a self-monitoring program such as keeping a log of food intake and exercise participation

Identify patient-specific barriers to the lifestyle changes

Distribute information that uses health messages associated with dyslipidemia that are easy to understand, interactive, and culturally sensitive

Design a program that is reasonable, gradual, and easily implemented

Source: National Institutes of Health, National Heart, Lung, and Blood Institute. Third report of the National Cholesterol Education Program (NCEP) Expert Panel on Detection, Evaluation, and Treatment of High Blood Cholesterol in Adults (Adult Treatment Panel III). NIH Publication No. 02-5215, September 2002. TLC, therapeutic lifestyle changes.

As with other diseases, adherence strategies are very important for patients with metabolic syndrome as lifestyle modifications are the primary focus of treatment and prevention. Several program adherence strategies have been identified in the dyslipidemia NCEP ATP III guidelines that have shown success in various studies.[1] A majority of the information comes from studies assessing weight-management therapy. In general, the literature emphasizes the importance of baseline assessment of dietary therapy as well as self-monitoring techniques of both dietary and exercise habits to improve program compliance.[1] In addition, offering health information that is culturally sensitive, interactive, and from reliable sources is important for improving adherence.[1] Suggestions to improve program adherence are listed in Table 14-3.

NUTRITION AND METABOLIC SYNDROME

Nutrition is an important aspect of treatment and prevention strategies for patients with metabolic syndrome. The NCEP ATP III dyslipidemia guidelines discuss in much detail several strategies for decreasing blood lipids and atherosclerotic risk through the use of a proper eating plan.[1] In addition, the AHA/NHLBI scientific statement on the diagnosis and management of metabolic syndrome also uses the NCEP ATP III guidelines in its nutritional recommendations.[2] Therefore, the nutritional recommendations in this chapter will follow those of the NCEP ATP III guidelines, which can also be found in Chapter 7.

Dietary modifications are the primary focus of the NCEP ATP III therapeutic lifestyle changes (TLC) therapy. The TLC diet is in general consistent with the Dietary Guidelines for Americans published by the U.S. Department of Agriculture and U.S. Department of Health and Human Services (http://healthierus.gov/dietaryguidelines/).[13] Lowering the LDL cholesterol is the first priority with diet modifications.[1] Once the patient has reached the LDL goal, emphasis on weight control and physical activity becomes the treatment priority.[1]

Lowering the LDL cholesterol through diet modifications can most successfully be accomplished by reducing the dietary intake of saturated fats, *trans* fatty acids, and cholesterol.[1,13] The NCEP ATP III guidelines recommend that total fat consumption not exceed 25 to 35% of the total daily caloric intake.[1,13] Most of the fat calorie consumption should be obtained from **unsaturated fatty acids.**[1,13,14] Polyunsaturated fats and monounsaturated fats make up the total of unsaturated fatty acids and should represent approximately 10 and 20%, respectively, of the total daily caloric intake.[1,14] The remaining amount of fat intake (less than 7% of total calories) can come from saturated fats.[1,14] In addition, NCEP ATP III further recommends that 50 to 60% of total calories come from carbohydrate and 15% from protein, and that there should be a daily fiber intake of 20 to 30 g.[1]

Saturated fats have proven to be closely associated with increases in total and LDL cholesterol.[1,14] Studies show that every 1% increase in calories of dietary **saturated fatty acids** correlates with a 2% increase in LDL cholesterol.[1,15,16] The opposite has also been shown to be true. Every 1% decrease in calories of dietary saturated fatty acids correlates with a 2% decrease in LDL cholesterol.[1,15–18] To limit the intake of saturated fatty acids, the American Heart Association recommends substituting unsaturated fatty acids in its place.[13,14] They have been shown to help reduce the amount of newly formed cholesterol and can help lower blood cholesterol levels when substituted for saturated fatty acids in the diet.[1,14] **Monounsaturated fatty acids** have also been shown to reduce blood cholesterol when consumed with a diet very low in saturated fats.[1,14]

A rise in LDL cholesterol levels has been associated with an increased dietary intake of *trans* fatty acids.[1,19–31] In addition, *trans* fatty acids have been associated with a higher risk for coronary heart disease.[1,32–35] It is recommended in NCEP ATP III to keep the intake of *trans* fatty acids low and to try to use liquid vegetable oil, soft margarine, and *trans* fatty acid–free margarine in place of stick margarine, butter, and shortening.[1]

The national average of dietary cholesterol intake in the United States is 256 mg/day.[1,36] Approximately one third of dietary cholesterol intake is obtained from the consumption of eggs.[1,37] It is recommended in the TLC diet that Americans consume an average of 200 mg or less of dietary cholesterol daily.[1] High consumptions of dietary cholesterol have been associated with an increased response in serum cholesterol.[1,38,39] In addition, higher intakes of dietary cholesterol have been associated with increases in LDL cholesterol, which then increases the risk for CHD.[1] Decreasing the intake of dietary cholesterol will decrease LDL cholesterol levels in most people.[1]

Plant stanols and sterols are also recommended in NCEP ATP III for patients with high serum cholesterol because they have been shown to reduce LDL cholesterol levels.[1] Studies have shown that plant-derived stanols and sterol esters at dosages of 2 to 3 g/day lower LDL cholesterol levels by 6 to 15% with a maximum LDL lowering effect occurring with 2 g/day.[1,40–46] Dietary consumption of plant stanols and sterols can be obtained from commercially available products containing plant sterols and stanols (i.e., margarines, juice).[1] A summary of the dietary recommendations listed in the NCEP ATP III guidelines is provided in Table 14-4.

PHYSICAL ACTIVITY AND METABOLIC SYNDROME

Increased physical activity is one of the cornerstones for the treatment of patients with metabolic syndrome. Physical activity has been shown to improve lipid profiles, reduce blood pressure, stabilize blood glucose levels, decrease and maintain a healthy body

TABLE 14–4 Dietary Recommendations for Patients With Metabolic Syndrome

Nutrient	Recommendation
Total calories	Balance calorie intake with expenditure to obtain appropriate body weight
Carbohydrate[a]	50–60% of total calorie intake
Fiber	20–30 g/day
Protein	Around 15% of total calorie intake
Monounsaturated fat	Up to 20% of total calorie intake
Polyunsaturated fat	Up to 10% of total calorie intake
Saturated fat	Less than 7% of total calorie intake
Total fat	25–35% of total calorie intake
Dietary cholesterol	Less than 200 mg/day

[a]Most carbohydrate intake should come from whole grains, fruits, and vegetables.
Source: National Institutes of Health, National Heart, Lung, and Blood Institute. Third report of the National Cholesterol Education Program (NCEP) Expert Panel on Detection, Evaluation, and Treatment of High Blood Cholesterol in Adults (Adult Treatment Panel III). NIH Publication No. 02-5215, September 2002.

weight, and decrease a patient's overall risk for cardiovascular disease.[1] It is recommended in the NCEP ATP III guidelines that physical activity be introduced to hyperlipidemic patients when TLC therapy is initiated and that the concept be reinforced when the treatment emphasis shifts to metabolic syndrome management.[1]

Specific recommendations for physical activity are not outlined in NCEP ATP III guidelines, but it is noted that healthcare professionals are to refer to the U.S. Surgeon General's Report on Physical Activities published in 1996 (http://www.surgeongeneral.gov/).[47,48] The recommendations in the AHA/NHLBI scientific statement on metabolic syndrome also follow the recommendations from the Surgeon General's report. The general recommendations made in the report emphasize moderate physical activity for 30 minutes per day on most, if not all, days of the week.[47,48] An emphasis should be placed on the amount of physical activity rather than the intensity of the activity, as sedentary people should incorporate greater amounts of physical activity into all aspects of daily life. Therefore, as patients can tolerate, the duration of physical activity should be increased to 60 minutes per day on most days of the week.

Accumulating physical activity during the course of a day (i.e., walking 10 minutes at a time, several times a day) is also recommended as an effective alternative to a one-time exercise session, and may even lead to greater exercise adherence.[47,48] It is important to note that sedentary people with preexisting disease should start at lower levels of exercise intensity and gradually build up to the desired level of activity and that people recently experiencing a coronary event (e.g., **myocardial infarction**) should exercise under direct supervision.[49]

For patients with metabolic syndrome, both aerobic and resistance training exercises should be incorporated into the patient's disease risk-reduction program. Aerobic exercise should be incorporated to reduce the overall risk for coronary heart disease, and resistance training exercises should be performed to enhance weight loss, if needed, and to reduce the risks associated with metabolic syndrome. Aerobic type

TABLE 14–5	Physical Activity Recommendations for Patients With Metabolic Syndrome
Goals	Promote healthy body weight Control dyslipidemia Control blood pressure Control blood glucose Reduce risk of cardiovascular disease
Type of activity	Large muscle activities (e.g., walking, jogging, bicycling, stairclimbing, dancing, basketball, volleyball, lawn mowing, gardening)
Intensity	Moderate level
Duration[a]	10–20 minutes (initially) 30–60 minutes (more advanced)
Frequency[a]	2–5 times per week (for initial 1–4 weeks) 6–7 times per week (after initial 4 weeks)
Resistance training	All major muscle groups 2 sets 15–20 repetitions 2–3 times per week (rest at least 48 hours between sessions)
Lifestyle activity	Increase overall daily physical activities through taking stairs instead of elevators, parking farther away in parking lots, walking the family pet, etc.

[a]Emphasize increasing duration rather than intensity.

Source: U.S. Department of Health and Human Services. Physical activity and health: a report of the Surgeon General. Atlanta: U.S. Department of Health and Human Services, Centers for Disease Control and Prevention, National Center for Chronic Disease Prevention and Health Promotion, 1996, 278 pages.

activities, among others, could include walking or jogging, bicycling, stairclimbing, dancing, basketball, and volleyball, as well as lawn mowing and gardening. Resistance training exercises are recommended to be performed on 2 days per week and can range from using stretch bands to weight-lifting exercises at a local health club. It is very important that the exercises recommended to patients be specific to their individual needs to optimize outcomes and adherence.[49] Suggested physical activity guidelines for patients with metabolic syndrome are provided in Table 14-5.

PHARMACY PRACTICE APPLICATION

Because metabolic syndrome incorporates several disease states and because the cornerstone of treatment is lifestyle modifications, pharmacists can play a very important role in the treatment of these patients. A pharmacist can pull together his or her skills in dyslipidemia, hypertension, diabetes, obesity, and cardiovascular disease prevention to help patients with metabolic syndrome. Even though there are no specific drugs recommended to treat metabolic syndrome itself, the pharmacist must incorporate drug knowledge from several other diseases, as well as lifestyle modifications, to treat these patients. As pharmacists are one of the most highly accessible healthcare providers and as approximately one third of Americans have metabolic syndrome, pharmacists are well positioned to make a difference in treating this population and decreasing overall cardiovascular risk.

CASE STUDY

L.L. is a 44-year-old white male truck driver who visits the pharmacy with his wife to pick up her medicine. L.L.'s wife expresses her concern for her husband's overall health as he has not seen a physician in 15 years. She would like to enroll L.L. in the pharmacy's wellness program, and L.L. reluctantly agrees. The assessments that L.L. will get tested for are fasting blood lipids, fasting blood glucose, blood pressure, body mass index and waist circumference, dietary analysis, physical activity level, and Framingham score.

During the course of a week, much information is gathered on L.L. He is a current smoker, 6'0", 273 lb, and is sedentary with a resting blood pressure of 138/90 mm Hg, a heart rate of 82 beats/min, and a waist circumference of 46 inches. In addition, L.L. drinks 6 to 10 beers per week, and his father had a heart attack at age 43 years. Point-of-care fasting blood lipids and glucose were as follows: total cholesterol = 240 mg/dL, LDL cholesterol = 185 mg/dL, HDL cholesterol = 25 mg/dL, triglycerides = 360 mg/dL, blood glucose = 108 mg/dL; and a baseline pedometer reading of 3,865 steps per day average was measured during the course of 1 week. Because he has not seen a physician in 15 years he has no diagnosed diseases and is not taking any medications. Results from his 4-day dietary analysis were as follows:

> *Total caloric intake per day = 3,426 calories*
> *Carbohydrates = 40% of total calories*
> *Monounsaturated fats = 12% of total calories*
> *Polyunsaturated fats = 12% of total calories*
> *Saturated fats = 24% of total calories*
> *Total fats = 48% of total calories*
> *Protein = 12% of total calories*
> *Total dietary cholesterol = 485 mg*
> *Fiber = 8 g*
> *Calcium = 473 mg/day*
> *Potassium = 3,800 mg/day*
> *Magnesium = 525 mg/day*
> *Sodium = 4,725 mg/day*

Case Activities

1. *Write an SOAP note for L.L.*
2. *List L.L.'s risk factors for cardiovascular disease and determine whether intervention is needed.*
3. *Design a program that includes nutrition, exercise, weight-loss, and smoking-cessation counseling for L.L. that will decrease his risk for cardiovascular disease.*

REFERENCES

1. National Institutes of Health, National Heart, Lung, and Blood Institute. Third report of the National Cholesterol Education Program (NCEP) Expert Panel on Detection, Evaluation, and Treatment of High Blood Cholesterol in Adults (Adult Treatment Panel III). NIH Publication No. 02-5215, September 2002.
2. Grundy SM, Cleeman JI, Daniels SR, et al. Diagnosis and management of the metabolic syndrome. An American Heart Association/National Heart, Lung, and Blood Institute Scientific Statement: executive summary. Circulation 2005;112:1–6.
3. American Heart Association. Heart Disease and Stroke Statistics—2006 Update. Available at: http://american-heart.org/downloadable/heart/113535864858055–1026_HS_Stats06book.pdf. Accessed January 28, 2006.
4. Khan R, Buse J, Ferrannini E, Stern M. The metabolic syndrome: time for a critical appraisal. Joint statement from the American Diabetes Association and the European Association for the Studies of Diabetes. Diabetes Care 2005;28:2289–2304.

5. Anderson LH, Martinson BC, Crain AL, et al. Health care charges associated with physical inactivity, overweight, and obesity. Preventing Chronic Disease 2005 Oct. Available at: http://www.cdc.gov.pcd/issues/2005/oct/04_0118.htm. Accessed October 31, 2005.

6. Chandola T, Brunner E, Marmont M. Chronic stress at work and the metabolic syndrome: prospective study. BMJ 2006;332:521–525.

7. Rosengren A, Hawken S, Ounpuu S, et al. Association of psychological risk factors with risk of acute myocardial infarction in 11,119 cases and 13,648 controls from 52 countries (the INTERHEART study): case-control study. Lancet 2004;364:953–962.

8. Marmot MG, Bosma H, Hemingway H, Brunner E, Stansfeld S. Contribution of job control and other risk factors to social variations in coronary heart disease. Lancet 1997;350:325–240.

9. Marmot MG, Davey Smith G, Stansfeld SA, et al. Health inequalities among British civil servants: the Whitehall II study. Lancet 1991;337:1387–1393.

10. Brunner EJ, Marmot MG, Nanchahal K, et al. Social inequality in coronary risk: central obesity and metabolic syndrome. Evidence from the WII study. Diabetologia 1997;40:1341–1349.

11. Siegrist J, Peter R. Chronic work stress is associated with atherogenic lipids and elevated fibrinogen in middle-aged men. J Intern Med 1997;242:149–156.

12. Peter R, Alfredsson L, Hammar N, Siegrist J, Theorell T, Westerholm P. High effort, low reward and cardiovascular risk factors in employed Swedish men and women—baseline results of the WOLF study. J Epidemiol Community Health 1998;52:540–547.

13. U.S. Department of Agriculture and U.S. Department of Health and Human Services. Nutrition and Your Health: Dietary Guidelines for Americans, 5th ed. Home and Garden Bulletin No. 232. Washington, D.C.: U.S. Department of Agriculture, 2000, 44 pages.

14. American Heart Association. Delicious Decisions. Available at: http://www.deliciousdecisions.org/. Accessed March 23, 2004.

15. Kris-Etherton PM, Yu S. Individual fatty acid effects on plasma lipids and lipoproteins: human studies. Am J Clin Nutr 1997;65(Suppl 5):1628S–1644S.

16. Mensink RP, Katan MB. Effects of dietary fatty acids on serum lipids and lipoproteins: a meta-analysis of 27 trails. Arterioscler Thromb 1992;12:911–919.

17. Obarzanek E, Hunsberger SA, Van Horn L, et al. Safety of a fat-reduced diet: the Dietary Intervention Study in Children (DISC). Pediatrics 1997;100:51–59.

18. Niinikoski H, Lapinleimu H, Viikari J, et al. Growth until three years of age in a prospective, randomized trial of a diet with reduced saturated fat and cholesterol. Pediatrics 1997;99:687–694.

19. Lichtenstein AH, Ausman LM, Jalbert SM, Schaefer EJ. Effects of different forms of dietary hydrogenated fats on serum lipoprotein cholesterol levels. N Engl J Med 1999;340:1933–1940.

20. Judd JT, Clevidence BA, Muesing RA, Wittes J, Sunkin ME, Podczasy JJ. Dietary trans fatty acids: effects of plasma lipids and lipoproteins of healthy men and women. Am J Clin Nutr 1994;59:861–868.

21. Judd JT, Baer DJ, Clevidence BA, et al. Effects of margarine compared with those of butter on blood lipid profiles related to cardiovascular disease risk factors in normolipemic adults fed controlled diets. Am J Clin Nutr 1998;68:768–777.

22. Noakes M, Clifton PM. Oil blends containing partially hydrogenated or interesterified fats: differential effects on plasma lipids. Am J Clin Nutr 1998;68:242–247.

23. Aro A, Jauhiainen M, Partanen R, Salminen I, Mutanen M. Stearic acid, trans-fatty acids, and dairy fat: effects on serum and lipoprotein lipids, apolipoproteins, lipoprotein (a), and lipid transfer proteins in healthy subjects. Am J Clin Nutr 1997;65:1419–1426.

24. Almendingen K, Jordal O, Kierulf P, Sandstad B, Pedersen JI. Effects of partially hydrogenated fish oil, partially hydrogenated soybean oil, and butter on serum lipoproteins and Lp[a] in men. J Lipid Res 1995;36:1370–1384.

25. Wood R, Kubena K, O'Brien B, Tseng S, Martin G. Effect of butter, mono- and polyunsaturated fatty acid-enriched butter, trans-fatty acid margarine on serum lipids and lipoproteins in healthy men. J Lipid Res 1993;34:1–11.

26. Wood R, Kubena K, Tseng S, Martin G, Crook R. Effect of palm oil, margarine, butter, and sunflower oil on the serum lipids and lipoproteins of normocholerolemic middle-aged men. J Nutr Biochem 1993; 4:286–297.

27. Nestel PJ, Noakes M, Belling GB, McArthur R, Clifton PM, Abbey M. Plasma cholesterol lowering potential of edible-oil blends suitable for commercial use. Am J Clin Nutr 1992;55:46–50.

28. Zock PL, Katan MB. Hydrogenation alternatives: effects of trans fatty acids and stearic acid versus linoleic acid on serum lipids and lipoproteins in humans. J Lipid Res 1992;33:399–410.

29. Katan MB, Zock, Mensink RP. Trans fatty acids and their effects on lipoproteins in humans. Ann Rev Nutr 1995;15:473–493.

30. Mensink RP, Katan MB. Effects of dietary trans fatty acids on high density and low density lipoprotein cholesterol levels in healthy subjects. N Engl J Med 1990;323:439–445.

31. Lichtenstein AH, Ausman LM, Carrasco W, Jenner JL, Ordovas JM, Schaefer EJ. Hydrogenation impairs the hypolipidemic effect of corn oil in humans: hydrogenation, trans fatty acids, and plasma lipids. Arterioscler Thromb 1993;13:154–161.

32. Willett WC, Stampfer MJ, Manson JE, et al. Intake of trans fatty acids and risk of coronary heart disease among women. Lancet 1993;341:581–585.

33. Pietinen P, Ascherio A, Korhonen P, et al. Intake of fatty acids and risk of coronary heart disease in a cohort of Finnish men: the Alpha-Tocopherol, Beta-Carotene Cancer Prevention Study. Am J Epidemiol 1997;145:876–887.

34. Hu FB, Stampfer MJ, Manson JE, et al. Dietary saturated fats and their food sources in relation to the risk of coronary heart disease in women. Am J Clin Nutr 1999;70:1001–1008.

35. Kromhout D, Menotti A, Bloemberg B, et al. Dietary saturated and trans fatty acids and cholesterol and 25 year mortality from coronary heart disease: the Seven Countries Study. Prev Med 1995;24:308–315.

36. Tippett KS, Cleveland LE. How current diets stack up: comparison of dietary guidelines. In: America's Eating Habits: Changes and Consequences. Washington, D.C.: U.S. Department of Agriculture, Economic Research Service, 1999:51–70.

37. Putnam J, Gerrior S. Trends in the U.S. food supply, 1970–1997. In: America's Eating Habits: Changes and Consequences. Washington, D.C.: U.S. Department of Agriculture, Economic Research Service, 1999:133–160.

38. Grundy SM, Barrett-Conner E, Rudel LL, Miettinen T, Spector AA. Workshop on the impact of dietary cholesterol on plasma lipoproteins and atherogenesis. Arteriosclerosis 1988;8:95–101.

39. National Research Council. Diet and Health: Implications for Reducing Chronic Disease Risk. Washington, D.C.: National Academy Press, 1989:171–201.

40. Hallikainen MA, Uusitupa MI. Effects of 2 low fat stanols ester containing margarines on serum cholesterol concentrations as part of a low fat diet in hypercholesterolaemic subjects. Am J Clin Nutr 1999;69:403–410.

41. Gylling H, Miettinen TA. Cholesterol reduction by different plant stanols mixtures and with variable fat intake. Metabolism 1999;48:575–580.

42. Gylling H, Radhakrishnan R, Miettinen TA. Reduction of serum cholesterol in postmenopausal women with previous myocardial infarction and cholesterol malabsorption indiced by dietary sitostanol ester margarine: women in dietary sitostanol. Circulation 1997;96:4226–4231.

43. Hendriks HFJ, Weststrate JA, van Vliet T, Meijer GW. Spreads enriched with three different levels of vegetable oil sterols and the degree of cholesterol lowering in normocholesterolaemic and mildly hypercholesterolaemic subjects. Eur J Clin Nutr 1999;53:319–327.

44. Miettinen TA, Puska P, Gylling H, Vanhanen H, Vartianen E. Reduction of serum cholesterol with sitostanol ester margarine in a mildly hypercholesterolaemic population. N Engl J Med 1995;333:1308–1312.

45. Vanhanen HT, Blomqvist S, Ehnholm C, et al. Serum cholesterol, serum precursors, and plant sterols in hypercholesterolemic subjects with different apoE phenotypes during dietary sitostanol ester treatment. J Lipid Res 1993;34:1535–1544.

46. Vuorio AF, Gylling H, Turola H, Kontula K, Ketonen P, Miettinen TA. Stanol ester margarine alone with simvastatin lowers serum cholesterol in families with familial hypercholesterolemia caused by FH-North Karelia mutation. Arterioscler Thromb Vasc Biol 2000;20:500–506.

47. American College of Sports Medicine. ACSM's Guidelines For Exercise Testing and Prescription, 6th ed. Philadelphia: Lippincott Williams & Wilkins, 2000:3–32.

48. U.S. Department of Health and Human Services. Physical activity and health: a report of the Surgeon General. Atlanta: U.S. Department of Health and Human Services, Centers for Disease Control and Prevention, National Center for Chronic Disease Prevention and Health Promotion, 1996, 278 pages.

49. Durstine JL, Moore GE, Thompson PD. Hyperlipidemia. In: Durstine JL ed. ACSM's Exercise Management for Persons With Chronic Diseases and Disabilities. Champaign, IL: Human Kinetics, 2003:142–148.

15

Cancer

At the end of this chapter the reader should be able to:

1. Explain the risks associated with cancer.
2. Summarize the prevention options for patients at risk for cancer.
3. Describe appropriate nutritional strategies for patients at risk for cancer.
4. Suggest appropriate exercises for patients at risk for cancer.
5. Formulate basic nutrition, exercise, weight-loss, and smoking-cessation programs for a patient at risk for cancer.

OVERVIEW OF CANCER

Cancer is a major public health concern in the United States. It is second only to cardiovascular disease as the most common cause of death.[1] Cancer, also referred to as a neoplasm, tumor, or malignancy, is not simply a single disease.[2] Rather, it is a group of more than 100 diseases that are characterized by an uncontrolled growth and spread of abnormal cells.[2,3] Most cancers can be categorized as either developing from epithelia (carcinoma), from cells of the blood (leukemia), from cells of the immune system (lymphoma), or from cells of connective tissue such as bone (sarcoma).[3] Each type of cancer can have unique developmental and treatment characteristics. Many, however, have similar prevention strategies, especially as they relate to lifestyle modifications. Because the developmental and treatment strategies of the many types of cancers can be so diverse, the focus of this chapter will be on prevention strategies that have been shown to be effective at mitigating the onset of certain types of cancers. It is not meant to discuss comprehensive treatment strategies, but rather to discuss ways in which individuals who may be at risk for developing certain types of cancers can lower their risks through lifestyle modification strategies.

PREVALENCE, ECONOMIC COSTS, AND HEALTH RISKS ASSOCIATED WITH CANCER

In 2006, cancer was estimated to account for approximately 564,000 deaths in the United States.[4] This represents approximately one quarter (25%) of the American population. In that same year, nearly 1.4 million Americans were diagnosed with cancer.[4] Slightly more men than women (51.5% versus 48.5%, respectively) are diagnosed with cancer each year. The most commonly diagnosed types of cancers are prostate, breast, lung, and colon. These four cancer sites also represent more than 50% of all cancer deaths.[4] The lifetime risk for developing any type of cancer is 46% in men and 38% in women.[5] The lifetime risk of dying of cancer is 24% in men and 20% in women.[5]

PATHOPHYSIOLOGY OF CANCER

Cancer begins when a single normal cell is transformed as a result of an initial event that damages or mutates the cell's DNA.[2] Cellular DNA that mutates can lead to the development of oncogenes, which are a type of gene that can lead to the development of cancer when it is present in certain forms or when it is overactive.[2] The genetic alterations of normal cells to oncogenes develop from normal genes called proto-oncogenes. These proto-oncogenes are responsible for many cellular signaling processes.[2] Therefore, mutations to these cells can disrupt normal cell growth signaling pathways, which can in turn lead to excessive cell growth and proliferation, and eventually a malignant transformation.[2]

Damage to cellular DNA is also related to the loss or inactivation of tumor suppressor genes.[2] Tumor suppressor genes are normal genes that suppress abnormal or unwanted cell division or growth.[2] Gene losses or mutations to the tumor suppressor genes result in the loss of the normal inhibition of cell division, therefore leading to cancer.[2]

There are several possible initial events that can cause damaged or mutated DNA cells.[2] These events can come from genetic, environmental, occupational, medication, and lifestyle activities factors. These initial events therefore become the risk factors that place patients at greater risk for developing cancer. A list of examples for each of the events is provided in Table 15-1.

CANCER PREVENTION AND TREATMENT

This section generally allows for some discussion on the proper treatment of the specific disease. However, as cancer treatment and medication use is such a broad topic it would be difficult to justifiably cover it in this section and is a bit beyond the scope of this chapter. Individuals interested in learning more about appropriate treatments for specific cancers are encouraged to pursue that in detail in other resources. Likewise, this section of the chapter usually lists medications used to treat the disease. This will also not be covered, but instead a table summarizing the effectiveness of lifestyle modification strategies on certain types of cancers is included (Table 15-2).

A strong component that places patients at increased risk for certain types of cancers is family history or genetics. Even though family history is not something that patients or healthcare professionals can control, reducing risk factors that are modifi-

TABLE 15–1	Environmental Risk Factors Leading to Cancer

Genetic conditions
Lifestyle
Tobacco use
Dietary factors
Physical inactivity
Obesity
Overconsumption of alcohol
Environmental
Ultraviolet radiation
Viruses
Ionizing radiation such as radon gas from the soil that contains uranium
Secondhand smoke
Occupational factors
Asbestos
Aniline dye
Benzene
Chromium
Nickel
Vinyl chloride
Medications
Alkylating agents
Azathioprine
Cyclophosphamide
Diethylstilbestrol
Estrogens
Phenacetin
Tamoxifen

Adopted from page 88-2, Table 88-1, Davis L, Lindley C. Neoplastic disorders and their treatment: general principles. In: Koda-Kimble MA, ed. Applied Therapeutics: The Clinical Use of Drugs, 8th ed. Philadelphia: Lippincott Williams & Wilkins, 2005:88.1–88.35.

able can decrease risk in patients who are genetically predisposed to certain types of cancers. Being diligent about avoiding elements in the environment and in certain occupations can help decrease risks for certain cancers. A good example of this is using sunscreen to avoid ultraviolet radiation that can lead to skin melanomas.[2] Another example is wearing protective equipment when working around asbestos to prevent lung cancer.[2]

Certain lifestyle modifications have also been shown to be effective at preventing many types of cancers. Lifestyle modifications primarily focus on tobacco cessation, **physical activity,** proper nutrition, maintaining a healthy body weight, and abstaining from excess or chronic alcohol consumption. For example, cigarette smoking is currently the single most significant modifiable risk factor for cancer.[2] It is estimated that tobacco smoking is responsible for 30% of all cancer deaths annually in the United States.[6] Additionally, other lifestyle-related factors such as **physical inactivity, obesity,** and improper nutrition combined accounted for approximately 30% of the expected cancer deaths in 2003.[2,7,8] Implementing lifestyle modification strategies in persons with and without cancer risk factors can have positive effects on preventing cancer.

TABLE 15–2 Effect of Lifestyle Modification Strategies on the Risk of Obtaining Certain Types of Cancers

Cancer Site	Decrease Cancer Risk		Increase Cancer Risk		
	Physical Activity	Healthy Eating	Tobacco Use	Obesity	Alcohol Consumption
Bladder		X	X[a]		
Blood		X			
Breast	X	X	a	X	X
Cervix			a		
Colon	X	X		X	X
Endometrium	X			X	
Esophagus		X	X	X	
Gallbladder				X	
Kidney				X	
Larynx		X	X		
Liver			X	X	
Lung	X	X	X[a]		
Nasal			a		
Oral cavity		X	X		X
Ovaries		X			
Pancreas		X	X		
Pharynx		X	X		
Prostate	X	X			
Rectum		X			
Skin		X			
Stomach		X		X	
Uterus				X	

[a]Indicates secondhand smoke risk.

Sources: National Cancer Institute. Cigarette smoking and cancer: questions and answers. National Cancer Institute, U.S. National Institutes of Health, 2004. Available at: http://www.cancer.gov/cancertopics/factsheet/Tobacco/cancer. Accessed March 30, 2006. National Cancer Institute. Physical activity and cancer: fact sheet. National Cancer Institute, U.S. National Institutes of Health, 2004. Available at: http://www.cancer.gov/cancertopics/factsheet/physical-activity-qa. Accessed March 30, 2006. National Cancer Institute. Eat 5 to 9 a day for better health. National Cancer Institute, U.S. National Institutes of Health, 2006. Available at: http://5aday.gov/. Accessed March 30, 2006. National Cancer Institute. Obesity and Cancer: Questions and Answers. National Cancer Institute, U.S. National Institutes of Health, 2004. Available at: http://www.cancer.gov/cancertopics/factsheet/Risk/obesity. Accessed March 30, 2006.

Tobacco Use

Cigarette smoking causes 87% of all annual lung cancer deaths, and lung cancer is the leading cause of cancer death in both men and women in the United States.[6] Additionally, cigarette smoking can lead to other types of cancers such as larynx, oral cavity and pharynx, esophageal, and bladder cancer.[6] Secondhand smoke has also been linked with lung cancer. It is estimated that 3,000 lung cancer deaths occur each year in the United States in non-smokers as a result of exposure to secondhand smoke.[9,10] Smoking cessation can have a major impact on the health of the individual by decreasing not only the risk for lung and other cancers, but also the risk of heart attack, **stroke, and chronic lung**

disease, among others.[6] It has been demonstrated that people who quit smoking before age 50 reduce their risk of dying in the next 10 years by half compared with people who continue to smoke.[6,11]

Physical Activity

Several studies have been able to show that individuals who participate in regular amounts of physical activity have a lower risk for developing several types of cancers. The most robust and convincing data come from research on colon and breast cancer. Studies have shown that colon cancer can be reduced by 40 to 50% in individuals who are physically active.[3,12–19] Women, both premenopausal and postmenopausal, who are physically active have up to a 40% reduced risk for developing breast cancer.[12] There is also good evidence to show that physical activity may have protective effects that guard against prostate, lung, and endometrial cancer. Other cancers such as ovarian, pancreatic, and stomach cancer may also be affected by physical activity participation, but more research is needed.[3,12] Of course, individuals who engage in regular physical activity reduce their risk not only for certain cancers but also for **cardiovascular disease,** stroke, and metabolic diseases, among others, as well.

NUTRITION AND CANCER

Proper nutrition affects nearly all aspects of promoting overall good health. Reducing cancer risk with proper nutrition has been demonstrated, especially in the area of consuming adequate amounts of fresh fruits and vegetables.[20] Studies have shown that individuals who consume the recommended five to nine daily servings of fruits and vegetables have a lower risk of developing several types of cancers. These cancers are lung, mouth, pharynx, esophagus, stomach, colon, and the rectum as well as cancers of the breast, pancreas, ovaries, larynx, and bladder.[20] Additionally, studies looking at the cancer protective effects of red wine have been able to show that consuming a glass of red wine per day reduces the incidence of prostate cancer by 50 to 60%.[21] Studies of other types of cancers such as leukemia, skin, and breast cancer have also shown positive effects of reducing risk with red wine consumption.[21] It should also be noted that studies looking at low-fat and omega-3 fatty acid consumption have not shown convincing evidence that they significantly reduce cancer risks.[22]

Obesity

During the previous two decades, the incidence of obesity has increased in the United States. As a result, Americans are now at greater risk for certain diseases than they were in the past, including cancer. Sedentary lifestyles and poor eating habits have led to nearly one third of Americans now being considered obese (body mass index $> 30\,\mathrm{kg/m^2}$). Obesity is now being linked with cancer of the colon, breast, endometrium, kidney, and esophagus, as well as cancers of the gallbladder, pancreas, and ovaries.[23,24] It is estimated that obesity and physical inactivity combined are responsible for 25 to 30% of the major cancers (i.e., colon, breast, endometrial, kidney, and esophagus).[24] It is recommended that obese individuals lose 5 to 10% of their total body weight by eating healthier and participating in regular physical activity to decrease their risk for these certain types of cancers (Table 15-2).[24]

Program Adherence

Because cancer prevention strategies can primarily focus on lifestyle changes, program adherence strategies must be implemented to give patients the best possible chance of being successful. Many times patients who will be participating in cancer prevention strategies will be relatively healthy, and in fact, may be free of any chronic diseases. Therefore, adherence strategies for this type of population should focus heavily on proper education of the importance of participating in these activities to reduce cancer risk as well as other risks such as cardiovascular disease. In addition, this population may be younger, and programs must be tailored to the specific needs of the patient and their lifestyle. A list of program adherence strategies for cancer prevention programs is listed in Table 15-3.[25]

Most of the research and recommendations for reducing cancer risk through proper nutrition has centered on widely accepted dietary guidelines and principles. As discussed above, the most robust evidence to support reducing cancer risk by changing eating habits is to consume the recommended five to nine servings of fruits and vegetables each day as recommended by the National Cancer Institute and the National Institutes of Health (http://www.cancer.gov/cancertopics/prevention-genetics-causes).[20] In addition, obesity has demonstrated that it increases cancer risk. Therefore, dietary changes that promote weight loss are also a nutritional strategy to lower cancer risk. Specific nutritional strategies to reduce cancer risk can come from simply adhering to the 2005 Dietary Guidelines for Americans (http://healthierus.gov/dietaryguidelines/) and emphasizing optimal daily caloric consumption to promote a healthy body weight.[26] Patients who are overweight or obese should follow weight-loss strategies outlined in the weight control and obesity chapters of this book. Individuals who are of normal weight will want to follow the general nutrition guidelines outlined in the nutrition chapter of this book as well as the 2005 Dietary Guidelines for Americans to reduce cancer risks. These strategies will lead to lowering the incidence of not only many types of cancers,

---

TABLE 15–3 Program Adherence Recommendations for Patients With Cancer

Recommend that multiple adherence strategies work better than a single approach

Establish weekly contact with patients for the first 4 weeks of the program, then monthly thereafter, to continually assess the patient's progress and troubleshoot problems

Set achievable goals

Obtain baseline assessment of overall food consumption

Obtain baseline assessment of physical activity

Institute a self-monitoring program such as keeping a log of food intake and exercise participation

Identify patient-specific barriers to the lifestyle changes

Distribute information that uses health messages associated with cancer prevention that are easy to understand, interactive, and culturally sensitive

Design a program that is reasonable, gradual, and easily implemented

Source: National Institutes of Health, National Heart, Lung, and Blood Institute. Third report of the National Cholesterol Education Program (NCEP) Expert Panel on Detection, Evaluation, and Treatment of High Blood Cholesterol in Adults (Adult Treatment Panel III). NIH Publication No. 02-5215, September 2002.

TABLE 15–4	Specific Dietary Recommendations to Reduce Cancer Risk
Nutrient	**Recommendation**
Total calories[a]	Approximately 500–1,000 kcal/day reduction from usual intake
Carbohydrate[b]	55% or more of total calories
Fiber	20–30 g/day
Protein	Approximately 15% of total calories
Monounsaturated fat	Up to 15% of total calories
Polyunsaturated fat	Up to 10% of total calories
Saturated fat	8–10% of total calories
Total fat	30% or less of total calories
Dietary cholesterol	<300 mg/day
Sodium chloride	No more than 100 mmol/day (approximately 2.4 g of sodium, or approximately 6 g of sodium chloride)
Calcium	1,000–1,500 mg/day

[a]This assumes weight loss is warranted, and it is recommended that alcohol not be consumed as part of the daily caloric intake as it will increase the total calories but has also been shown to be associated with obesity in epidemiologic studies.

[b]Most carbohydrate intake should come from whole grains, fruits, and vegetables. Five to nine servings of fruits and vegetables are recommended each day.

Source: HHS Publication No. HHS-ODPHP-2005-01-DGA-A. Dietary Guidelines for Americans 2005, U.S. Department of Health and Human Services, U.S. Department of Agriculture. Available at: http://healthierus.gov/dietaryguidelines. Accessed March 30, 2006.

but also other diseases and will promote overall good health. Table 15-4 lists recommended guidelines for reducing cancer risk.

PHYSICAL ACTIVITY AND CANCER

Much has been studied about the effects of regular amounts of physical activity on reducing the risks of many types of cancers. Like nutrition, the kind of physical activity that has demonstrated lower cancer rates is the same as what is recommended for overall good health to the general public. Additionally, physical activity is a key component of weight-loss programs, which can also decrease cancer risks. The American Cancer Society and the American College of Sports Medicine recommend that adults engage in at least moderate-intensity activity for 30 minutes or more on 5 or more days of the week to reduce the risk of many types of cancer.[3,27] These organizations further state that there is evidence to show that 45 minutes or more of moderate to vigorous intensity activity on 5 or more days per week may further enhance reductions in the risk of breast and colon cancer.[3,27] Children and adolescents should engage in at least 60 minutes of moderate to vigorous intensity physical activity per day on at least 5 days of the week.[3,27] Individuals who require weight loss should follow the physical activity recommendations outlined in the weight control and obesity chapters of this book. Physical activity recommendations for individuals wanting to lower their cancer risk are provided in Table 15-5.[28]

TABLE 15–5	Physical Activity Recommendations to Reduce Cancer Risks
Goals	Reduce cancer risk Promote healthy body weight Promote overall good health and reduce risk of other diseases
Type of activity	Large muscle activities (e.g., walking, jogging, bicycling, stairclimbing, dancing, basketball, volleyball, lawn mowing, gardening)
Intensity[a]	Moderate to vigorous level
Duration[a]	10–20 minutes (initially) 30–60 minutes (more advanced)
Frequency	2–5 times per week (for initial 1–4 weeks) 6–7 times per week (after initial 4 weeks)
Resistance training	All major muscle groups 2 sets 15–20 repetitions 2–3 times per week (rest at least 48 hours between sessions)
Lifestyle activity	Increase overall daily physical activities through taking stairs instead of elevators, parking farther away in parking lots, walking the family pet, etc.

[a]Emphasize increasing duration rather than intensity for patients needing to lose weight.
Source: U.S. Department of Health and Human Services. Physical activity and health: a report of the Surgeon General. Atlanta: U.S. Department of Health and Human Services, Centers for Disease Control and Prevention, National Center for Chronic Disease Prevention and Health Promotion, 1996, 278 pages.

Exercise for Cancer Survivors and Effects on Quality of Life

Much of the physical activity research relating to its effects on cancer has focused on the prevention aspect. Recently, however, more research has been done to see whether physical activity can aid in the recovery efforts of cancer survivors. Many of the studies have tested aerobic exercise programs, but a few have looked at aerobic plus resistance training programs, especially with regard to quality-of-life enhancement.[3] Studies have consistently demonstrated that enhanced physical activity has many beneficial outcomes on the quality of life of cancer survivors. These studies demonstrate that cancer survivors who participate in regular physical activity improve exercise capacity, muscular strength, body weight and composition, flexibility, fatigue, nausea, diarrhea, pain, physical well-being, functional well-being, depression, anxiety, vigor, anger, mood, self-esteem, satisfaction with life, and overall quality of life.[3] As a result of these studies, physical activity is recommended as a therapy modality for treating fatigue in patients who have survived cancer.[3,29]

Because cancer pathophysiology and treatments are so diverse and complex from one type of cancer to another, exercise recommendations for cancer patients can vary widely depending on cancer site, treatment protocols, responses to treatment, and baseline fitness levels. Optimal modes, frequency, duration, and intensity of an exercise prescription are largely unknown for most cancers because of the lack of research in the area. It is generally thought that walking and cycling on a stationary bicycle are the safest modes of activity. Walking is the preferred exercise for cancer survivors because it is most closely related to activities of daily living.[3,30] Most studies thus far have tested moderate levels of intensity performed on 3 to 5 days per week for 20 to 30 minutes per session. The American College of Sports Medicine states that this exercise prescription appears to be most appropriate for cancer patients but acknowledges that modifications will be needed for each patient and more research in this area is needed.[3]

Several exercise precautions should be considered when prescribing exercise to cancer survivors. Cancer survivors should avoid activity if certain laboratory values such as hemoglobin levels, absolute neutrophil counts, and platelet counts are not within normal levels. Also, symptoms such as fever, dizziness, and ataxia may warrant avoiding exercise and signal other problems. One of the most important precautions is the presence of metastatic bone disease. Bone metastases in the lower extremities and spine can cause pain and increase fracture risks while exercising, and therefore patients who experience pain, especially in the hip, while exercising should be referred back to their cancer care team. Other precautions include ensuring proper hydration and exercise as tolerated with symptoms of nausea, dyspnea, and fatigue.[3] More research in this area is needed as to specific exercises and amounts of exercise for patients with cancer. It is well accepted, however, that exercise can improve cancer survivors' quality of life and therefore should be considered by the cancer care team.

PHARMACY PRACTICE APPLICATION

The pharmacy practice community setting is an ideal place to promote general health and wellness to the public. Individuals who patronize pharmacies most likely have some kind of medical condition and are concerned about the quality of their health or the health of a family member or loved one. Because of the large volume of individuals who patronize pharmacies on a regular basis, pharmacists have a large and captive audience for which to offer informational material and programs that promote wellness and public health. Cancer prevention can be part of this heath promotion. As stated throughout this chapter, specific strategies that can reduce the risks for many types of cancers are very similar to the recommendations that promote overall good health. Therefore, pharmacies can offer programs in smoking cessation, weight loss, physical activity, and proper nutrition to individuals who may not necessarily have a chronic disease as a means of preventing cancer and other diseases such as cardiovascular disease, stroke, and diabetes. Pharmacies should try to convey an image to the public that they are a resource for preventing diseases as well as treating them. Pharmacists should be viewed as knowledgeable healthcare professionals who also prevent patients from getting sick along with helping patients recover once they are sick. This public persona can be realized if more pharmacists and pharmacies gain the skills in disease prevention and offer programs in these areas.

CASE STUDY

G.D. is a 25-year-old male who comes to the pharmacy to buy an over-the-counter anti-inflammatory medication to treat a sore shoulder that was injured while waterskiing. He notices the advertisements within the pharmacy that promote an overall wellness program that can lower the risks for cancer and other diseases. G.D. has a family history of cancer and would like to know more about the program. After assessing and interviewing G.D., the pharmacist discovers that

G.D. has no past or current medical history (other than a sore shoulder), follows no specific eating regimen, is active in playing many types of sports like basketball 2 to 3 times per week but does not participate in a structured exercise program, does not smoke or drink alcohol regularly, has a height of 6′4″, and weighs 195 lb, with a resting blood pressure of 110/70 mm Hg and a heart rate of 60 beats per minute.

G.D. is interested in knowing more information about ways in which he can reduce his risks for cancer and would like to enroll in the program. G.D. completes a 3-day dietary analysis, and it reveals the following information:

> *Average caloric intake per day = 3,500 calories*
> *Carbohydrates = 58% of total calories*
> *Monounsaturated fats = 8% of total calories*
> *Polyunsaturated fats = 5% of total calories*
> *Saturated fats = 12% of total calories*
> *Total fats = 25% of total calories*
> *Protein = 17% of total calories*
> *Total dietary cholesterol = 330 mg*
> *Fiber = 16 g*
> *Calcium = 1,500 mg/day*
> *Potassium = 4,800 mg/day*
> *Magnesium = 600 mg/day*
> *Sodium = 2,800 mg/day*

Case Activities

1. *Write an SOAP note for G.D.*
2. *List G.D.'s risk factors for cancer.*
3. *Design a program that includes nutrition and exercise recommendations for G.D. that will decrease his risk for cancer.*

REFERENCES

1. Mokdad AH, Marks JS, Stroup DF, Gerberding JL. Actual causes of death in the United States, 2000. JAMA 2004;291:1238–1245.
2. Davis L, Lindley C. Neoplastic disorders and their treatment: general principles. In: Koda-Kimble MA, ed. Applied Therapeutics: The Clinical Use of Drugs, 8th ed. Philadelphia: Lippincott Williams & Wilkins, 2005:88.1–88.35.
3. Nieman DC, Courneya KS. Immunological conditions. In: Kaminsky LA, et al., eds. ACSM's Resource Manual for Guidelines for Exercise Testing and Prescription, 5th ed. Baltimore: Lippincott Williams & Wilkins, 2006:536–542.
4. American Cancer Society: Cancer Facts and Figures 2006. Atlanta: American Cancer Society. Available at: http://www.cancer.org/downloads/stt/CAFF06EsCsMc.pdf. Accessed March 30, 2006.
5. Ries LAG, Eisner MP, Kosary CL, et al., eds. SEER Cancer Statistics Review, 1975–2002. Bethesda, MD: National Cancer Institute. Available at: http://seer.cancer.gov/csr/1975_2002/, based on November 2004 SEER data submission, posted to the SEER web site 2005. Accessed February 13, 2007.
6. National Cancer Institute. Cigarette smoking and cancer: questions and answers. National Cancer Institute, U.S. National Institutes of Health, 2004. Available at: http://www.cancer.gov/cancertopics/factsheet/Tobacco/cancer. Accessed March 30, 2006.
7. American Cancer Society. Cancer Facts and Figures 2003. Atlanta: American Cancer Society, 2003.
8. Calle EE, Rodriguez C, Walker-Thurmond K, Thun MJ. Overweight, obesity, and mortality from cancer in a prospectively studied cohort of U.S. adults. N Engl J Med 2003;348:1625–1638.
9. National Cancer Institute. Secondhand smoking: questions and answers. National Cancer Institute, U.S. National Institutes of Health, 2005. Available at: http://www.cancer.gov/cancertopics/factsheet/Tobacco/ETS. Accessed March 30, 2006.

10. National Cancer Institute. Cancer Progress Report 2003. Public Health Service, National Institutes of Health, U.S. Department of Health and Human Services, 2004. Available at: http://progressreport.cancer.gov/. Accessed March 30, 2006.

11. International Agency for Research on Cancer. Tobacco smoke and involuntary smoking. Lyon, France: International Agency for Research on Cancer, 2002. Available at: http://www-cie.iarc.fr/htdocs/indexes/vol83index.html. Accessed March 30, 2006.

12. National Cancer Institute. Physical activity and cancer: fact sheet. National Cancer Institute, U.S. National Institutes of Health, 2004. Available at: http://www.cancer.gov/cancertopics/factsheet/physical-activity-qa. Accessed March 30, 2006.

13. Wu AH, Paganini-Hill A, Ross RK, Henderson BE. Alcohol, physical activity, and other risk factors for colorectal cancer: a prospective study. Br J Cancer 1987;55:687–694.

14. Levi F, Pasche C, Lucchini F, Tavani A, La Vecchia C. Occupational and leisure-time physical activity and the risk of colorectal cancer. Eur J Cancer Prev 1999;8:487–493.

15. Tang R, Wang JY, Lo SK, Hsieh LL. Physical activity, water intake, and risk of colorectal cancer in Taiwan: a hospital-based case-control study. Int J Cancer 1999;82:484–489.

16. Martinez ME, Giovannucci E, Spiegelman D, Hunter DJ, Willett WC, Colditz, GA. Leisure-time physical activity, body size, and colon cancer in women. J Natl Cancer Inst 1997;89:948–955.

17. Slattery ML, Potter J, Caan B, et al. Energy balance and colon cancer—beyond physical activity. Cancer Res 1997;57:75–80.

18. Tavani A, Braga C, La Vecchia C, et al. Physical activity and risk of cancers of the colon and rectum: an Italian case-control study. Br J Cancer 1999;79:1912–1916.

19. Slattery ML, Schumacher MC, Smith KR, West DW, Abd-Elghany N. Physical activity, diet, and risk of colon cancer in Utah. Am J Epidemiol 1988;128:989–999.

20. National Cancer Institute. Eat 5 to 9 a day for better health. National Cancer Institute, U.S. National Institutes of Health, 2006. Available at: http://5aday.gov/. Accessed March 30, 2006.

21. National Cancer Institute. Red wine and cancer prevention: fact sheet. National Cancer Institute, U.S. National Institutes of Health, 2002. Available at: http://www.cancer.gov/cancertopics/factsheet/red-wine-and-cancer-prevention. Accessed March 30, 2006.

22. National Cancer Institute. Cancer prevention. National Cancer Institute, U.S. National Institutes of Health, 2002. Available at: http://www.cancer.gov/cancertopics/prevention-genetics-causes/prevention. Accessed March 30, 2006.

23. National Cancer Institute. Obesity and cancer: questions and answers. National Cancer Institute, U.S. National Institutes of Health, 2004. Available at: http://www.cancer.gov/cancertopics/factsheet/Risk/obesity. Accessed March 30, 2006.

24. Vainio H, Bianchini F. IARC Handbooks of Cancer Prevention. Vol. 6: Weight Control and Physical Activity. Lyon, France: IARC Press, 2002.

25. National Institutes of Health, National Heart, Lung, and Blood Institute. Third report of the National Cholesterol Education Program (NCEP) Expert Panel on Detection, Evaluation, and Treatment of High Blood Cholesterol in Adults (Adult Treatment Panel III). NIH Publication No. 02-5215, September 2002.

26. HHS Publication No. HHS-ODPHP-2005-01-DGA-A. Dietary Guidelines for Americans 2005, U.S. Department of Health and Human Services, U.S. Department of Agriculture. Available at: http://healthierus.gov/dietaryguidelines. Accessed March 30, 2006.

27. Friedenreich CM. Physical activity and cancer prevention: from observational to interventional research. Cancer Epidemiol Biomarkers Prev 2001;10:287–301.

28. U.S. Department of Health and Human Services. Physical activity and health: a report of the Surgeon General. Atlanta: U.S. Department of Health and Human Services, Centers for Disease Control and Prevention, National Center for Chronic Disease Prevention and Health Promotion, 1996, 278 pages.

29. Jacobsen PB, Thors CL. Fatigue in the radiation therapy patient: current management and investigations. Semin Radiat Oncol 2003;13:372–380.

30. Jones LW, Courneya KS. Exercise counseling and programming preferences of cancer survivors. Cancer Pract 2002;10:208–215.

CHAPTER 16

Osteoporosis

OBJECTIVES

At the end of this chapter the reader should be able to:

1. Explain the risks associated with osteoporosis.
2. Summarize the prevention and treatment options for osteoporosis.
3. Describe appropriate nutritional strategies for patients at risk for and with osteoporosis.
4. Suggest appropriate exercises for patients at risk for and with osteoporosis.
5. Formulate a basic nutrition and exercise program for a patient at risk for osteoporosis.

OVERVIEW OF OSTEOPOROSIS

Osteoporosis by definition means "porous bone."[1] It is characterized by low bone mass and a structural deterioration of bone tissue resulting in bone fragility and an increased risk of fractures of the hip, spine, and wrist.[1] Like women, men are also afflicted by osteoporosis, but the disease can be prevented and effectively treated, especially with lifestyle modifications.[1]

Bone diseases, like osteoporosis, have a major impact on the American population as a whole and especially on the individuals and families that are affected by the disease.[2] It is often called a "silent" disorder until it causes one or more fractures.[2] Individuals and families affected by osteoporosis that results in bone fractures must deal with the complications that follow such as ill health, disability, reduced quality of life, and possibly even death.[2] Therefore, taking the necessary steps to prevent this "silent" disease is an important individual patient health concern as well as a public health concern.

PREVALENCE, ECONOMIC COSTS, AND HEALTH RISKS ASSOCIATED WITH OSTEOPOROSIS

Osteoporosis affects approximately 44 million Americans age 50 years and older.[3] Although men experience osteoporosis, 80% of Americans with the disease are women. In addition, women who are white or Asian have a higher prevalence of osteoporosis than women who are black or Hispanic.[4]

Osteoporotic fractures led to more than 500,000 hospitalizations, more than 800,000 emergency room encounters, and more than 2.6 million physician office visits in 1995 in the United States.[2] In addition, nearly 180,000 individuals were placed in nursing homes in 1995 as a result of osteoporotic fractures.[2] Hip fractures are by far the most devastating type of fracture. Approximately 26% of individuals suffering hip fractures become disabled in the year after the fracture, and approximately 20% of these individuals require long-term nursing home care.[2]

The costs related to fractures resulting from osteoporosis are expensive. Studies show that the annual direct care expenditures for osteoporotic fractures range from $12.2 to $17.2 billion.[2] Men account for 18% of this amount, or approximately $3.2 billion per year.[2] Because hip fractures are so devastating, they account for 63% ($11.3 billion) of osteoporotic medical care costs. The treatment for each hip fracture is approximately $30,100 to $43,400 in 2002 U.S. dollars.[2] Hospital care and nursing home care account for a majority of the total direct costs associated with osteoporotic fractures.[2]

PATHOPHYSIOLOGY OF OSTEOPOROSIS

As individuals progress through life, bone is continuously changing through a dynamic process called remodeling.[4–6] The process of remodeling is important to our bone health because it helps to maintain the mechanical integrity of bone to keep it strong and resist injury such as fractures. In the remodeling process, older fatigued and damaged bone is replaced by new bone. **Osteoclasts** are cells that are responsible for the degradation (also called resorption) of old bone.[4–6] **Osteoblasts** are cells that are responsible for building new bone to replace the bone that has been removed by the osteoclasts.[4–6] Osteoclasts work by eroding portions of the bone surface, which creates cavities. These cavities are then filled with a collagen matrix from the osteoblasts that then mineralizes to form new bone.[4–6]

During childhood and adolescence, new bone formation occurs more rapidly than old bone is removed.[4] The formation of new bone occurs at a faster pace than bone degradation until peak bone mass is attained at around the age of 30 years.[4] After this peak, the bone remodeling process becomes less efficient. Each subsequent remodeling process that occurs results in small deficits in bone formation, which begin to accumulate with aging.[4] The accumulation of these deficits results in decreased bone mass and an overall weakened bone that is more susceptible to fractures. Depending on genetics and environmental factors, bone loss generally occurs at a rate of 0.5 to 1.0% until perimenopause in women.[4] During perimenopause, women lose bone at a rate of approximately 1.0% per year. During menopause, if estrogen is not replaced, women lose bone at a rate of 9 to 13% during the first 5 years. Some researchers have found that women lose 20 to 30% of their lifetime bone density during the early postmenopausal period.[7] Bone loss then returns to rates similar to those of premenopause after women adapt to the hormonal deficiency.[4] Men also experience bone loss as they

TABLE 16–1   Environmental Risk Factors Leading to Osteoporosis

Physical inactivity

Smoking

Low calcium and vitamin D intake

Excessive alcohol intake

Decreased mobility

Eating disorder (anorexia nervosa)

Advanced age

Family history for osteoporosis

Female gender

Caucasian or Asian

Small stature

Low body weight (<125 pounds)

Early menopause or oophorectomy

Abnormal absence of menopause

Certain diseases: chronic liver disease, chronic liver failure, hyperthyroidism, primary hyperparathyroidism, Cushing's syndrome, gastrointestinal resection, malabsorption

Certain medications: corticosteroids, long-term anticonvulsants (phenytoin, phenobarbital), excessive use of aluminum-containing antacids, long-term high-dose heparin, furosemide, excessive levothyroxine therapy

Sources: National Institutes of Health. Osteoporosis overview. National Institutes of Health, Osteoporosis and Related Bone Diseases, National Resource Center, June 2005. Available at: http://www.niams.nih.gov/bone/hi/overview.htm. Accessed March 9, 2006; Parent-Stevens L, Sagraves R. Gynecologic and other disorders of women. In: Koda-Kimble MA, ed. Applied Therapeutics: The Clinical Use of Drugs, 8th ed. Philadelphia: Lippincott Williams & Wilkins, 2005:48.1–48.47.

age. By age 65 to 70 years, men and women are losing bone at the same rate, and the resorption of calcium decreases in both sexes.[8]

Several risk factors are associated with placing individuals at higher risk for osteoporosis. Some of the risks can be modified through lifestyle changes and medications whereas others are non-modifiable. Table 16-1 lists risk factors for the development of osteoporosis.

OSTEOPOROSIS DISEASE PREVENTION AND TREATMENT

As stated in the pathophysiology of osteoporosis, bone loss naturally occurs as we age, leading to higher risks for fractures. Additionally, many factors have been identified that place women and men at greater risk for osteoporosis. Identifying patients who might be at risk for osteoporosis and assisting them to become proactive to prevent the disease can maintain high quality-of-life standards and can save patients and the healthcare system money.

Several strategies have been identified that can help individuals reach optimal peak bone mass and continue building new bone tissue with age to prevent osteoporosis. These strategies include adequate calcium and vitamin intake, adequate **physical activity,** maintaining a healthy body weight, smoking abstinence, alcohol control, avoiding long-term use of medications known to increase risk of osteoporosis, taking medications known to lower osteoporosis risk, and teaching fall prevention.[1] An appropriate eating plan and proper physical activity will be covered in more detail in the following sections.

Excess body weight is many times a culprit to ensuing disease. For osteoporosis, however, it is just the opposite. Patients with excessively low body weight are the ones who are at increased risk for osteoporosis. It is always important to talk to patients about maintaining a "healthy" body weight. Unfortunately, a majority of our society is overweight and therefore healthcare providers tend to focus more attention, with respect to body weight, on patients who are overweight and obese. Healthcare providers must always keep in mind that underweight patients can also be at risk for certain diseases like osteoporosis.

It is well known that smoking causes undesirable effects to the heart and lungs. Smoking, however, is also bad for bone health. Women who smoke have lower estrogen levels compared with non-smokers and they often go into menopause earlier.[1] In addition, smokers may also absorb less calcium from their food than non-smokers. These factors place smokers at a higher risk for osteoporosis, and therefore smoking abstinence and smoking cessation programs should be emphasized as a means to decrease osteoporosis risk. Likewise, excessive alcohol intake in the amount of 2 to 3 ounces a day can damage the skeleton, even in young women and men. Individuals who drink heavily are more prone to bone loss and fractures, because of both poor nutrition and the increased risk for falling.[1]

Several medications can increase osteoporosis risk. Avoiding unnecessary long-term use of these medications can help to prevent the disease. Patients who are stabilized on these medications and who should therapeutically avoid switching to alternative medications should diligently use lifestyle modification therapy to prevent osteoporosis. Additionally, adding medications known to treat osteoporosis may be done as a preventive measure in patients at high risk for osteoporosis. Several drugs have been studied and proven to work effectively at preventing or treating osteoporosis. A list of these drugs is provided in Table 16-2.

Preventing falls is a special concern for patients with osteoporosis or those at high risk for the disease as they increase the likelihood of bone fractures. Pharmacists and other healthcare providers can talk with patients about several factors that can put patients at risk for falls. It is important for patients with osteoporosis to be able to identify situations that may put them at risk for falls and to avoid or modify these situations. Falls can be caused by impaired vision or balance, diseases that affect mental or physical functioning, certain medications such as sedatives and antidepressants, and environmental factors.[2] Such environmental factors can include slippery sidewalks and floors, wet or icy conditions, uneven terrain, items that can be tripped over such as floor rugs, small toys, shoes, and electrical cords, non-supportive shoes, wearing stockings that may be slippery, stairwells without handrails, climbing into and out of the shower or bathtub without grab bars, and step stools, among others.[2]

TABLE 16–2   **Medications Used to Treat or Prevent Osteoporosis**

Calcium products
Vitamin D
Estrogens
Calcitonin
Oral bisphosphonates
Parathyroid hormone
Selective estrogen receptor modulator

TABLE 16–3 Program Adherence Recommendations for Patients With Osteoporosis

Ensure the patient has a clear understanding of the risks for osteoporosis and the strategies to prevent the disease

Recommend that multiple adherence strategies work better than a single approach

Establish weekly contact with patients for the first 4 weeks of the program, then monthly thereafter, to continually assess the patient's progress and troubleshoot problems

Set achievable goals

Obtain baseline assessment of calcium and vitamin D intake as well as overall food consumption

Institute a self-monitoring program such as keeping a log of food intake and exercise participation

Identify patient-specific barriers to the lifestyle changes

Distribute information that uses health messages associated with osteoporosis that are easy to understand, interactive, and culturally sensitive

Design a program that is reasonable, gradual, and easily implemented

Source: National Institutes of Health, National Heart, Lung, and Blood Institute. Third report of the National Cholesterol Education Program (NCEP) Expert Panel on Detection, Evaluation, and Treatment of High Blood Cholesterol in Adults (Adult Treatment Panel III). NIH Publication No. 02-5215, September 2002.

As with other diseases in which lifestyle changes are important for the prevention and treatment of the disease, adherence to these changes is very important. A patient-centered healthcare model and health information that is culturally sensitive, interactive, and from reliable sources are important for improving adherence rates. Table 16-3 lists common suggestions for improving program adherence to osteoporosis prevention.[9]

NUTRITION AND OSTEOPOROSIS

Although calcium is a very important nutrient for strong bones, optimal bone health is dependent on many nutrients. For this reason the Surgeon General of the United States recommends a well-balanced eating plan from a variety of foods to achieve optimal bone health.[2] The 2005 Dietary Guidelines for Americans (http://healthierus.gov/dietaryguidelines/) and the DASH (Dietary Approaches to Stop Hypertension) Eating Plan (http://www.nhlbi.nih.gov/guidelines/) are both excellent examples of well-balanced eating plans.[10,11] The DASH Eating Plan can be good for both bone and heart health, although bone outcomes from the DASH Eating Plan have not been specifically tested.[2] The DASH Eating Plan emphasizes fruits, vegetables, low-fat or fat-free dairy foods, whole grains, fish, poultry, and nuts. This makes the DASH Eating Plan rich in calcium, magnesium, protein, and potassium while also being low in fat, cholesterol, and sodium. Dietary recommendations from the DASH Eating Plan are listed in Table 16-4.

Calcium

Calcium has been shown in many studies to be an important nutrient for optimal bone health as low calcium intake is associated with low bone mass, rapid bone loss, and high fracture rates.[2] The U.S. Surgeon General's Report on Bone Health and Osteoporosis (http://www.surgeongeneral.gov/) recommends that adequate calcium intake differ

TABLE 16–4	Dietary Recommendations for Patients With Osteoporosis	
Nutrient	**Nutrient Target**
Fat (% of total kcal)	27%
Saturated	6%
Monounsaturated	13%
Polyunsaturated	8%
Carbohydrates (% of total kcal)	55%
Protein (% of total kcal)	18%
Cholesterol	150 mg/day
Fiber	31 g/day
Potassium	4,700 mg/day
Magnesium	500 mg/day
Calcium	1,240 mg/day
Sodium	1,500 mg/day

Source: U.S. Department of Health and Human Services, National Institutes of Health. Facts about the DASH eating plan. Publication No. 03-4082, May 2003.

by age.[2] The recommended amounts of calcium are meant to be applied to individuals without disease. Those with osteoporosis or other chronic diseases may need more calcium, but data are not conclusive as to the recommended amounts.[2]

Adequate calcium intake should begin during childhood. It is recommended that children between the ages of 1 and 3 years should have 500 mg/day and children 4 to 8 years of age should have 800 mg/day of calcium. Interestingly, children and adolescents between the ages of 9 and 18 years have the highest recommended calcium intake of any age group. These individuals should consume 1,300 mg/day because this is a period during which bones grow rapidly.[2] Further, adults between the ages of 19 and 50 years should consume 1,000 mg/day whereas adults older than age 51 should consume 1,200 mg/day. The U.S. Surgeon General lists the highest tolerable calcium intake to be 2,500 mg/day, an amount that is the same for all individuals older than 1 year of age.[2]

Most Americans obtain a majority of their calcium from dairy products.[2] Combined with the amount of calcium in a "normal" American diet, adding just three 8-ounce glasses of milk each day is enough to meet the recommended daily requirements for most adults.[2] Dairy products that are low-fat or non-fat are good choices because they allow for the full amount of calcium but avoid high fat and calorie intake. In addition to low-fat dairy products such as milk, yogurt, cheese, and ice cream, good dietary sources of calcium include dark green leafy vegetables, such as broccoli, collard greens, bok choy, and spinach; sardines and salmon with bones; tofu; almonds; and foods fortified with calcium, such as orange juice, cereals, and breads.[1]

National nutrition surveys indicate that many Americans consume less than half the amount of calcium they need to build and maintain healthy bones.[1] A simple calculation can be done to estimate a patient's current calcium intake. The calculation is as follows:[2]

- Start with 290 for females, regardless of age, or males aged 60 years or greater
- Start with 370 for males younger than the age of 60 years
- Add 300 mg for each 8-ounce serving of milk or equivalent calcium-rich food (e.g., yogurt, cheese, fortified orange juice, broccoli)

- For patients taking calcium supplements or multivitamins containing calcium, add the total daily amount of calcium from the source
- Compare this total to the recommended amounts listed above

Healthcare practitioners can also teach patients to read food labels to estimate the amount of calcium that a particular food may have. This is relatively easy to do. The amount of calcium listed on food labels is stated as a percentage of the daily value of recommended calcium intake for most adults, which is 1,000 mg/day.[2] So, for example, a 1-cup serving of yogurt may list the calcium content as 30%. To convert the % Daily Value (DV) into milligrams, simply multiply the 30% by 10 or add a "0," which equals 300 mg of calcium for the serving size of 1 cup of yogurt.[2] Foods that contain 20% or more of the % DV are considered high in calcium and those that contain 5% or less of the % DV are considered low in calcium content.

Vitamin D

Vitamin D plays an important role in bone health in that it allows for the calcium to be absorbed adequately.[2] Too little vitamin D will not allow for the calcium to be absorbed and can lead to overall poor bone health. There are two sources of vitamin D, sunlight and diet.[2] Many people are able to obtain enough vitamin D naturally via sunlight, especially during summer months. Studies, however, show that vitamin D production decreases in the elderly, in individuals who are housebound, and during the winter months. For these reasons, some people may need to enhance their vitamin D intake with dietary supplements. The recommended amount of vitamin D is 400 to 800 IU per day.[2]

Other Nutrients

In addition to calcium and vitamin D, adequate amounts of other nutrients such as phosphorus and magnesium are also important for optimal bone health and can be inadequate in the "typical" American diet.[2] Phosphorus can be obtained from meats, cereals, and milk. Magnesium can be obtained from green leafy vegetables, whole grains, nuts, and dairy products. Fortunately, Americans generally consume adequate amounts of other important micronutrients that are important for good bone health such as vitamins K and C, copper, manganese, zinc, and iron.[2]

PHYSICAL ACTIVITY AND OSTEOPOROSIS

Physical activity is one of the cornerstones for good bone health and for the prevention of osteoporosis and bone fractures. The general physical activity recommendations set forth by the U.S. Surgeon General of 30 minutes/day (60 minutes for children) of moderate-intensity physical activity on most days of the week remains the foundation of physical activity recommendations for all Americans (http://www.surgeongeneral.gov/).[2] There are, however, specific aspects of physical activity for osteoporosis prevention that go beyond the general physical activity recommendations. These aspects largely focus on activities that impose a greater load on the skeleton than it is accustomed to during regular daily activities or even low-impact aerobic exercise activities. Physical activity is the only intervention that can potentially increase both bone mass and strength and reduce the risk of falling in older adults.[12]

Bone Health and Overtraining in Women

It has been known for many years that physical activity is good for bone health. With all the positive health outcomes associated with physical activity, it is sometimes hard to imagine negative outcomes associated with exercise. Of course, more is not always better, and we must always keep in mind that a balanced approach to all that we do should be the goal. Physical activity is no exception to this rule.

It is not uncommon to have patients who exercise too much and eat too little. Some athletes and highly active individuals tend to exercise to extremes. Some women can exercise to such extremes that they become amenorrheic or miss menstrual periods. It is common for these women to see this as a sign of successful training or a great answer to a monthly inconvenience.[13] It should, however, be a warning sign that they may be putting themselves at an increased risk for osteoporosis. Amenorrhea is often a sign of decreased estrogen levels. Low estrogen levels can lead to low bone mineral density and predispose these women to osteoporosis, even at a young age.[13]

There are reports of women in their 20s who have become amenorrheic secondary to high levels of physical activity who actually have bone mineral densities that are similar to those for women in their 80s.[13] Even if these women do not experience fractures at a young age, the low estrogen levels during these peak bone-building years can have lifelong effects. Studies have shown that bone growth that is lost during the peak bone-growth years may never be regained.[13] This then predisposes these women to osteoporosis when they get older.

Healthcare professionals should be aware of warning signs of women who are overtraining. These warning signs can include missed or irregular menstrual periods; extreme or "unhealthy-looking" thinness; extreme or rapid weight loss; behaviors that reflect frequent dieting such as eating very little, not eating in front of others, trips to the bathroom after meals, preoccupation with thinness, or possible increase in chewing gum among others; several intense bouts of exercise in the same day; anxiety about missing an exercise session; exercising despite illness; unusual amount of self-criticism; and indications of significant psychological and physical stress such as depression, inability to concentrate, feeling cold all the time, problems sleeping, fatigue, and constantly talking about their body weight.[13] Healthcare professionals who observe several of these warning signs should attempt to refer these patients to professionals trained in psychological and obsessive behaviors.

Emphasizing proper nutrition and physical activity to patients is important because it has been shown to decrease the risks for many diseases and improve mortality. It is important also to emphasize to patients that a balance must be maintained to achieve optimal health both physically and mentally. Pharmacists and other health-care professionals should be aware of the warning signs and symptoms of individuals who may be out of balance with physical activity and exercising too much.

There are a few principles about the osteogenic effects of exercise training programs that healthcare professionals should be aware of and talk to their patients about during physical activity counseling sessions. First, research has shown that only the skeletal sites that are exposed to a change in loading forces undergo adaptation to those forces.[12] In other words, doing activities that impose an increased load to the bones of the lower body will only affect the bones in the lower body (e.g., hips) and not those of the upper body (e.g., wrist). Second, the adaptive response that occurs as a result of the increased bone load occurs only when the loading stimulus exceeds that of the patient's usual loading conditions.[12] Therefore, the bones of the lower extremities will not have beneficial adaptations to simply standing for long periods of time or possibly even walking. The patient must perform higher impact activities like jogging, rope jumping, or resistance training for significant bone adaptations to occur. In addition, continued adaptation requires a progressively increasing overload to the bone to experience continued bone strength improvements.[12] Third, in adults the benefits of physical activity on bone health may not persist if the physical activity is significantly reduced.[12] Therefore, if a physical activity program is discontinued, the gains that were made in bone mineral density appear to be lost. This phenomenon, however, does not appear to be the same for children. Some evidence suggests that exercise-induced gains to bone mineral density obtained during childhood are maintained into adulthood.[12] This area, however, is still not well understood.[12]

During adulthood, the primary goal of physical activity should be to maintain bone mass through the use of bone-loading activities.[12] It is still unclear whether adults are able to significantly increase bone mineral density through exercise training.[12] Research that has shown increases in bone mineral density have come from high-intensity weight-bearing endurance or resistance training exercises.[12] Observational studies, however, have reported that patients who are physically active can lower their age-related decline in bone mineral density and the relative risk for fractures even when the activity is not particularly vigorous.[12] Animal studies have shown that fracture risk can be decreased even with no changes in bone mineral density, but non-observational human studies in this area are lacking. Several small studies have shown that bone health is favorably influenced by participating in high-level physical activity if the activity is weight-bearing in nature.

It should be noted that medications to prevent osteoporosis may still be indicated for postmenopausal women who are regularly physically active.[12] As a result of the current information that is known regarding the preservation of bone health during adulthood through the use of physical activity, the American College of Sports Medicine has offered several exercise recommendations. These recommendations are listed in Table 16-5.

PHARMACY PRACTICE APPLICATION

As with most chronic diseases, pharmacists can play a significant role not only in treating the disease but also in preventing it as well. Preventing osteoporosis may not be on the forefront of many pharmacists' minds because osteoporosis is not as significant a disease as others like **cardiovascular disease** and **cancer** and because those individuals for whom prevention strategies are most effective may not appear to be unhealthy or at risk. Yet the U.S. Surgeon General has named osteoporosis a significant public health concern and called all healthcare professionals, including pharmacists, to assist patients in its prevention.[2] Pharmacists should be aware of the risk factors that lead to osteoporosis, especially those that are medication related, and be able to identify patients in whom preventive strategies can be used. Pharmacists are in an ideal position to identify and talk with patients about osteoporosis prevention because of their exposure and frequent contact with their patients and the public. As with all chronic diseases, pharmacists can play a significant role in the treatment and the prevention of these diseases.

There are several examples published in the literature of pharmacists providing osteoporosis screening, risk assessments, and health information to patients.[14–17] Many of the successful projects have used risk assessment questionnaires and patient-appropriate health information to increase awareness of the disease. In addition, some have used

TABLE 16–5 Physical Activity Recommendations for the Prevention of Osteoporosis

Goals	Maintain bone mass
	Prevent falls and fractures
	Improve overall health and fitness level to decrease risks for chronic diseases
	Increase strength in upper and lower body
	Maintain a high quality of life
Type of activity	Weight-bearing endurance (e.g., jogging, at least intermittently during walking, stair climbing), activities that involve jumping (e.g., basketball, volleyball), and resistance training or weight training (specifically multijoint exercises of both upper and lower body)
Intensity	Moderate to high in terms of bone-loading forces
	Moderate in terms aerobic activities
Duration	20–30 minutes initially of a combination of weight-bearing endurance activities plus resistance training activities
	30–60 minutes optimally of a combination of weight-bearing endurance activities plus resistance training activities
Frequency	3–5 times per week for weight-bearing endurance activities
	2–3 times per week for resistance training activities
Lifestyle activity	Increase overall daily physical activities through taking stairs instead of elevators, parking farther away in parking lots, walking the family pet, etc.

Source: U.S. Department of Health and Human Services. Physical activity and health: a report of the Surgeon General. Atlanta: U.S. Department of Health and Human Services, Centers for Disease Control and Prevention, National Center for Chronic Disease Prevention and Health Promotion, 1996, 278 pages.

portable ultrasound bone mineral density analyzers to offer patients an estimate of their risk for osteoporosis and an opinion whether they should be referred to their physician for further analysis.

One particular study sponsored by the American Pharmacists Association, called Project ImPACT: Osteoporosis, is a good example of community-based pharmacists operating a successful osteoporosis screening and treatment program in conjunction with physicians.[17] Project ImPACT: Osteoporosis was conducted in a 29-store chain pharmacy in which interventions with patients took place with an initial visit to screen patients and provide health promotion information and to refer patients who required physician follow-up. The second phase of the project was a collaborative community health management service focused on osteoporosis monitoring and management conducted in the pharmacy. Lastly, the project demonstrated that patients as well as third-party payers were willing to pay for these services offered by pharmacists. The project results showed that 532 patients were screened, and the investigators were able to contact 305 of these patients for follow-up interviews 3 to 6 months later.[17] Of the patients screened, 37% were high risk, 33% were moderate risk, and 30% were low risk. A total of 78% of the patients indicated that they had no prior knowledge of their risk for future fractures. Additionally, 37% of patients in the moderate- and high-risk categories scheduled and completed a physician visit, and 24% of those patients were started on osteoporosis therapy after the screening.[17] Project ImPACT: Osteoporosis is an excellent example of pharmacists providing health promotion and disease prevention to patients and successfully collaborating with patients and physicians to do so.

CASE STUDY

L.K. is a 27-year-old female who comes to the pharmacy to pick up an over-the-counter analgesic medication. She notices an advertisement for the osteoporosis screening and prevention service that the pharmacy offers. L.K. inquires with the pharmacist about the service. During the conversation the pharmacist discovers that L.K. is interested in learning more about osteoporosis prevention because her grandmother has the disease and it has been very debilitating for her and her family. L.K. has no current diseases or health issues, but she is sedentary and smokes one pack per day. She occasionally drinks alcohol, follows no specific eating plan, does not regularly drink milk, and is 5' 1" tall and weighs 105 lb. L.K. has a resting blood pressure of 110/68 mm Hg and a heart rate of 75 beats/min, and has never had a blood lipid screening to her recollection. She expresses interest in receiving further counseling on osteoporosis prevention and sets up a time with the pharmacist to come back for the appointment. Her 3-day dietary analysis reveals the following:

> *Average caloric intake per day = 1,750 calories*
> *Carbohydrates = 54% of total calories*
> *Monounsaturated fats = 12% of total calories*
> *Polyunsaturated fats = 9% of total calories*
> *Saturated fats = 10% of total calories*
> *Total fats = 31% of total calories*
> *Protein = 15% of total calories*
> *Total dietary cholesterol = 280 mg*
> *Fiber = 18 g*
> *Calcium = 580 mg/day*
> *Potassium = 4,000 mg/day*
> *Magnesium = 480 mg/day*
> *Sodium = 2,500 mg/day*

Case Activities

1. *Write an SOAP note for L.K.*
2. *List L.K.'s risk factors for osteoporosis.*
3. *Design a program to reduce L.K.'s risk for osteoporosis that includes nutrition, physical activity, and smoking cessation.*

REFERENCES

1. National Institutes of Health. Osteoporosis overview. National Institutes of Health, Osteoporosis and Related Bone Diseases, National Resource Center. June 2005. Available at: http://www.niams.nih.gov/bone/hi/overview.htm. Accessed March 9, 2006.
2. U.S. Department of Health and Human Services. Bone health and osteoporosis: a report of the Surgeon General. Rockville, MD: U.S. Department of Health and Human Services, Office of the Surgeon General, 2004.
3. National Osteoporosis Foundation: America's bone health: the state of osteoporosis and low bone mass. Washington, D.C.: National Osteoporosis Foundation, 2002.
4. Nichols DL, Essery EV. Osteoporosis and exercise. In: Kaminsky LA, et al, eds. ACSM's Resource Manual for Guidelines for Exercise Testing and Prescription, 5th ed. Baltimore: Lippincott Williams & Wilkins, 2006:489–499.
5. Parent-Stevens L, Sagraves R. Gynecologic and other disorders of women. In: Koda-Kimble MA, ed. Applied Therapeutics: The Clinical Use of Drugs, 8th ed. Philadelphia: Lippincott Williams & Wilkins.2005:48.1–48.47.
6. O'Connell MB, Seaton TL. Osteoporosis and osteomalacia. In: Dipiro JT, ed. Pharmacotherapy: A Pathophysiologic Approach, 6th ed. New York: McGraw-Hill, 2005:1645–1669.

7. Hedlund LR, Gallagher JC. The effect of age and menopause on bone mineral density of the proximal femur. J Bone Miner Res 1989;4:639–646.

8. National Institutes of Health. Osteoporosis in men. National Institutes of Health, Osteoporosis and Related Bone Diseases, National Resource Center. August 2005. Available at: http://www.niams.nih.gov/bone/hi/osteoporosis_men.htm. Accessed March 9, 2006.

9. National Institutes of Health, National Heart, Lung, and Blood Institute. Third report of the National Cholesterol Education Program (NCEP) Expert Panel on Detection, Evaluation, and Treatment of High Blood Cholesterol in Adults (Adult Treatment Panel III). NIH Publication No. 02-5215, September 2002.

10. HHS Publication No. HHS-ODPHP-2005-01-DGA-A, Dietary Guidelines for Americans 2005, U.S. Department of Health and Human Services, U.S. Department of Agriculture. Available at: http://healthierus.gov/dietaryguidelines. Accessed February 13, 2007.

11. U.S. Department of Health and Human Services, National Institutes of Health. Facts about the DASH eating plan. Publication No. 03-4082, May 2003.

12. Kohrt WM, Bloomfield SA, Little KD, Nelson ME, Yingling VR. American College of Sports Medicine: Position stand: physical activity and bone health. Med Sci Sports Exerc 2004;36:1985–1996.

13. National Institutes of Health. Fitness and bone health for women: the skeletal risk of overtraining. National Institutes of Health, Osteoporosis and Related Bone Diseases, National Resource Center, November 2005. Available at: http://www.niams.nih.gov/bone/hi/fitness_bonehealth.htm. Accessed March 9, 2006.

14. Naunton M, Peterson GM, Jones G. Pharmacists provided quantitative heel ultrasound screening for rural women at risk for osteoporosis. Ann Pharmacother 2006;40:38–44.

15. Law AV, Shapiro K. Impact of a community pharmacist directed clinic in improving screening and awareness of osteoporosis. J Eval Clin Pract 2005;11:247–255.

16. Summers KM, Brock TP. Impact of pharmacist led community bone mineral density screening. Ann Pharmacother 2005;39:243–248.

17. Goode JV, Swiger K, Bluml BM. Regional osteoporosis screening, referral, and monitoring program in community pharmacies: findings from Project ImPACT: osteoporosis. J Am Pharm Assoc 2004;44:152–160.

CHAPTER 17

Osteoarthritis

OBJECTIVES

OBJECTIVES

At the end of this chapter the reader should be able to:

1. Explain the risks associated with osteoarthritis.
2. Summarize the prevention and treatment options for patients with osteoarthritis.
3. Describe appropriate nutritional strategies for patients at risk for and with osteoarthritis.
4. Suggest appropriate exercises for patients at risk for and with osteoarthritis.
5. Formulate a basic nutrition and exercise program for a patient with osteoarthritis.

OVERVIEW OF OSTEOARTHRITIS

There are more than 100 different types of arthritic diseases and conditions.[1] The most common form of arthritis is **osteoarthritis,** also called **degenerative joint disease.**[2] Osteoarthritis is localized to the affected joint and presents on examination as a defect of the articular cartilage of that joint. An inflammatory response is usually present with osteoarthritis but is localized to the affected joint and is not widespread as in other forms of arthritis.

PREVALENCE, ECONOMIC COSTS, AND HEALTH RISKS ASSOCIATED WITH OSTEOARTHRITIS

The prevalence of osteoarthritis in the United States is conservatively estimated to be at 21 million Americans or approximately 12% of the population.[3] Overall, arthritis is the leading cause of disability in the United States, affecting about one third of the population. Disability from arthritis results in 750,000 hospitalizations and 36 million outpatient visits each year.[1] The economic costs associated with arthritis are estimated to be at $51 billion in medical care costs each year and a total of $81 billion when lost productivity is included.[1]

PATHOPHYSIOLOGY OF OSTEOARTHRITIS

As stated above, osteoarthritis is a degeneration of the articular cartilage as well as the underlying subchondral bone of a joint.[2] Osteoarthritis can occur in any joint, but it is most commonly diagnosed in the knees, hips, hands, and spine. During the arthritic process the surface of the cartilage becomes pitted, which results in changes of the joint spacing or margins as well as changes in the subchondral bone.[2,4,5] Osteoarthritis is therefore characterized by narrow joint spacing, absence of articular cartilage, increased bone density, and stiffness of the subchondral bone and bone spur formation along the joint margins.[2,4–6]

The cause of osteoarthritis is largely unknown. Many speculate that both biomechanical and inflammatory mechanisms play an important role in the development and progression of the disease.[2] From a biomechanical viewpoint, weight-bearing joints such as the knees and hips can be compromised by structural factors such as obesity or neuromuscular abnormalities.[2] These factors can alter the joint dynamics and cause force changes on the joints that increase the load that the joint must bear. Some suggest that the inability of the joint to absorb these greater loads during activities of daily living causes a series of events that lead to the degeneration of joint.[2,7]

In the knee, increased loads may cause microcracks in subchondral tissue that result in a thinning of the overlying articular cartilage.[2,7] This thinning then leads to increased stress and eventual degradation of the cartilage, which in turn increases the subchondral bone density and decreases the shock-absorbing capability of the trabecular bone of the joint.[2,7] This process results in a feedback loop that creates even greater loads on the joint, creating even further joint degradation.

Inflammation may also play a significant role in the development and progression of osteoarthritis. The inflammatory cytokine interleukin-1β (IL-1β) has been shown in studies to be present in joints of patients with osteoarthritis and is thought to play a role in mediating joint inflammation and cartilage degradation.[2,8] Likewise, the inflammatory markers interleukin-6 (IL-6), tumor necrosis factor α (TNF-α), and C-reactive protein (CRP) have been shown to be higher in serum concentrations of patients with hip or knee osteoarthritis compared with individuals without osteoarthritis.[2,9,10]

The major symptoms of osteoarthritis are pain and stiffness. The clinical consequences of osteoarthritis can be severe. Joint cartilage degradation leads to pain, which usually results in a decline in **physical activity** that in turn leads to a loss in **muscular strength,** loss of physical functioning, and disability.[2] The loss of muscular strength and physical functioning often leads to the inability of patients to participate in activities of daily living that require ambulation, lifting, and carrying. This often results in a loss of independence and a decreased quality of life.[1,2,4,5,11–13] Therefore, the ability to prevent osteoarthritis and especially the ability to remain active in patients with existing osteoarthritis is extremely important for overall health and quality of life (Table 17-1).

OSTEOARTHRITIS PREVENTION AND TREATMENT

Treatment for osteoarthritis can be difficult. To date, there are no treatments available that affect the underlying disease process.[2] No pharmacologic agent is currently known to prevent, delay the progression of, or reverse the pathologic changes that occur in

TABLE 17–1   Environmental Risk Factors Leading to Osteoarthritis

Increased age
Overweight and obesity
Joint injury
Joint overuse from certain vocational or sport activities
Quadriceps muscle weakness
Genetic predisposition
Developmental abnormalities

Source: Chen SW, Gong WC. Rheumatic disorders. In: Koda-Kimble MA, ed. Applied Therapeutics: The Clinical Use of Drugs, 8th ed. Philadelphia: Lippincott Williams & Wilkins, 2005:43.1–43.42.

patients with osteoarthritis.[4] The primary goal of therapy is aimed at pain relief.[2,4,5] Several pharmacologic agents have been approved and used to treat the symptoms associated with osteoarthritis.[4,5] Additionally, **exercise** and weight control have also been used to treat the symptoms of osteoarthritis, especially in patients with knee osteoarthritis.[2] A list of the medications commonly used to treat osteoarthritis is provided in Table 17-2.

The causes of osteoarthritis that are related to lifestyle and vocational habits are overweight and **obesity,** quadriceps muscle weakness, and chronic overuse of particular joints. Therefore, osteoarthritis prevention strategies would mostly focus on weight control, muscular fitness, and conscious efforts to avoid overuse of certain joints.

As stated in many of the chapters of this book, overweight and obesity can play a significant role in the development and progression of several diseases. Carrying excess body weight for several years can increase the load on weight-bearing joints, especially the knees. Obese individuals often develop osteoarthritis in their knees simply as a result of carrying an excess load during daily living activities for many years. Patients who can maintain a healthy body weight through healthy eating and regular physical activity can not only fight off several cardiovascular and metabolic diseases but also lower their risk for osteoarthritis. Additionally, obese patients who are not physically active often develop weak quadriceps muscles in relation to the muscles in the back of the legs and buttocks because of alterations in body weight distribution. This, in turn, leads to biomechanical changes of knee load distribution, which can also increase the risk for osteoarthritis, especially in the knees.[2] This gives further evidence to emphasize to patients about maintaining a healthy body weight through physical activity that incorporates muscular fitness activities as well as aerobic fitness activities.

In one particular study, weight loss between 7.5 and 11% of body weight in patients with osteoarthritis significantly improved self-reported function compared with patients who had little or no weight loss.[2] Another study showed that a 5% decrease in body weight was associated with decreased inflammatory markers such as CRP, IL-6, and TNF-α that are thought to contribute to overall inflammation and joint cartilage degradation.[2,14]

TABLE 17–2   Medications Used to Treat Osteoarthritis

Oral analgesics
Non-steroidal anti-inflammatory drugs (NSAIDs)
Topical analgesics
Nutritional supplements

Source: Chen SW, Gong WC. Rheumatic disorders. In: Koda-Kimble MA, ed. Applied Therapeutics: The Clinical Use of Drugs, 8th ed. Philadelphia: Lippincott Williams & Wilkins, 2005:43.1–43.42.

It is currently unknown, however, whether weight loss directly affects inflammatory markers or whether the physical activity and progression of the disease affect these markers. Further research in this area is needed.

Certain occupations and sporting activities can increase the risk for osteoporosis simply by constant use of certain joints. For example, individuals who use frequent hand or wrist movements for their occupation may increase their risk for developing osteoarthritis in the joints of the hands and wrists. Likewise, athletes such as runners can develop osteoarthritis in their knees and hips after many years of running, even if they are not overweight. This overuse phenomenon can have a significant impact on the lives of the individuals that it affects. Counseling individuals to make small body position adjustments at work or to cross train (alternate activities) during physical activity may help to avoid the onset of osteoarthritis. It is important to note that some individuals may develop osteoarthritis even if they are not overweight or obese, alter body positions during work activities, and participate in cross-training activities.

Adherence strategies to weight loss and physical activity programs are important to allow the individual the best possible opportunity to be successful in the program. Behavior modification strategies such as effective communication and identification of participation barriers can help improve program adherence. Patients living with osteoarthritis may often have barriers to participating in activities that involve supporting the body weight, such as jogging or other high-impact activities. Patients who participate in these types of activities can experience increased pain, which often leads to decreased adherence. Therefore, special attention must be paid to suggesting activities that make the patient's symptoms improve rather than worsen. Table 17-3 lists suggestions that can enhance weight-loss and physical activity programs for patients at risk for or with osteoarthritis.[15]

NUTRITION AND OSTEOARTHRITIS

There are no specific dietary recommendations that have proven to be effective to prevent or treat the development or progression of osteoarthritis. Nutritional recommendations for patients at risk for or with osteoarthritis primarily focus on maintaining and achieving a healthy body weight. Osteoarthritic patients who are overweight or obese

---

TABLE 17–3　Program Adherence Recommendations for Patients With Osteoarthritis

Recommend that multiple adherence strategies work better than a single approach

Establish weekly contact with patients for the first 4 weeks of the program, then monthly thereafter, to continually assess the patient's progress and troubleshoot problems

Set achievable goals

Obtain baseline assessment of overall food consumption

Obtain baseline assessment of physical activity

Institute a self-monitoring program such as keeping a log of food intake and exercise participation

Identify patient-specific barriers to the lifestyle changes

Distribute information that uses health messages associated with osteoarthritis that are easy to understand, interactive, and culturally sensitive

Design a program that is reasonable, gradual, and easily implemented

Source: National Institutes of Health, National Heart, Lung, and Blood Institute. Third report of the National Cholesterol Education Program (NCEP) Expert Panel on Detection, Evaluation, and Treatment of High Blood Cholesterol in Adults (Adult Treatment Panel III). NIH Publication No. 02-5215, September 2002.

should focus prevention and treatment strategies on weight loss to help improve their symptoms associated with the disease.

Dietary therapy is a key component of weight-loss and weight-maintenance therapy, as most overweight and obese persons will need adjustments in caloric intake to lose weight.[16] The dietary therapy component of weight loss focuses on teaching patients how to modify their individual diet to decrease calorie intake. It is very important that calorie reduction recommendations are not too aggressive and are done with the goal of slow and progressive weight loss through moderate calorie reduction. In addition, the composition of the diet should be balanced and structured in a way that decreases other possible risk factors such as **hypertension, dyslipidemia,** and **diabetes mellitus.**[16]

Successful dietary therapy is dependent on modifying the patient's diet to create a **caloric deficit** while allowing for all the necessary dietary allowances and also maintaining food preferences of the patient. This can be challenging but is achievable through detailed patient consultation. The patients must be involved in this process. It is often helpful to give patients several appropriate choices and allow the patients to choose the eating plan. This allows them to self-monitor their intake and improves compliance. The keys to success for dietary therapy are to:

1. Educate the patients regarding the calorie value of foods they are choosing as well as the composition (carbohydrate, fats, and protein) by reading the nutrition label
2. Avoid overconsumption of high-calorie foods
3. Reduce portion size
4. Maintain adequate water intake[16]

Specific dietary composition recommendations for weight loss are listed in Table 17-4.

TABLE 17–4   **Dietary Recommendations for Overweight and Obese Patients With Osteoarthritis**

Nutrient	Recommendation
Total calories[a]	Approximately 500–1000 kcal/day reduction from usual intake
Carbohydrate[b]	55% or more of total calories
Fiber	20–30 g/day
Protein	Approximately 15% of total calories
Monounsaturated fat	Up to 15% of total calories
Polyunsaturated fat	Up to 10% of total calories
Saturated fat	8–10% of total calories
Total fat	30% or less of total calories
Dietary cholesterol	<300 mg/day
Sodium chloride	No more than 100 mmol per day (approximately 2.4 g of sodium, or approximately 6 g of sodium chloride)
Calcium	1,000–1,500 mg/day

[a]It is recommended that alcohol not be consumed as part of the daily caloric intake as it will not only increase the total calories but has also been shown to be associated with obesity in epidemiologic studies.
[b]Most carbohydrate intake should come from whole grains, fruits, and vegetables.
Source: The Practical Guide. Identification, Evaluation, and Treatment of Overweight and Obesity in Adults. Bethesda, MD: National Institutes of Health, U.S. Department of Health and Human Services, 2000. NIH Publication No. 00-4084.

PHYSICAL ACTIVITY AND OSTEOARTHRITIS

Many patients and healthcare providers with osteoarthritis have the misconception that physical activity is harmful and should be avoided. These beliefs come from the fact that joint movements can many times result in pain with osteoarthritis, and physical activity creates more movement and therefore should be avoided. These beliefs are false and, in fact, the opposite is true. Patients with osteoarthritis who participate in regular physical activity often report less pain and greater abilities to perform activities of daily living.[2]

Patients with knee osteoarthritis have reported that short-term walking programs improve aerobic capacity, walking time, and self-reported function.[2,17,18] Likewise, long-term walking programs in patients with knee osteoarthritis have reported reduced disability and pain, improved balance, and improved physical performance when compared with a control group.[2,19] Additionally, patients who participate in resistance training exercises along with walking programs experience even greater improvements in physical functioning, increases in strength, and decreased pain relative to those who do not participate in resistance training.[2,20,21]

The American College of Sports Medicine (ACSM) recommends physical activity in patients with arthritis that is consistent with general physical activity guidelines for cardiorespiratory, resistance, and flexibility activity recommendations.[22] The primary goals for physical activity should be to both increase joint functionality and improve **physical fitness.** Initial phases of the program may require low-intensity and low-duration of activity (5 to 10 minutes) for patients who are deconditioned, but it is recommended that a single exercise session begin with **flexibility** exercises for the affected joints, progress to resistance training activities, and end with aerobic activities. The aerobic activities can be either weight-bearing or non–weight-bearing, but those that are weight-bearing should not be vigorous, high impact, and highly repetitive in nature.[22] In fact, the ACSM recommends that it is important for patients with osteoarthritis to alternate modes of activity (cross-training) to avoid highly repetitive movement on the affected joints. It is important to note that continuous weight-bearing activity (e.g., walking) may initially be difficult for patients with knee osteoarthritis. Recommending short bouts of exercise with frequent resting periods may improve pain symptoms and adherence as the activity duration builds up to 30 to 40 minutes.[2] Additionally, exercise should not be performed if patients experience persistent fatigue, increased weakness, decreased range of motion, increased joint swelling, and continuing pain that lasts more than 1 hour after exercise.[22] Table 17-5 lists specific recommendations for exercise programming in patients with osteoarthritis.

People With Arthritis Can Exercise (PACE)

Promoting healthy lifestyle behaviors in the pharmacy practice setting is important to increase public awareness of various disease prevention and treatment strategies and to promote the initiative that pharmacists can care for patients in ways other than just dispensing medications when they are ill. The promotion of healthy behaviors does not have to be difficult or even expensive. Many organizations and government agencies have done a great deal of work in developing educational materials and literature to increase awareness about various diseases and treatment strategies. Arthritis is no exception.

The Arthritis Foundation has established a program to increase awareness and promote the benefits of participation in regular physical activity as a means of managing arthritis and the symptoms associated with the disease.[23] The program is called People With Arthritis Can Exercise (PACE). The PACE program is a community-based, non-clinical program that is designed specifically for individuals with one of the more than 100 forms of arthritis. The program is designed for individuals who may or may not have physical limitations but is especially helpful for patients with joint motion or strength limitations who are currently sedentary as a result of these limitations.

The specific goals of the PACE program are to relieve stiffness, increase endurance, and improve posture; restore or maintain joint range of motion and muscle strength; and increase flexibility of the structures surrounding the joint. Although the program includes activities designed to improve certain physical parameters, the community-based nature of the program and group exercise experience also encourage peer interaction and socialization with others who have the same conditions. The PACE program has been successfully implemented at wellness centers, community centers, churches, gyms, assisted-living facilities, senior centers, and other community recreational centers throughout the United States.[23]

The PACE program is generally organized by the state chapters of the Arthritis Foundation where PACE instructors are specifically trained to lead such exercise classes. Pharmacists can get involved by contacting their state Arthritis Foundation chapter to learn more about the program, to find out where PACE program classes are offered in their area, and to ask for brochures that they can give to their patients with arthritis as a means to promote physical activity and as an additional treatment strategy. Disease management programs such as this offer healthcare professionals such as pharmacists an excellent opportunity to promote healthy living with little investment in time or resources. More information can be found about the PACE program at the Arthritis Foundation website: http://www.arthritis.org.

TABLE 17–5   Physical Activity Recommendations for Patients With Osteoarthritis

Goals	Improve functional status by increasing or maintaining activities of daily living, improving quality of life, and possibly returning to work for patients who previously could not do so because of osteoarthritis Improve cardiorespiratory fitness Improve muscular strength Increase or maintain pain-free range of motion Decrease joint stiffness Improve balance and walking gait Lose weight if needed
Type of activity	Aerobic activity[a] (walking, bicycling, swimming, water aerobics), resistance training (all major muscle groups, 8–10 exercises, 2–3 repetitions initially building to 10–12 repetitions, 2–3 days per week, use pain tolerance to set resistance), and flexibility of all major muscle groups 5–7 days per week
Intensity	Light to moderate
Duration	20–60 minutes (initially 5–10 for deconditioned patients and those with increased osteoarthritic pain)
Frequency	3–5 days per week for exercise program but maintaining a high level of activities of daily living through lifestyle activities on most days of the week
Lifestyle activity	Increase overall daily physical activities through taking stairs instead of elevators, parking farther away in parking lots, walking the family pet, etc.

[a]Use a cross-training method of alternating activities and avoid exercises that are vigorous, high-impact, and highly repetitive.

Source: Messier SP. Arthritic disease and conditions. In: Kaminsky LA, et al., eds. ACSM's Resource Manual for Guidelines for Exercise Testing and Prescription, 5th ed. Baltimore: Lippincott Williams & Wilkins, 2006:500–513.

PHARMACY PRACTICE APPLICATION

Pharmacists can have a highly effective role in assisting patients with osteoarthritis. First, as a highly accessible healthcare provider, pharmacists can recognize patients who may be at risk for osteoarthritis and offer educational material to increase awareness of the disease. Second, patients with osteoarthritis often need support to be able to cope with the disease. Pharmacists can assist patients by recommending both pharmacologic and non-pharmacologic treatments that can improve pain symptoms, activities of daily living, and quality of life. Properly educating patients about safe and effective treatments and offering continued follow-up in a collaborative effort with the patient's physician and physical therapist can lead to higher adherence rates and to the achievement of the patient and program goals.

CASE STUDY

E.P. is a 73-year-old female (5′6″ tall and 190 lb) who regularly visits the pharmacy to pick up medications for herself and her husband. She inquires about the informational brochure that was attached to her last prescription about pain management for osteoarthritis. E.P. has a medical history of knee osteoarthritis and hypertension for which she takes acetaminophen 1,000 mg every 6 to 8 hours and hydrochlorothiazide 50 mg daily, respectively. She is sedentary, and a non-smoker and non-drinker, and tries to follow a low-sodium diet to "improve her blood pressure." Her current blood pressure is under control at 116/78 mm Hg, and she has a heart rate of 76 beats per minute. She states that she doesn't really like to take medication and would like to know how she can improve her knee pain in ways other than taking more medicine. She decides to enroll in the pharmacy's osteoarthritis disease management program. The results of her 4-day dietary analysis are as follows:

> *Average caloric intake per day = 2,150 calories*
> *Carbohydrates = 50% of total calories*
> *Monounsaturated fats = 12% of total calories*
> *Polyunsaturated fats = 11% of total calories*
> *Saturated fats = 10% of total calories*
> *Total fats = 33% of total calories*
> *Protein = 17% of total calories*
> *Total dietary cholesterol = 250 mg*
> *Fiber = 20 g*
> *Calcium = 1,000 mg/day*
> *Potassium = 4,500 mg/day*
> *Magnesium = 500 mg/day*
> *Sodium = 2,000 mg/day*

Case Activities

1. *Write an SOAP note for E.P.*
2. *List E.P.'s risk factors for osteoarthritis and cardiovascular disease.*
3. *Design a program that includes nutrition, exercise, and weight-loss recommendations for E.P. that will help her manage her osteoarthritis as well as decrease her risks for cardiovascular disease.*

REFERENCES

1. Centers for Disease Control and Prevention: Targeting arthritis: the nation's leading cause of disability. Atlanta: Department of Health and Human Services, 2004. Available at: http://www.cdc.gov/nccdphp/publications/aag/arthritis.htm. Accessed March 23, 2006.

2. Messier SP. Arthritic disease and conditions. In: Kaminsky LA, et al., eds. ACSM's Resource Manual for Guidelines for Exercise Testing and Prescription, 5th ed. Baltimore: Lippincott Williams & Wilkins, 2006: 500–513.

3. Lawrence RC, Helmick CG, Arnett FC, et al. Estimates of the prevalence of arthritis and selected musculoskeletal disorders in the United States. Arthritis Rheum 1998;41:778–799.

4. Chen SW, Gong WC. Rheumatic disorders. In: Koda-Kimble MA, ed. Applied Therapeutics: The Clinical Use of Drugs, 8th ed. Philadelphia: Lippincott Williams & Wilkins, 2005:43.1–43.42.

5. Hansen KE, Elliott ME. Osteoarthritis. In: Dipiro JT, ed. Pharmacotherapy: A Pathophysiologic Approach, 6th ed. New York: McGraw-Hill, 2005:1685–1703.

6. Martin DF. Pathomechanics of knee osteoarthritis. Med Sci Sports Exer 1994;26:1429–1434.

7. Burr DB, Radin EL. Microfractures and microcracks in subchondral bone: are they relevant to osteoarthritis? Rheum Dis Clin North Am 2003;29:675–685.

8. Messier SP, Loeser RF, Mitchell MN, et al. Exercise and weight loss in obese older adults with knee osteoarthritis: A preliminary study. J Am Geriatr Soc 2000;48:1062–1072.

9. Otterness IG, Swindell AC, Zimmerer RO, et al. An analysis of 14 molecular markers for monitoring osteoarthritis: segregation of the markers into clusters and distinguishing osteoarthritis at baseline. Osteoarthritis Cartilage 2000;8:180–185.

10. Spector TD, Hart DJ, Nandra D, et al. Low-level increases in serum C-reactive protein are present in early osteoarthritis of the knee and predict progressive disease. Arthritis Rheum 1997;40:723–727.

11. Felson DT, Naimark A, Anderson J, et al. The prevalence of knee osteoarthritis in the elderly. The Framingham Osteoarthritis Study. Arthritis Rheum 1987;30:914–918.

12. Brunning RD, Materson RS. A rational program of exercise for patients with osteoarthritis. Semin Arthritis Rheum 1991;21:33–43.

13. Jokl P. Prevention of disuse muscle atrophy in chronic arthritides. Rheum Dis Clin North Am 1990;16:837–844.

14. Nicklas BJ, Ambrosius W, Messier SP, et al. Diet-induced weight loss, exercise and chronic inflammation in older, obese adults. A randomized, controlled clinical trial. Am J Clin Nutr 2004;79:544–551.

15. National Institutes of Health, National Heart, Lung, and Blood Institute. Third report of the National Cholesterol Education Program (NCEP) Expert Panel on Detection, Evaluation, and Treatment of High Blood Cholesterol in Adults (Adult Treatment Panel III). NIH Publication No. 02-5215, September 2002.

16. The Practical Guide. Identification, Evaluation, and Treatment of Overweight and Obesity in Adults. Bethesda, MD: National Institutes of Health, U.S. Department of Health and Human Services, 2000, NIH Publication No. 00-4084.

17. Kovar PA, Allegrante JP, MacKenzie CR, et al. Supervised fitness walking in patients with osteoarthritis of the knee. A randomized, controlled trial. Ann Intern Med 1992;116:529–534.

18. Minor MA, Hewett JE, Webel RR, et al. Efficacy of physical conditioning exercise in patients with rheumatoid arthritis and osteoarthritis. Arthritis Rheum 1989;32:1396–1405.

19. Ettinger WH Jr, Burns R, Messier SP, et al. A randomized trial comparing aerobic exercise and resistance training with a health education program in older adults with knee osteoarthritis. The Fitness Arthritis and Seniors Trial (FAST). JAMA 1997;277:25–31.

20. Fisher NM, Gresham G, Pendergast DR. Effects of quantitative progressive rehabilitation program applied unilaterally to the osteoarthritic knee. Arch Phys Med Rehabil 1993;74:1319–1326.

21. Fisher NM, Pendergast DR. Effects of a muscle exercise program on exercise capacity in subjects with osteoarthritis. Arch Phys Med Rehabil 1994;75:792–797.

22. Franklin BA, Whaley MH, Howley ET. American College of Sports Medicine. Other clinical conditions influencing exercise prescription. In: ACSM's Guidelines for Exercise Testing and Prescription, 6th ed. Philadelphia: Lippincott Williams & Wilkins, 2000:205–207.

23. Arthritis Foundation. Available at: http://www.arthritis.org. Accessed March 23, 2006.

CHAPTER 18

Chronic Lung Disease

At the end of this chapter the reader should be able to:

1. Explain the risks associated with the chronic lung diseases such as asthma and chronic obstructive pulmonary disease.
2. Summarize the prevention and treatment options for patients with asthma and chronic obstructive pulmonary disease.
3. Describe appropriate nutritional strategies for patients with asthma and chronic obstructive pulmonary disease.
4. Suggest appropriate exercises for patients with asthma and chronic obstructive pulmonary disease.
5. Formulate a basic nutrition and exercise program for a patient with asthma or chronic obstructive pulmonary disease.

OVERVIEW OF CHRONIC LUNG DISEASE

The topic of **chronic lung disease** can include many different pulmonary disorders such as **asthma, chronic obstructive pulmonary disease (COPD), chronic bronchitis, emphysema,** chronic rhinitis, cystic fibrosis, and drug-induced pulmonary diseases.[1–4] This chapter, however, will focus on asthma and COPD as these are two of the most common chronic lung diseases. Asthma is a disease characterized by wheezing, breathlessness, chest tightness, and nighttime or early morning coughing.[5] It is the most common long-term disease in children.[5] COPD refers to a group of pulmonary diseases, including emphysema, chronic bronchitis, and in some cases asthma, that cause airflow blockage and breathing-related problems.[6] This chapter will focus on these two lung disorders from the perspective of managing the disease symptoms through lifestyle modifications and ways in which to remain physically active with a chronic lung disease.

PREVALENCE, ECONOMIC COSTS, AND HEALTH RISKS ASSOCIATED WITH ASTHMA AND COPD

In 2001, more than 20 million Americans had asthma.[5] Of these individuals, 12 million (60%) had experienced an asthma attack in the previous year.[5] Asthma is linked to approximately 100 million days missed from work or school each year, as well as 470,000 hospital visits annually.[7] Additionally, asthma accounts for approximately 5,000 deaths per year in the United States.[7] It is estimated that asthma costs more than $12 billion annually in the United States, with an estimated societal burden of $640 per patient per year.[1,2]

COPD is one of the leading causes of death, illness, and disability in the United States.[6] In 2000, COPD accounted for 119,000 deaths, 726,000 hospitalizations, and 1.5 million hospital emergency department visits.[6] Additionally, 8 million COPD outpatient treatments occurred in 2000, with 10 million adults diagnosed that same year.[6] During the previous 25 years, however, the proportion of the U.S. population aged 25 to 54 years (both male and female) with mild to moderate COPD has declined.[6] This suggests that hospitalizations and deaths associated with COPD may begin to decrease in the coming years.[6] In 2000, the economic burden of COPD was approximately $23 billion in the United States and in 2002 it was about $32 billion.[4]

PATHOPHYSIOLOGY OF CHRONIC LUNG DISEASE

Asthma

Asthma is characterized by reversible airflow obstruction that can occur at any time in an individual, but most patients are diagnosed with asthma by age 5.[2] Genetic studies of patients with asthma strongly suggest that there is a genetic predisposition.[2] An individual who has a parent with asthma is three to six times more likely to develop asthma than is a person who does not have a parent with asthma.[5]

Asthma is a chronic inflammatory disorder and is caused by a complex interaction between inflammatory cells and mediators.[1] Cellular elements involved in the inflammatory process include mast cells, eosinophils, T lymphocytes, neutrophils, epithelial cells, and others. In persons susceptible to asthma, the inflammatory process usually occurs as a result of exposure to triggers or events that begin the process. These triggers are commonly an allergy to certain environmental elements or chemicals. After exposure to a trigger, an asthma attack can occur as a result of airway inflammation and a hyperreactivity of the bronchial smooth muscles, which causes variable degrees of airway obstruction.[1,2]

COPD

COPD is a disease that progresses with time and is characterized by limited airflow that is not completely reversible. Like asthma, inflammation plays a significant role in the progression of COPD. An inflammatory response in the lungs can occur in patients with COPD as a result of noxious particles or gases.[4] The two most common pulmonary disorders comprising COPD are chronic bronchitis and emphysema.[4] Chronic bronchitis is a disorder of excessive mucus secretion into the bronchial tree that is accompanied by a chronic cough.[3,4] Emphysema is a pulmonary disorder in which there is abnormal enlargement of the airspaces in the lungs with permanent damage to the bronchial walls.[4]

Because much of the lung damage associated with COPD is in and distal to the bronchial tree, COPD is said to be a disease of small airways and parenchymal destruction.[3] The chronic inflammatory process in the lungs occurs as a result of environmental, behavioral, and genetic factors.[3] Lung inflammation occurs as a result of neutrophils, macrophages, and lymphocytes, as well as inflammatory chemical mediators.[4] These cells and mediators are redundant and complementary and lead to widespread destruction of lung tissue.[4] A list of the risk factors leading to both asthma and COPD is provided in Table 18-1.

CHRONIC LUNG DISEASE PREVENTION AND TREATMENT

Many of the risk factors associated with asthma and the development of COPD are related to allergens and exposure to cigarette smoke. Therefore, disease prevention strategies should focus on avoiding environmental allergens and chemicals, as well as

TABLE 18–1   Environmental Risk Factors Leading to Asthma and COPD

Asthma	COPD
Airborne pollens	Tobacco smoke
Household dust mites	Occupational chemicals
Animal dander	Genetic predisposition
Cockroach allergen	
Mold	
Tobacco smoke	
Secondhand tobacco smoke	
Outdoor air pollution	
Wood smoke	
Cold air	
Exercising in cold, dry climate	
Respiratory infections	
Gastroesophageal reflux	
Anxiety	
Stress	
Anger	
Some foods and food additives	
Drug allergies (e.g., aspirin)	
Occupational triggers (i.e., various chemicals)	

Sources: U.S. Department of Health and Human Services, National Institutes of Health, National Heart, Lung and Blood Institute. Clinical Practice Guidelines. Expert Panel 2: Guidelines for the diagnosis and management of asthma. NIH Publication No. 97-4051, July 1997; U.S. Department of Health and Human Services, National Institutes of Health, National Heart, Lung and Blood Institute, National Asthma Prevention Program. Clinical Practice Guidelines. Expert Panel 2: Guidelines for the diagnosis and management of asthma. Update on selected topics 2002. NIH Publication No. 02-5074, June 2003. COPD, chronic obstructive pulmonary disease.

TABLE 18–2   Medications Used to Treat Asthma and COPD

β_2 agonists (asthma and COPD)
Corticosteroids (asthma and COPD)
Anticholinergics (asthma and COPD)
Antimicrobial agents (asthma and COPD)
Methylxanthines (asthma and COPD)
Leukotriene receptor antagonists (asthma)
α_1-Antitrypsin replacement therapy (COPD)
Other alternative therapies (asthma and COPD)

Sources: U.S. Department of Health and Human Services, National Institutes of Health, National Heart, Lung and Blood Institute. Clinical Practice Guidelines. Expert Panel 2: Guidelines for the diagnosis and management of asthma. NIH Publication No. 97-4051, July 1997; U.S. Department of Health and Human Services, National Institutes of Health, National Heart, Lung and Blood Institute, National Asthma Prevention Program. Clinical Practice Guidelines. Expert Panel 2: Guidelines for the diagnosis and management of asthma. Update on selected topics 2002. NIH Publication No. 02-5074, June 2003. COPD, chronic obstructive pulmonary disease.

smoking abstinence. In addition, it is important for patients with asthma and COPD to be compliant with their prescribed medications that treat their disease. Of the 5,000 asthma-related deaths that occur each year, most can be prevented with proper medication usage and prevention strategies.[7] The treatment and prevention guidelines for asthma can be accessed at http://www.nhlbi.nih.gov/guidelines/. Categories of medications used to treat asthma and COPD are listed in Table 18-2.

Theophylline and Physical Activity

Some drugs have specific characteristics that make them susceptible to interacting with physical activity. A drug–exercise interaction can occur from a pharmacodynamic or a pharmacokinetic perspective.[8] Drugs like β-blockers used to treat hypertension and other illnesses can have a pharmacodynamic interaction with exercise in that they decrease cardiac output, which leads to the inability to exercise at a high level of intensity. Pharmacokinetic interactions between exercise and certain drugs occur when the act of performing exercise alters the pharmacokinetic parameters of the drug.

Theophylline is a bronchodilator used to treat asthma and COPD.[8] Extra care must be taken when administering theophylline because it is said to have a narrow therapeutic range. Side effects that can occur when theophylline blood levels are outside the therapeutic range can be significant. Theophylline toxicity can produce symptoms such as sinus tachycardia, nausea, vomiting, diarrhea, and headache.[8] Underdosing theophylline can result in acute respiratory attacks. Factors that affect the pharmacokinetic parameters of theophylline, such as half-life and drug clearance, should be closely monitored to ensure toxicity symptoms do not occur while maintaining adequate asthma control.[8]

One particular study has shown that pharmacokinetic parameters of theophylline can be altered by exercise.[8] Participants in the study demonstrated that exercising at various intensities and room temperatures significantly affected theophylline half-life and clearance.[8] Plasma half-life significantly increased when participants exercised at 30% of their maximum oxygen consumption ($\dot{V}o_2$ max) at both 22 and 40°Celsius as well as at 50% $\dot{V}o_2$ max at 22° Celsius compared with control patients ($P < 0.05$).[8] Additionally, plasma theophylline clearance significantly decreased during these same parameters when compared with the control group ($P < 0.05$).[8]

Caution should be taken when patients exercise while taking theophylline. Healthcare providers should maintain adequate theophylline blood levels by dosing the medication properly and providing quality patient counseling. Patients who are highly active and taking theophylline may want to monitor blood levels more frequently to ensure proper levels and be aware of signs and symptoms that would indicate theophylline toxicity.

Smoking is a significant modifiable risk factor for both asthma and COPD. Children who are exposed to cigarettes through secondhand smoke are more likely to develop asthma and experience asthma attacks. Nearly 85 to 90% of cases of COPD have developed as a result of a current or past history of cigarette smoking.[3,9] Cigarette smoking is the most common risk for COPD because it causes lung function to decline more quickly with age compared with those who do not smoke. In non-smokers, forced expiratory volume in 1 second (FEV_1) decreases by approximately 20 to 30 mL per year after age 35. In smokers, FEV_1 decreases at a rate of 50 to 120 mL per year during this same time frame.[3] Some smokers can experience a decline that is more significant than others as a result of genetic and other environmental factors.[3] Smoking-cessation programs are a major recommendation for patients and family members of patients with asthma and COPD.

Exercise and **physical activity** in certain environments have been shown to be risks for asthma and lead to **exercise-induced asthma (EIA)** or **exercise-induced bronchospasm (EIB).** Many studies show that 70 to 90% of patients with asthma experience EIA.[2] EIA is characterized by a transient airway obstruction that usually occurs 5 to 15 minutes after physical exertion and especially occurs in environments that are cold or dry.[10] The symptoms of EIA can include shortness of breath, wheezing, coughing, chest discomfort, or a combination that last up to 30 minutes after exercise has stopped.[10] A significant stimulus for EIA is increased ventilation while exercising, but the pathophysiology of the syndrome is largely unknown. EIA is thought to be related to a loss of respiratory heat, increased osmolality as a result of respiratory water loss, or associated vascular events.[10] Most patients susceptible to EIA experience the symptoms when the exercise intensity exceeds 75% of maximal heart rate.[10] Some asthmatic patients, however, may experience EIA during very mild exertion.[10] Other individuals may only experience asthma symptoms during and after exercising, while being symptom-free all other times.

The key to preventing EIA is ensuring asthma medications are adequately controlled.[2,10] In addition, exercising in climates that are not at temperature or humidity extremes can decrease the susceptibility of EIA. Patients with asthma and EIA can experience all the physical benefits from exercise as those without asthma and EIA when symptoms are well controlled with medications. Asthmatic patients who are acutely sensitive to EIA at moderate or greater exercise intensities may be limited in their ability to increase their exercise capacity or fitness levels, but are still able to exercise for longer durations at lower intensities.[10] Although physical activity may provoke an asthmatic episode, it is still recommended to be incorporated into the management plan of these patients.[10]

As patients with COPD age and the disease progresses with time, lung function declines and often leads to decreased physical activity. This leads to deconditioning and the loss of the ability to perform many daily tasks.[11] Although patients with COPD can experience reduced exercise tolerance and exertional dyspnea with enhanced physical activity, participating in physical activity can potentially have multiple benefits such as improved physical endurance and fitness level; improved ventilatory endurance efficiency; improved cardiovascular conditioning; improved oxygen transport, extraction, endurance, and efficiency of skeletal muscles; reduced blood flow requirement to respiratory muscles, which will then increase blood flow available to working limb muscles; desensitization to the perception of dyspnea and fear of exertion; and improved quality of life.[11] Patients with COPD who regularly exercise can significantly enhance their feeling of well-being even if large increases in fitness levels do not occur.[11] Maintaining a high quality of life by avoiding disabilities is a major goal in patients with COPD in which enhanced physical activity levels can make a significant difference.

A disease prevention program that incorporates lifestyle modification for a patient with asthma or COPD would primarily focus on smoking cessation and enhanced physical activity. Strategies to improve adherence to these components are similar to those of other diseases. It is important to keep in mind that patients with COPD can benefit from physical activity even if they do not significantly improve their fitness levels. The focus of improvements should be on quality of life. Participating in a physical activity program may be difficult, especially in the beginning as a result of reductions in exercise tolerance and exertional dyspnea. Pharmacists should recommend physical activity to these patients with the collaboration and support of the patient's physician, respiratory therapist, occupational therapist, and other healthcare professionals. Support from other professionals can improve patient safety and adherence and optimize program outcomes. Table 18-3 lists suggestions to improve patient adherence to lifestyle modification strategies.[12]

NUTRITION AND CHRONIC LUNG DISEASE

Nutritional recommendations for the prevention of asthma primarily focus on avoiding foods and food additives that may be possible triggers for an asthma attack. It is not well documented that food allergens are a trigger for asthma. It is known, however, that

TABLE 18–3 Program Adherence Recommendations for Patients With Asthma and COPD

Collaborate with the patient's physician and respiratory therapist

Recommend that multiple adherence strategies work better than a single approach

Establish weekly contact with patients for the first 4 weeks of the program, then monthly thereafter, to continually assess the patient's progress and troubleshoot problems

Set achievable goals

Obtain baseline assessment of physical activity

Institute a self-monitoring program such as keeping a log of exercise participation

Identify patient-specific barriers to the lifestyle changes

Distribute information that uses health messages associated with asthma and COPD that are easy to understand, interactive, and culturally sensitive

Design a program that is reasonable, gradual, and easily implemented

Source: National Institutes of Health, National Heart, Lung, and Blood Institute. Third report of the National Cholesterol Education Program (NCEP) Expert Panel on Detection, Evaluation, and Treatment of High Blood Cholesterol in Adults (Adult Treatment Panel III). NIH Publication No. 02-5215, September 2002. COPD, chronic obstructive pulmonary disease.

food additives, specifically sulfites, can trigger an asthma attack. Foods such as beer, wine, dried fruit, and open salad bars have particularly high amounts of metabisulfites.[2] Patients sensitive to these foods should avoid them to prevent asthma exacerbations.

Additionally, a healthy and balanced eating plan should be recommended to patients with asthma and COPD as described in the 2005 Dietary Guidelines for Americans (http://www.healthierus.gov/dietaryguidelines/) and outlined in Chapter 1 of this book.[13] Nutritional counseling for patients with chronic lung diseases is general and is the same as that recommended for all adults to obtain proper nutrients while maintaining a healthy caloric balance. One study has reported that a diet that is high in salt can result in decreased lung function and diffusion capacity after exercise.[3] Following the sodium amounts recommended in the 2005 Dietary Guidelines should prevent such occurrences. A dietary analysis can be conducted on patients with chronic lung disease to assess nutritional intake compared with the 2005 Dietary Guidelines for Americans. Recommendations should be made on an individual patient basis to achieve ideal outcomes for each patient. Table 18-4 lists nutritional recommendations from the 2005 Dietary Guidelines for Americans.

PHYSICAL ACTIVITY AND CHRONIC LUNG DISEASE

Physical activity guidelines for patients with asthma are the same as those recommended by the American College of Sports Medicine (ACSM) and the Centers for Disease Control and Prevention (CDC) for healthy sedentary individuals.[10] The goals for a physical activity program are to increase fitness level (Vo_2 max), become less sensitive to dyspnea, develop more efficient breathing patterns, and maintain or enhance activities of daily living.[10] The one major difference in the exercise prescription for patients with asthma compared with patients without asthma is in the measurement of exercise intensity. The ACSM recommends that patients with asthma use the **Borg rating of perceived exertion (RPE)** scale to assess the intensity of breathlessness associated with physical activity rather than

TABLE 18–4	Dietary Recommendations for Patients With Asthma and COPD
Nutrient	**Recommendation**
Carbohydrate*a*	55% or more of total calories
Fiber	20–30 g/day
Protein	Approximately 15% of total calories
Monounsaturated fat	Up to 15% of total calories
Polyunsaturated fat	Up to 10% of total calories
Saturated fat	8–10% of total calories
Total fat*b*	20–35% or less of total calories
Dietary cholesterol	<300 mg/day
Sodium chloride	2,300 mg/day or less

*a*Most carbohydrate intake should come from whole grains, fruits, and vegetables.
*b*Keep *trans* fatty acid consumption as low as possible.
Source: HHS Publication No. HHS-ODPHP-2005-01-DGA-A. Dietary Guidelines for Americans 2005, U.S. Department of Health and Human Services, U.S. Department of Agriculture. Available at: http://www.healthierus.gov/dietaryguidelines. Accessed February 13, 2007.
COPD, chronic obstructive pulmonary disease.

using heart rate.[10] (Refer to Table 2-3 in Chapter 2 to see the Borg RPE scale.) Patients should become familiar with the Borg RPE scale as a means of measuring their exercise intensity because it can help decrease fears of difficulty in breathing while exercising, especially when it is combined with an optimal medication regimen and close measurements of peak flow using a peak flowmeter.[10] Peak flow measurements should be assessed before exercise to indicate whether EIA is fully controlled and whether additional medication is required. Patients who are susceptible to EIA should not underestimate the importance of measuring their peak flow before exercising as a means of preventing EIA.[10]

Each patient with asthma, depending on severity, will have a different maximal work rate at which they are able to tolerate exercise. Patients should be encouraged to exercise at a work rate that is relative to their maximal exercise tolerance. Younger asthmatic patients wishing to maximally improve their fitness level should try to exercise at an intensity that is close to their maximal exercise tolerance. Asthmatic patients who are older and who also have concomitant diseases may want to exercise at an intensity in the moderate range relative to their maximal exercise tolerance. Working with patients to discover what their maximal work rate is and then scaling exercise intensity relative to that work rate and to their personal goals are critical to designing an optimal physical activity program. Patients with severe asthma or those who are very sedentary may begin a physical activity program by participating in resistance training exercises only. Resistance training, especially circuit training, can improve muscular fitness, as well as have a positive effect on cardiovascular fitness and activities of daily living for patients with severe asthma who are not yet able to participate in an aerobic training program. Table 18-5 offers recommendations for a physical activity program for a patient with asthma.

Patients with COPD are encouraged to participate in physical activity as a means of maintaining and enhancing their quality of life, as well as for preventing other diseases such as **cancer** and **cardiovascular disease.**[11] Physical activity programs for patients with COPD should be highly individualized and flexible to adjust to clinical status changes. Medical condition changes should warrant a reassessment of physical activity program and goals.[11]

An important point to note about recommending physical activity to patients with COPD is that it should always be done in collaboration with the patient's physician, respiratory therapist, and occupational therapist. Doing so ensures that the patient's safety is secured, medications are optimal, and activities of daily living and quality of life are at the highest possible level for each individual patient. Like patients with asthma, the exercise intensity should be measured by using the Borg RPE scale and should be relative to the patient's respiratory capabilities. The goal for duration should be to sustain 20 to 30 minutes of activity, but initially may need to be done in intervals of 5 to 10 minutes until physical adaptations are made.[11] The type, or mode, of activity can be walking, cycling, swimming, or other aerobic activities, but should be one that is enjoyable for the patient and should directly improve the ability of the patient to perform daily activities.[11] Maintaining and improving a high quality of life is a major outcome of a physical activity program for patients with COPD; therefore, the activities that are performed should directly reflect their daily lifestyle activities. Table 18-5 offers recommendations for a physical activity program for a patient with COPD.

PHARMACY PRACTICE APPLICATION

Optimal medication therapy is of major importance for patients with asthma and COPD. Optimal medication therapy allows patients to perform daily activities without

TABLE 18–5 Physical Activity Recommendations for Patients With Asthma and COPD

Goals	Improve functional status by increasing or maintaining activities of daily living and improving quality of life (especially for COPD) Improve cardiorespiratory fitness Become less sensitive to dyspnea Develop more efficient breathing patterns Improve muscular strength
Type of activity	Aerobic activity[a] (walking, bicycling, swimming, water aerobics), resistance training (all major muscle groups, 15–20 repetitions, 2–3 days per week, with low resistance, and flexibility of all major muscle groups 3 days per week)
Intensity	Light to moderate (Borg RPE 11–13)
Duration[b]	20–30 minutes (initially 5–10 for COPD and deconditioned patients) 30–60 minutes for younger asthmatic patients
Frequency	1 to 2 sessions per day, 3 to 7 days per week for exercise program, but maintain a high level of activities of daily living through lifestyle activities on most days of the week
Lifestyle activity	Increase overall daily physical activities by performing household duties of cleaning, vacuuming, dusting, yard work, etc.

[a]For patients with COPD, perform activities that will help directly improve activities of daily living.
[b]Emphasize duration over intensity.
Sources: Clark CJ. Asthma. In: Durstine JL, Moore GE, eds. ACSM's Exercise Management for Persons With Chronic Diseases and Disabilities, 2nd ed. Champaign, IL: Human Kinetics, 2003:105–110; Cooper CB. Chronic obstructive pulmonary disease. In: Durstine JL, Moore GE, eds. ACSM's Exercise Management for Persons With Chronic Diseases and Disabilities, 2nd ed. Champaign, IL: Human Kinetics, 2003:92–104.
COPD, chronic obstructive pulmonary disease; RPE, rating of perceived exertion.

symptoms, decreases medical office and hospital visits, and decreases costs associated with the diseases. Pharmacists can have a significant impact on the health and outcomes of patients with chronic lung disease by ensuring optimal medication therapy. The Asheville Project on asthma is an excellent example of how pharmacists can positively affect the outcome of patients with asthma.[14]

The Asheville Project for patients with asthma set out to assess clinical, humanistic, and economic outcomes of a medication therapy management program that was run by pharmacists.[14] The study consisted of 207 adult asthmatic patients who were followed by pharmacists and other healthcare professionals for 5 years. The project interventions consisted of education from a certified asthma educator and regular long-term follow-up by pharmacists, which included scheduled consultations, monitoring, and recommendations to physicians. Pharmacists were reimbursed for their medication therapy management by health plans.[14]

The results of the study showed that all objective and subjective measures of asthma control improved and were sustained for 5 years. Emergency department visits and hospitalization visits decreased from 9.9 to 1.3% and from 4.0 to 1.9%, respectively.[14] In addition, the percentage of patients with an asthma action plan to manage their disease increased from 63 to 99%. Economic costs associated with asthma management were also greatly influenced. Even though the amount of money spent on asthma medications increased, direct costs savings averaged $725 per patient per year and indirect cost savings were estimated to be $1,230 per patient per year.[14] This was because of decreased asthma-related medical claims, decreased emergency department visits and hospitalizations, and a decrease in the number of work days that were missed because of asthma.[14]

The Asheville Project on asthma is an excellent example of the significant impact that pharmacists can make on the health outcomes of patients with asthma and be financially reimbursed while doing so. Patients who receive education and long-term medication therapy management services can demonstrate significant improvements in controlling their asthma. Pharmacists can play a significant role in managing patients' asthma medications, as well as counseling them on lifestyle modifications that can improve their overall health. Working closely with other healthcare providers will ensure that patients receive optimal care in the safest possible manner.

CASE STUDY

R.O. is a 14-year-old female with no history of chronic diseases. She does not take any chronic medications, but occasionally takes a non-prescription medication in the spring to help with seasonal allergies. She is trying out for her high school track team for the first time and is having symptoms of wheezing, coughing, and shortness of breath during and shortly after each training session. Her coach told her that she is just out of shape and it will get better with more training. R.O.'s mother came to the pharmacy to refill her own asthma prescription and inquired about the possibility of her daughter having asthma also based on her symptoms. She is 5' 3" tall, weighs 100 lb, has a resting blood pressure of 110/60 mm Hg, and a heart rate of 74 beats/min.

Case Activities

1. *Write an SOAP note for R.O.*
2. *List R.O.'s risk factors for asthma.*
3. *Write an exercise prescription for R.O. that she can use after track season is over.*

REFERENCES

1. Self TH. Asthma. In: Koda-Kimble MA, ed. Applied Therapeutics: The Clinical Use of Drugs, 8th ed. Philadelphia: Lippincott Williams & Wilkins, 2005:23.1–23.43.
2. Kelly HW, Sorkness CA. Asthma. In: Dipiro JT, ed. Pharmacotherapy: A Pathophysiologic Approach, 6th ed. New York: McGraw-Hill, 2005:503–535.
3. Williams DH, Kradjan WA. Chronic obstructive pulmonary disease. In: Koda-Kimble MA, ed. Applied Therapeutics: The Clinical Use of Drugs, 8th ed. Philadelphia: Lippincott Williams & Wilkins, 2005:24.1–24.28.
4. Bourdet SV, Williams DH. Chronic obstructive pulmonary disease. In: Dipiro JT, ed. Pharmacotherapy: A Pathophysiologic Approach, 6th ed. New York: McGraw-Hill, 2005:537–556.
5. Centers for Disease Control and Prevention. Asthma FAQ: basic facts about asthma. Department of Health and Human Services, Centers for Disease Control and Prevention, August 2003. Available at: http://www.cdc.gov/asthma/faqs.htm. Accessed April 6, 2006.
6. Centers for Disease Control and Prevention. COPD: facts about chronic obstructive pulmonary disease. Department of Health and Human Services, Centers for Disease Control and Prevention, August 2003. Available at: http://www.cdc.gov/nceh/airpollution/copd/copdfaq.htm. Accessed April 6, 2006.
7. Peno-Green LA, Cooper CB. Treatment and rehabilitation of pulmonary diseases. In: Kaminsky LA, et al., eds. ACSM's Resource Manual for Guidelines for Exercise Testing and Prescription, 5th ed. Baltimore: Lippincott Williams & Wilkins, 2006:452–469.
8. Lenz TL, Lenz NJ, Faulkner MA. Potential interactions between exercise and drug therapy. Sports Med 2004;34:293–306.
9. Fabbri LM, Hurd SS, GOLD Scientific Committee. Global strategy for the diagnosis, management and prevention of chronic obstructive pulmonary disease (COPD): 2003 update. Eur Respir J 2003;22:1–2. Available at: http://www.goldcopd.com. Accessed April 6, 2006.

10. Clark CJ. Asthma. In: Durstine JL, Moore GE, eds. ACSM's Exercise Management for Persons With Chronic Diseases and Disabilities, 2nd ed. Champaign, IL: Human Kinetics. 2003:105–110.

11. Cooper CB. Chronic obstructive pulmonary disease. In: Durstine JL, Moore GE, eds. ACSM's Exercise Management for Persons With Chronic Diseases and Disabilities, 2nd ed. Champaign, IL: Human Kinetics, 2003:92–104.

12. National Institutes of Health, National Heart, Lung, and Blood Institute. Third report of the National Cholesterol Education Program (NCEP) Expert Panel on Detection, Evaluation, and Treatment of High Blood Cholesterol in Adults (Adult Treatment Panel III). NIH Publication No. 02-5215, September 2002.

13. HHS Publication No. HHS-ODPHP-2005-01-DGA-A, Dietary Guidelines for Americans 2005, U.S. Department of Health and Human Services, U.S. Department of Agriculture. Available at: http://healthierus.gov/dietaryguidelines. Accessed February 13, 2007.

14. Bunting BA, Cranor CW. The Asheville Project: long-term clinical, humanistic, and economic outcomes of a community-based medication therapy management program for asthma. J Am Pharm Assoc 2006;46:133–147.

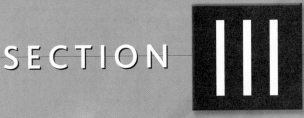

SECTION III

Special Populations

INTRODUCTION

Section III consists of three chapters that broadly discuss disease prevention in the specific population groups of children and youth, older adults, and women and minorities. The information provided in Section III is intended to supplement the disease states presented in Section II. The reader may take the information presented in any, or perhaps all, of the chapters in Section III and practically use it for designing a wellness program for patients with a specific chronic disease who may also have other important factors (e.g., pregnancy) to consider when designing that program. There are no specific case studies implemented in this section, but rather the information is meant to enhance the cases already presented in the previous section. It is not necessary for the chapters in this section to be read in the order in which they are presented. Additionally, the reader will need to have a firm grasp of the information presented in Section I before understanding the information in Section III.

Children and Youth

At the end of this chapter the reader should be able to:

1. Recall how the prevalence of obesity in children has increased to an epidemic in recent decades.
2. Outline the risks associated with childhood obesity.
3. Summarize several solutions aimed at decreasing the incidence of childhood obesity.

The primary focus of this text is on disease prevention. The ideal place to begin the disease prevention process is with children. There have been dramatic improvements in the prevention of disease, illness, and injury in children in the United States during the past century.[1] Vaccines have targeted diseases that were common to children, and measles, polio, diphtheria, tetanus, rubella, and haemophilus influenza have nearly been eliminated.[1] In addition, improvements in community sanitation, water systems to include fluoridation, vitamin and mineral supplementation, child safety seats, seat belts, and bicycle helmets have also significantly contributed to improving the health outcomes and preventing disease in our children.[1] Unfortunately, a new modern childhood epidemic now exists. This epidemic is childhood **obesity.** Many factors contribute to the alarming rise in childhood obesity. This chapter will focus on the factors leading to childhood obesity and the ways in which healthcare providers, especially pharmacists, can help to slow the progression of this national public health concern. Further information about this topic can be found by referencing the comprehensive study performed by the Institute of Medicine (IOM) on Preventing Childhood Obesity published in 2005 (http://www.iom.edu/).[1]

CHILDHOOD OBESITY

The IOM defines the term epidemic as "a condition that is occurring more frequently and extensively among individuals in the community or population than is expected."[1] The term childhood obesity epidemic fits the current situation as there has been a significant rise in childhood obesity since the early 1970s. The prevalence of childhood obesity during the past three decades has more than doubled in children between the ages of 2 and 5 years and adolescents 12 to 19 years.[1] The prevalence has more than tripled in children between the ages of 6 and 11 years.[1] In 2003, approximately 9 million children older than 6 years of age were considered to be obese.[1] The obesity epidemic is affecting both girls and boys and is occurring in all age, race, and ethnic groups throughout the United States.[1,2]

Adult obesity is defined as having a **body mass index (BMI)** of 30 kg/m² or greater. Childhood obesity is defined a bit differently, however. The IOM uses the term childhood obesity to refer to children and youth between the ages of 2 and 19 years who have a BMI equal to or greater than the 95th percentile of age- and gender-specific BMI charts developed by the Centers for Disease Control and Prevention (CDC).[1] Data between 1999 and 2000 show that approximately 10% of children aged 2 to 5 years were above the 95th percentile for BMI, which is twice the expected percentage.[1] Additionally, more than 15% of 6- to 19-year-old children were above the 95th percentile, three times the expected percentage.[1,2]

Childhood obesity is prevalent among all age, race, and ethnic groups in the United States, but certain population subgroups are at particularly high risk. Population subgroups such as Hispanic, non-Hispanic black, and Native American children have a disproportionately high rate of obesity compared with children in the general population.[1,2] Additionally, children of low socioeconomic status and children who live in the southern region of the United States have higher rates of obesity compared with children in the rest of the U.S. population.[1] It is speculated, but not yet confirmed, that the factors causing obesity in these children are more pronounced in their communities and population subgroups, or that these children are more sensitive to the factors leading to obesity or may be less able to avoid the contributing factors.[1]

Causes of Childhood Obesity

As described in other chapters of this book, the principal causes of obesity are most commonly attributable to a simple imbalance in caloric intake and **energy** expenditure. To explain why childhood obesity is now an epidemic is far more complicated. The causes of the obesity epidemic in our children are related to a complex interaction of social, environmental, and health policy issues that directly and indirectly influence caloric intake and energy expenditure.[1] These influences during the past three to four decades have collectively created an environment that promotes children to become overweight and obese. Specific environmental changes that have occurred include the following:

1. Family pressures to acquire and prepare food in less time and to minimize food costs, leading to the consumption of convenience food items that are high in **calories** and fat
2. Reduced access and affordability in some communities of fresh fruits, vegetables, and other nutritious foods

3. Urban and suburban designs of communities that do not allow for, or discourage, walking and other physical activities
4. Decreased opportunities for **physical activity** during and after school, and decreased opportunities to walk or bike to and from school
5. An increase in the electronic age of computers, video games, and television that compete for leisure time physical activities such as playing outdoors[1]

CHILDHOOD OBESITY PREVENTION

Prevention strategies for obesity in children are much the same as those for adults: Eat healthier foods and obtain more physical activity. Establishing an action plan to combat this problem will take a concentrated and coordinated effort from the federal, state, and local governments, the industry and media, healthcare professionals, community organizations, school systems, and parents and families.

Federal, State, and Local Government Involvement

The IOM recommends that government at all levels make the prevention of obesity in children a national priority by providing coordinated leadership that includes interdepartmental government collaboration and research funding, particularly for high-risk populations and communities.[1] Specific federal government recommendations from the IOM for confronting the epidemic include the following:

1. Establishing an interdepartmental task force to coordinate federal actions
2. Developing nutrition standards for foods and beverages sold in schools
3. Funding state-based nutrition and physical activity grants with strong evaluation components
4. Developing guidelines regarding advertising and marketing to children and youth by convening a national conference
5. Expanding funding for prevention intervention research, experimental behavioral research, and community-based population research
6. Strengthening and supporting surveillance, monitoring, and evaluation efforts[1]

Additionally, the IOM recommends that state and local governments expand and promote opportunities for physical activity in the community and work with communities to support partnerships and networks that expand the availability of and access to healthful foods.[1]

Industry and Media Involvement

The food, restaurant, and entertainment industry, as well as the media, have a significant influence on the types and quantities of foods children and adults consume. Food and beverage sales to young consumers alone were more than $27 billion in 2002. Food consumption outside the home has increased dramatically in the past three decades. Between 1970 and 1999 the amount of household income spent on away-from-home foods rose from 25 to 50% of total food spending.[1] In 1977, children consumed 20% of their calories from away-from-home foods and in 1996 this rose to 32%.[1] Food and beverage advertisers collectively spend $10 to $12 billion per year marketing products to children and youth.[1] Of this amount, $3 billion is spent on packaging designed for children.[1]

The IOM recommends that industry and media develop healthier food and beverage products and packaging innovations. Additionally they should expand consumer nutrition information and provide more clear and consistent media messages.[1] Providing young consumers and their parents and families with the knowledge and skills to make informed food choices is a key strategy in preventing obesity in children.[1]

Healthcare Provider Involvement

Healthcare professionals, including pharmacists, can have a significant influence on patients when it comes to obesity prevention. Because pharmacists are widely accessible to patients and their children, there are many opportunities for interventions. As healthcare advisors to both children and their parents, pharmacists and other healthcare professionals can make key suggestions regarding nutrition and physical activity throughout children's lives.[1] The IOM recommends that healthcare professionals routinely track BMI in children and youth, and offer appropriate counseling and guidance to children and families.[1] A specific discussion on the pharmacist's role in preventing and treating childhood obesity is provided later in this chapter.

Community Organization Involvement

The community environment that supports and promotes disease prevention, including a healthy body weight, is vitally important to combating the childhood obesity epidemic. Communities can encourage physical activity to children and youth by providing safe environments to walk, bike, run, play games, and participate in other events that encourage physical activity.[1] Community developments of streets and neighborhoods often place needs of motorized vehicles over those of pedestrians and bicyclists. Funding to encourage physical activity through examining zoning ordinances and priorities for capital investment should be encouraged at the community local government level. Additionally, local communities can develop ways in which to promote healthy eating habits through enhanced public education and by providing food sources to obtain fresh fruits, vegetables, and other nutritious foods at reasonable costs. The IOM recommends that communities provide opportunities for healthful eating and physical activity in existing and new community programs, particularly for high-risk populations.[1]

School System Involvement

Most children generally spend about half of their day in school, and some even more through before and after school programs and daycares. For this reason, schools are a primary location for promoting healthy eating and physical activity habits. Formal education programs can be offered in the classrooms that teach students healthy eating habits and the importance of physical activity. Outside of the classroom, activities such as physical education can promote energy expenditure, release stress, and develop physical activity habits that can be carried into adulthood. Unfortunately, many schools are cutting physical education classes because of budget constraints even though it is recommended that children participate in 60 minutes or more of moderate to vigorous physical activity each day.[1] Additionally, many "competitive foods" that are high in calories and low in nutritional value are now offered in school cafeterias, vending machines, and school stores and at school fundraisers.[1] Presently, federal standards on the sale of competitive foods in schools are only minimal.

Schools have many opportunities for teaching students to learn and practice healthful eating and physical activity behaviors. Coordinated changes in curriculum, in-school advertising environment, school health services, and after school programs are all ways that schools can help stop the epidemic of childhood obesity.[1] The IOM recommends that schools (1) improve the nutritional quality of foods and beverages sold in schools as part of school-related activities; (2) increase the opportunities for more frequent, intensive, and engaging physical activity during and after school; (3) develop, implement, and evaluate innovative pilot programs for both staffing and teaching about wellness, healthful eating, and physical activity, and (4) conduct annual assessments of students' weight, height, and gender- and age-specific BMI percentile and make information available to parents.[1]

Family Involvement

Parents (including the primary caregivers) have the most significant influence in developing the values, attitudes, and behaviors of their children. Because of this, parents can and should be the primary role model for healthy behaviors.[1] Parents can establish a family culture that promotes healthy eating and physical activity that become a part of everyday life for everyone in the family. Parents make the decisions as to which foods are purchased and available to the children, determine the setting for foods eaten in the home, and make daily decisions on recreational opportunities and many other day-to-day activities that influence the health of the family.[1] Many times it is difficult for individuals to make healthy decisions on their own, but creating family habits around healthy eating and physical activity can make it easier for everyone to achieve and maintain a healthy weight. Parents can use strategies such as planning regular family time that involves physical activity or make fruit readily available to the family to promote overall good health.

A few strategies that may help parents to promote healthy lifestyle behaviors within their family include limiting television and video game time, providing more fresh fruits and vegetables during family meals, skipping desserts, taking a family walk around the neighborhood after dinner instead of turning on the televisions, and planning family vacations around physical activities such as hiking, bicycling, or swimming. It is important to remember that implementing healthy behavior strategies into a family that is not accustomed to such a lifestyle should be done with small, easy changes over time. Family walks two to three times per week is a good place to begin, and offering fresh strawberries over angel food cake rather than cutting dessert all together may help the implementation of healthy behaviors occur more easily. Several different types of family health promotion strategies should be tried rather than concentrating only on one or two. Families often require a variety of activities and foods to suit everyone's preferences.

The IOM makes several recommendations for parents to promote healthy eating behaviors and regular physical activity for their children. Parents should provide healthy food and beverage choices for children by carefully considering nutrient quality and calorie density. Parents can also educate their children to make healthy food choices and choose healthy portion sizes so that when children become older they can be responsible for their own healthy eating habits. Parents should also serve as role models for their children by choosing to eat healthy, and by exercising with their children.

PHYSICAL ACTIVITY

A cornerstone for obesity prevention in children is adequate amounts of physical activity. The current recommendation for physical activity in school-aged children (6 to 18 years) is participation in accumulated 60 minutes or more per day of moderate to vigorous intensity physical activity that is enjoyable and developmentally appropriate.[3] Moderate to vigorous intensity activity is defined as 5 to 8 METs (**metabolic equivalents**), and the total **exercise** time can be accumulated throughout the day.[3] Activities such as brisk walking, bicycling, and active outdoor playing ordinarily reach this MET level and can be achieved during physical education, recess, intramural sports, and before and after school programs, as well as at home playing outdoors.[3] For children and youth who are currently physically inactive, an incremental approach to achieving the 60-minute-per-day goal is recommended.[3] These children and youth should increase their activity level by 10% each week until the goal duration is reached.[3]

Studies have shown that increasing physical activity levels to the recommended amounts can significantly decrease many risk factors such as adiposity, **metabolic syndrome,** elevated **triglycerides,** low **high-density lipoprotein (HDL)** cholesterol levels, **hypertension,** and low cardiovascular fitness that can lead to future heart disease.[3] In fact, evidence shows that high school-aged girls who are physically active are more than twice as likely to be active as adults and experience a 39% lower risk for heart disease as adults compared with sedentary high school-aged girls when they become adults.[4] Additionally, physical activity has been shown to improve students' academic performance and self-concept and possibly decrease anxiety and depression.[3]

The CDC recommends that all students between kindergarten and grade 12 participate in daily quality physical education.[3] Both physical education and recess allow children and youth the opportunity to attain physical activity goals and do not compromise academic performance.[3] Not only does daily physical education not hinder academic performance but it has been shown to have a positive influence on concentration, memory, and classroom behavior.[3] It was discovered in 2000 that only 8% of elementary schools, 6.4% of middle or junior high schools, and 5.8% of senior high schools provide daily physical education for the entire school year for all students in each grade.[1] The IOM recommends that schools ensure that all children and youth participate in a minimum of 30 minutes of moderate to vigorous physical activity during the school day. Additionally, the IOM recommends that physical activity opportunities available through schools be expanded to meet the needs and interests of all students.[1]

One of the keys for children to attain 60 minutes or more of physical activity each day is to make physical activity a priority within the family environment. Family time can be active time by riding bikes or walking to a restaurant to eat instead of driving, celebrating birthdays by playing a game of soccer, volleyball, or kickball, attending the children's sporting events to cheer them on, and having the children attend the parents' sporting events to cheer their parents.[5] Families can limit the amount of time watching television, or do something active like stretching, yoga, sit-ups, or weight lifting while watching television.[5] Family pets, such as dogs, can also make a great activity promoter for the family. Taking the family dog for a walk around the neighborhood each day is a great way for the whole family to increase their physical activity level. Countless activities and opportunities are available for families to increase physical activity levels. Each family should experiment with several strategies to find the ones that will fit their family the best.

NUTRITION

A consensus statement from the American Heart Association (endorsed by the American Academy of Pediatrics) on dietary recommendations for children and adolescents was published in September 2005 and is considered to be the dietary guidelines for children and youth.[6] The atherosclerotic process begins when individuals are in their youth and eventually culminates in heart disease and **stroke** during the third and fourth decades of life.[6] The intent of the nutrition guidelines for children and adolescents is to prevent the development of cardiovascular risk factors from the beginning, rather than controlling them once they are present in adults.[6] This concept is called **primordial prevention.**[6] Optimal nutrition and physical activity are discussed in the guidelines as the central strategies for primordial prevention.[6]

The dietary recommendations for individuals 2 years of age and older are generally very similar and have been discussed in Chapter 1 of this book. The recommendations primarily focus on a high intake of fruits and vegetables, whole grains, low-fat and non-fat diary products, beans, fish, and lean meats and an adequate intake of micronutrients.[6] Additionally, a low intake of saturated and *trans* fats, **cholesterol,** and added sugar and salt is also recommended.[6] Caloric intake that is appropriate to maintain a healthy body weight along with physical activity has a similar recommendation between children and adults.[6]

Adequate calorie intake to maintain a healthy body weight will obviously change as children grow into adults. The nutritional guidelines for children and adolescents recommend that children who are 1 year old consume approximately 900 kcal/day, and children 2 to 3 years old consume approximately 1,000 kcal/day, with a corresponding fat intake of 30 to 40% and 30 to 35%, respectively, of total calories.[6] Females 4 to 8 years, 9 to 13 years, and 14 to 18 years should consume 1,200, 1,600, and 1,800 kcal/day, respectively, with a corresponding fat intake in all age groups of 25 to 35%.[6] Males in these same age groups should consume 1,400, 1,800, and 2,200 kcal/day, respectively, with the same recommendations for fat intake. It should be noted that for youth 3 years of age and older, these calorie estimates are based on a sedentary lifestyle, and adjustments should be made for physically active children.[6] Additionally, the guidelines state that these calorie recommendations are a starting point for dietary counseling, and specific recommendations should be made on an individual basis.[6]

The guidelines also recommend that children younger than 1 year old receive breast milk for at least the first 4 to 6 months and ideally for the first 12 months.[6] The transition from dairy products after the age of 2 years should be made to low-fat milk and other dairy products, as high-fat dairy products can be a major source of saturated fat and cholesterol in individuals older than 2 years of age. Also, sweetened beverage intake contributes significantly to total calorie intake and should be limited.[6]

The guidelines make an effort to stress the importance of individualized counseling of older children and adolescents as it is important to accommodate the range of contemporary lifestyles that exist today.[6] Parental role modeling is also important in establishing children's food choices and in offering the best possible health outcomes for the entire family. Focusing on the general nutrition guidelines, consuming food in moderation, and participating in physical activity will give children the greatest opportunity for primordial prevention and disease prevention in general.

THE PHARMACIST'S ROLE IN CHILDHOOD OBESITY

Pharmacists can make a significant impact with patients in not only treating diseases but preventing them as well. Healthcare professionals, including pharmacists, have a unique opportunity in preventing disease in children in that they can prevent the risk factors that cause diseases (primordial prevention), rather than just modifying existing risk factors as is often the case in adults. Pharmacists can use the same approaches that have been discussed in previous chapters of this book, such as proper nutrition and adequate amounts of physical activity, when working with children and youth to prevent obesity. The major difference when working with children is that their parents must also believe in and participate in the interventions that are taking place. Children will naturally follow the lead of the parents so it is imperative that if a child needs to lose weight, the child's parents support the process and are willing to make the necessary changes at home to accomplish the goals that are set. As stated several times throughout this chapter, preventing childhood obesity is multifactorial, but the greatest influence is in the child's home. Making a healthy lifestyle of proper nutrition and physical activity should be a family affair that is cultivated early on during the child's development and is something that every family member values.

Pharmacists are also leaders within the community and can play a role in community government and schools to affect policy that can decrease the incidence of childhood obesity. Additionally, the pharmacy is an excellent place within the community to educate the public. Pharmacists can offer printed educational material and educational classes on health promotion to its patrons and their families about many types of disease, including childhood obesity. Because of the exposure that pharmacies and pharmacists have to the community, they are excellent recourses for health promotion activities and information. Preventing disease in children can be a very rewarding experience for healthcare professionals as children are regarded as one of our most precious resources.

REFERENCES

1. Koplan JP, Liverman CT, Kraak VI, eds. Institute of Medicine. Preventing Childhood Obesity: Health in Balance. Washington, D.C.: The National Academies Press, 2005.
2. Ogden CL, Flagel KM, Carroll MD, Johnson CL. Prevalence and trends in overweight among US children and adolescents, 1999–2000. JAMA 2002;288:1728–1732.
3. Strong WM, Malina RM, Blimkie CJR, et al. Evidence based physical activity for school-aged youth. J Pediatr 2005;146:732–737.
4. Conroy MB, Cook NR, Manson JE, Buring JE, Lee IM. Past physical activity, current physical activity, and the risk of coronary heart disease. Med Sci Sports Exerc 2005;37:1251–1256.
5. U.S. Department of Health and Human Services. We can! Ways to enhance children's activity and nutrition. U.S. Department of Health and Human Services, National Institutes of Health. NIH Publication No. 05-5273, June 2005.
6. Gidding SS, Dennsion BA, Birch LL, et al. Dietary recommendations for children and adolescents. A guide for practitioners. Consensus statement from the American Heart Association. Circulation 2005;112:2061–2075.

CHAPTER 20

Older Adults

OBJECTIVES

At the end of this chapter the reader should be able to:

1. Recall the significance of the aging of the American population.
2. Summarize the benefits of increased physical activity and proper nutrition in older adults.
3. Outline the pharmacist's and other healthcare professional's role in promoting a healthy lifestyle to older adults.

OVERVIEW

From the turn of the 20th century to the turn of the 21st century, life expectancy from birth increased from 48 years to 72 years in men and from 51 to 80 years in women.[1] Life expectancy from age 65 also increased from 12 to 17 years in men and from 12 to 20 years in women.[1] Between 1950 and 2004 the total resident population of the United States increased from 150 to 294 million people.[1] This represents an annual growth rate of 1% during those years.[1] At the same time, the number of individuals 65 years of age and older grew two times faster than the general population and increased in number from 12 to 36 million persons.[1] Additionally, the number of individuals 75 years of age and older grew almost three times faster than the general population and increased in numbers from 4 to 18 million persons.[1] It is projected that from now until the year 2050 the rate of population growth in the United States will be slower for all age groups compared with the previous 50 years, but the older age groups will continue to grow more than twice as rapidly as the general population.[1]

As people age, the need for greater medical care also increases. In 2002, more than 36 million U.S. adults older than age 65 incurred healthcare expenditures.[1] This represents more than 96% of the people in this age group. The average annual healthcare expense per person for U.S. adults older than age 65 in 2002 was $7,797.[1] This compares with $2,557 during the same year for those younger than age 65.[1]

The need for disease prevention in older adults is obvious. The average lifespan of the U.S. population is increasing and will continue to do so in the projected future. Preventing disease will not only help cut healthcare expenditures, but more importantly, can increase the overall quality of life in older adults. Some think that older adults do not need to participate in activities that can help prevent disease because they may already have one or more diseases or believe that it is too late and not worth the effort. The major goal in participating in disease prevention strategies such as **physical activity,** smoking cessation, and weight loss in older persons is for the maintenance and enhancement of quality of life. For some older adults the goal may be to increase life years but, for most, high quality-of-life years is the most important outcome. It is important to think about the ultimate goal of disease prevention strategies and to personalize these goals when working with older adults. This chapter will look at the impact of aging on health and discuss specific nutrition and physical activity recommendations that can help older adults maintain and improve quality of life.

IMPACT OF AGING

It is often assumed that as the body ages, it naturally becomes less healthy and requires more medical care simply as a result of the aging process. Is this really caused by aging alone, or is it also related to the effects of a more sedentary lifestyle? It is true that certain physiologic changes occur as a result of aging, but a lifetime of healthy living can help to prevent many of the health-related issues that occur later in life.

Studies have shown that maximal cardiac output in persons 65 years old is 10 to 30% lower than in young adults.[2] This is primarily because of decreases in maximal heart rate and maximal stroke volume in the older adults.[2] Studies have also shown that resting **cardiac output** and stroke volume decrease with age at a decline of about 1% per year from the third to ninth decades of life.[2] Interestingly, however, when studies carefully screen for **coronary heart disease,** it has been shown that left ventricular function (using resting ejection fraction as an index) and stroke volume do not decrease with age.[2,3] Therefore, because resting heart rate is not affected by age, these data suggest that resting cardiac output does not decline with age but rather is dependent on the health of the individual.[2] This supports the thought that resting cardiac output can be maintained by preventing diseases such as coronary heart disease.

Studies have also shown that aerobic capacity, assessed as **maximal oxygen uptake ($\dot{V}O_2$ max),** also decreases at a rate of 1% per year between ages 25 and 75 years.[2,4,5] The decline in aerobic capacity that is observed, however, is significantly affected by the amount and intensity of physical activity of the individual.[2] Other factors that can limit the ability of individuals to perform **exercise,** and therefore limit aerobic capacity, are physical limitations resulting from a sedentary lifestyle, loss of coordination, lack of familiarity of required skills, and disabling diseases such as arthritis and **obesity.**[2,6,7]

Other physiologic changes that occur as a result of aging are increased arterial stiffness, loss of lung compliance, muscle atrophy, decreased joint flexibility, increased body fat, and bone loss.[2] Much evidence exists to show that lifestyle changes such as **physical inactivity** contribute to many of these occurrences. For example, **basal metabolic rate** has been shown to decrease by approximately 5% per decade throughout adulthood, leading to increased levels of body fat and obesity. Evidence, however, shows that this is mostly related to decreased physical activity as people age.[2]

As discussed in Chapter 16, bone loss commonly occurs with increasing age and is greatly dependent on genetic factors, weight-bearing physical activity, nutrition, and the aging process itself. Women begin to lose bone mass between 30 and 35 years of age at a rate of 0.75 to 1% per year.[2,8] Men generally begin to lose bone mass between 50 and 55 years of age at an initial rate of 0.4% per year.[2,8] Proper medication, nutrition, and physical activity are important factors for preventing bone loss in both men and women.

NUTRITION AND AGING

The general nutrition guidelines discussed in the 2005 Dietary Guidelines for Americans (http://healthierus.gov/dietaryguidelines/) should be the basis for nutritional counseling in older adults.[9] This age group does, however, have certain qualities that necessitate specific nutritional recommendations aside from those of the general population. Nutritional recommendations for older adults emphasize the need for plenty of water, an eating plan high in grain products, vegetables, and fruits and low in saturated fats and cholesterol, moderate use of sugar, salt, and alcohol, and physical activity that improves functional abilities and is in balance with caloric intake needs.[9,10] Nutrients such as calcium, vitamin D, and vitamin B_{12} are also important for older adults to consume.[9,10]

The caloric needs of individuals often decrease with advancing age. This is most often because of decreased physical activity (caloric expenditure), which in turn decreases the amount of **calories** required each day. This change in caloric need can affect older adults in different ways. Some older adults continue to eat the same amount of calories each day even though physical activity levels have decreased, resulting in a positive caloric balance and weight gain. Others decrease caloric intake to a point where it is difficult to maintain adequate nutrient intake.[10] In either case it is important to work with the individual needs of the patient so that enough calories are consumed to maintain a healthy body weight and to ensure that appropriate amounts of essential nutrients are consumed. A conscious decision to choose foods that are fortified with calcium and vitamins D and B_{12} should be made.

The fluid needs of an older adult, especially those who are elderly, should be closely monitored as some older adults may have decreased thirst sensation.[10] Fluid needs may be affected by the amount of physical activity, certain medications, renal function, and ambient temperature.[10] Adequate amounts of fluid are important to prevent constipation, a common problem in older adults. It is recommended that older adults drink about 2 quarts (about 2 L) of fluid each day. Fluid sources can come from beverages as well as from foods such as soup, fruit, and others.[10] Alcohol should not be included as fluid intake because of the diuretic effect. Beverages that contain high amounts of caffeine should also be limited for the same reason.[10]

In many older adults, vitamin B_{12} from food sources is not efficiently absorbed as a result of atrophic gastritis, estimated to affect 10 to 30% of U.S. adults older than 60 years of age.[10] To prevent vitamin B_{12} deficiencies in older adults, the 2005 Dietary Guidelines for Americans recommend that adults older than age 50 consume vitamin B_{12} in its crystalline form. It can be obtained from either oral supplements or from food fortified with vitamin B_{12}, such as fortified cereals.[9] The recommended daily allowance (RDA) for vitamin B_{12} is 2.4 µg/day.[10]

PHYSICAL ACTIVITY

A great deal of evidence exists to support the notion that increased physical activity in older adults is extremely beneficial. As people age, it is common to decrease the amount of physical activity that is performed each day. This can be owing to several reasons such as time constraints with work, family, and other obligations, disinterest, and illness and disease. Deconditioning is a partial or complete reversal of the physiologic adaptations that occur from exercise.[2] Almost everyone is affected by reductions in physical activity and deconditioning at one time or another during their lives. Deconditioning can result from cessation or decreased physical activity, bed rest as a result of illness or disease, casting, paralysis, and aging itself.[2] The important point to understand about deconditioning is that it can be reversed through increased physical activity regardless of age. Physical activity in older adults that includes both aerobic and resistance training yields important health benefits for healthy aging, such as reductions in risk factors associated with diseases, improved health status, increased life expectancy, prevention of muscle loss and strength usually associated with aging, improved bone health, improved postural stability decreasing the risk for falls, and increased **flexibility** and joint range of motion, as well as preserved cognitive function, decreased depression symptoms, improved self-concept of personal control and **self-efficacy,** and improved quality of life.[11]

Cardiovascular Function

Maximal cardiovascular function, or $\dot{V}O_2$ max, decreases 5 to 15% per decade after the age of 25 years.[11] It is clear, however, that older adults, like younger adults, can experience that same 10 to 30% increase in $\dot{V}O_2$ max that results from prolonged endurance training.[11] As is the same in both groups, the magnitude of the increase in $\dot{V}O_2$ max is dependent on the training intensity.[11] Additionally, evidence shows that older adults can improve exercise efficiency to a greater degree than younger adults.[12] The American College of Sports Medicine recommends that aerobic exercise training be performed in older adults similar to the general physical activity recommendations for all adults.[11] Older adults should, however, perform activity at light to moderate intensities and emphasize increasing duration rather than intensity.[11] Activities of daily living that maintain and improve functional abilities are strongly recommended to maintain independence.[11]

Resistance Training

A reduction in muscle strength is a common occurrence of aging. Research shows that muscle strength declines by approximately 15% per decade in the sixth and seventh decades of life and about 30% in the decades thereafter.[11] The overwhelming majority of the loss in muscle strength during these years is caused by an age-related decrease in muscle mass.[11] Unfortunately this decrease in muscle strength results in significant consequences in functional capacity for older adults.

Strength training exercise studies in older adults have found that older men and women show similar or greater strength gains compared with younger individuals.[11] **Muscular strength** increases at levels two to three times that of baseline can be accomplished after a 3- to 4-month training program. It is clear, however, that if the intensity of the exercise is low, only modest strength gains are experienced compared with moderate- to high-intensity resistance training.[11] Additionally, resistance training that is incorporated with activities of daily living (ADL) has been shown to give even greater self-efficacy for older adults performing ADLs.[13] Therefore resistance training that is focused on increasing muscle strength and functionality that is specific to the individual patient's needs is recommended as a means of maintaining independence and a high quality of life.[2]

THE PHARMACIST'S ROLE

All healthcare providers have a responsibility for promoting health and preventing disease in their patients. This is especially true for older adult patients as they may be more vulnerable to certain medical conditions compared with younger patients. Much evidence supports an increase in physical activity and proper nutrition in older adults as a means of ensuring and maintaining high-quality health. Pharmacists have traditionally played an important role in the health of older adults by ensuring proper medication usage. Pharmacists can also play an important role in health promotion with these patients by encouraging and counseling on proper nutrition and physical activity.

Several important points should be considered when counseling older adults about physical activity. As stated many times throughout this book, pharmacists and other healthcare professionals should not work alone when promoting health. Healthcare professionals should rely on the strengths of their colleagues and work in collaboration to provide the best outcome for the patient. Many older adults have one or more chronic diseases, such as **cardiovascular disease,** that may affect their ability to exercise. Therefore, collaboration with the patient's physician should be done before prescribing specific activities for that patient. Additionally, exercises should initially be recommended at a low intensity and progress more slowly for older adults compared with younger adults. The emphasis should be placed on increasing the activity duration rather than on increasing the exercise intensity. Resistance training activities have been shown to be of significant benefit for older adults. Finding creative ways to provide resistance with household items, such as empty laundry detergent bottles filled with sand or water, can help patients save money on weight equipment as well as help to improve activities of daily living around the house.

The focus of enhancing lifestyle activities for older adults should be on improving the patient's quality of life and the management of existing diseases. Like all programs, careful planning and goal setting based on the particular outcomes of the patient are important to program adherence. Patient safety should always be at the forefront of treatment for healthcare professionals when working with older adults. A collaborative working relationship between the patient and all of the healthcare professionals involved is key to a successful program.

REFERENCES

1. U.S. Department of Health and Human Services. Health, United States, 2005 with chartbook on trends in the health of Americans. U.S. Department of Health and Human Services. Centers for Disease Control and Prevention, National Center for Health Statistics. DHHS Publication No 2005-1232, November 2005.
2. Graves BS, Whitehurst M, Findley BW. Physiologic effects of aging and deconditioning. In: Kaminsky LA, et al., eds. ACSM's Resource Manual for Guidelines for Exercise Testing and Prescription, 5th ed. Baltimore: Lippincott Williams & Wilkins, 2006:79–92.
3. Rodeheffer RJ, Gerstenblith G, Becker LC, et al. Exercise cardiac output is maintained with advancing age in healthy human subjects: cardiac dilation and increased stroke volume compensate for a diminished heart rate. Circulation 1984;69:203–213.

4. Jackson AS, Wier LT, Ayers GW, et al. Changes in aerobic power of women ages 20-64 yr. Med Sci Sports Exerc 1996;28:844–891.

5. Shvartz E, Reibold RC. Aerobic fitness norms for males and females aged 6-75 years: A review. Aviat Space Environ Med 1990;61:3–11.

6. Fitzgerald PL. Exercise for the elderly. Med Clin North Am 1995;69:189–196.

7. Ike RW, Lampmann RM, Castor CW. Arthritis and aerobic exercise. Phys Sportsmed 1989;17:128–139.

8. Shephard RJ. Aging. Physical Activity and Health, Champaign, IL: Human Kinetics, 1997.

9. HHS Publication No. HHS-ODPHP-2005-01-DGA-A. Dietary Guidelines for Americans 2005, U.S. Department of Health and Human Services, U.S. Department of Agriculture. Available at: http://healthierus.gov/dietaryguidelines. Accessed April 27, 2006.

10. Russell RM, Rasmussen H, Lichtenstein AH. Modified food guide pyramid for people over seventy years of age. J Nutr 1999;129:751–753.

11. Mazzeo RS, Cavanagh P, Evans WJ, et al. ACSM position stand on exercise and physical activity for older adults. Med Sci Sports Exerc 1998;30:992–1008.

12. Woo JS, Derleth C, Stratton JR, Levy WC. The influence of age, gender and training on exercise efficiency. J Am Coll Cardiol 2006;47:1049–1059.

13. Martin Ginis KA, Latimer AE, Brawley LR, Jung ME, Hicks AL. Weight training to activities of daily living: helping older adults make a connection. Med Sci Sports Exerc 2006;38:116–121.

CHAPTER 21

Women and Minorities

At the end of this chapter the reader should be able to:

1. Summarize specific diseases in women in which disease prevention strategies can be particularly beneficial to decrease the risks for those diseases.
2. Explain the importance of physical activity during pregnancy.
3. Recall the prevalence of certain diseases in minority populations.

OVERVIEW

Traditional research in medicine has primarily focused on using male subjects. This has resulted in knowing little about women and minority populations and the inability to make inferences about the general population. In the past decade, however, more research has been published involving women and minority populations to give healthcare professionals a broader and more complete view of the treatment and prevention of diseases. Campaigns to increase awareness, such as the "Go Red for Women" campaign by the American Heart Association, have helped women and minorities gain the attention of the general population and researchers in disease prevention efforts. This chapter will discuss several disease prevention issues that are specific to women and minority populations.

DISEASE PREVENTION IN WOMEN

Cardiovascular Disease

In the past, it was thought that **cardiovascular disease (CVD)** was a disease that was only prevalent in men. This is far from the truth. Cardiovascular disease is the number one killer among women as well. In the United States alone, almost 500,000 women die each year of CVD.[1] This number exceeds the number of CVD deaths in men.[1] More than 38 million women had CVD in 2003, which accounts for more than one third of all women in the United States.[1] **Coronary heart disease (CHD)** accounted for the majority (almost one half) of CVD deaths in women in 2003.[1] The prevalence of significant risk factors that affect women and lead to CVD include **hypertension** (36.6 million), high total **cholesterol** (51.5 million), high low-density lipoprotein (LDL) cholesterol (37 million), overweight or **obesity** (66.9 million), and **diabetes mellitus** (7.1 million).[1] Additionally, only 29% of women reported regular leisure-time **physical activity** in 2004.[1]

The need for the implementation of prevention strategies in women is great. In 2004, the American Heart Association published guidelines for the prevention of cardiovascular disease in women (http://www.americanheart.org/presenter.jhtml? identifier=2781).[2] The focus of these guidelines is on establishing cardiovascular risk assessment in women using the Framingham Point Score Table (see Appendix A) and then establishing and implementing appropriate treatments based on the Framingham score. Patients who are at high risk (>20% risk) should be treated most aggressively. Regardless of the patient's risk score, however, the guidelines recommend the same lifestyle modification interventions. These interventions include smoking cessation, physical activity, a heart-healthy diet, and body-weight maintenance or reduction.[2]

The physical activity recommendation for women is the same as that proposed for the population in general, which is 30 minutes of accumulated moderate-intensity physical activity on most, preferably all, days of the week (http://www.surgeongeneral.gov/).[2,3] Heart-healthy dietary recommendations for women include an eating plan that is concentrated on fruits, vegetables, whole grains, low-fat or non-fat dairy products, fish, legumes, and sources of protein low in saturated fat. Additionally, women should consume no more than 10% of total **calories** from saturated fats, limit cholesterol intake to less than 300 mg/day, and limit *trans* **fatty acid** intake.[2] Consistently encouraging women not to smoke or to avoid environmental smoke is recommended as well as maintaining a body weight that will achieve a **body mass index (BMI)** of 18.5 to 24.9 kg/m² and a waist circumference of less than 35 inches.[2]

Other, non-lifestyle CVD prevention issues that should be mentioned include the use of hormone therapy, antioxidant supplements, and the routine use of aspirin. The guidelines consider hormone-replacement therapy to be a class III CVD intervention, which means that it is considered not useful or effective and may be harmful.[2] Combined estrogen plus progestin hormone therapy as well as other forms of menopausal hormone therapy, such as unopposed estrogen, should not be initiated or continued to prevent CVD in postmenopausal women.[2] Additionally, antioxidant vitamin supplements should not be used to prevent CVD, and routine use of aspirin therapy should not be used in low-risk women to prevent CVD.[2] It is important to note, however, that ongoing trials exist in these areas, and healthcare professionals should be aware of new information as it becomes available to make the best clinical decisions.

Overwhelming evidence supports the use of many types of CVD prevention strategies in both women and men.[2] Healthcare professionals should attempt to implement the necessary interventions in their patients. Because of the rapidly evolving nature of CVD medicine and the publication of new information, all healthcare professionals should stay abreast of the latest research to provide their patients the best possible care and information.

Cancer

Cancer is a major public health concern in the United States. It is second only to cardio-vascular disease as the most common cause of death.[4] Women have 48.5% of all cancers diagnosed each year and have a 38% lifetime risk of developing cancer.[5] The lifetime risk of dying of cancer is 20% in women.[6] The most common types of cancer in women are breast, lung, colon, and uterine cancer, and those that claim the most lives are lung, breast, colon, and pancreatic cancer.[5]

Certain lifestyle modifications have been shown to be effective at preventing many types of cancers. Lifestyle modifications primarily focus on tobacco cessation, physical activity, proper nutrition, maintaining a healthy body weight, and abstaining from excess or chronic alcohol consumption. Cigarette smoking is currently the single most significant modifiable risk factor for cancer.[7] It is estimated that tobacco smoking is responsible for 30% of all cancer deaths annually in the United States.[8] Additionally, other lifestyle-related factors such as **physical inactivity,** obesity, and improper nutrition combined accounted for approximately 30% of the expected cancer deaths in 2003.[7,9,10]

Breast cancer is the leading cause of cancer in women, accounting for nearly 213,000 new cases in 2006.[5] Research has shown that the lifestyle modifications of physical activity, healthy eating, tobacco avoidance (including secondhand smoke), maintaining a healthy body weight, and moderation in alcohol consumption can all help to prevent the incidence of breast cancer. Lung cancer can be prevented with physical activity, healthy eating, and tobacco avoidance. Colon cancer can likewise decrease in prevalence with physical activity, healthy eating, maintaining a healthy body weight, and moderation in alcohol consumption. Much can be done to decrease the incidence of many types of cancers by implementing lifestyle modification strategies. Educating women about the benefits should be a priority for all healthcare providers.

Diabetes Mellitus

Diabetes mellitus is a serious health concern for both women and men in the United States. It is a unique problem for women compared with men because diabetes can affect both a mother and her unborn children.[11] More than 15 million Americans have diabetes, and more than half (8.1 million) are women.[11] Approximately 90 to 95% of women with diabetes have **type 2 diabetes mellitus,** and about 1.85 million women of reproductive age (18 to 44 years) have diabetes, of which 500,000 do not know they have the disease.[11] Children exposed to diabetes in the womb have a greater likelihood of becoming obese during childhood and adolescence and of developing type 2 diabetes later in life.[11] Gestational diabetes is a type of diabetes that occurs only during preg-nancy and is caused by hormones produced by the placenta.[11] Gestational diabetes occurs in 2.5 to 4% of women in the United States during pregnancy.[11] It usually ends after the baby is born, but women who have gestational diabetes have up to a 45% reoc-currence with the next pregnancy and up to a 63% risk of developing type 2 diabetes later in life.[11]

Diabetes is a major risk factor of cardiovascular disease. Several prevention strate-gies can be implemented that can help to decrease the prevalence of CVD in women with either type 1 or type 2 diabetes. The strategies include physical activity, healthy nutrition, smoking cessation, and weight loss for type 2 patients.[11] Healthcare professionals should give special focus to young women and women of child-bearing age who have diabetes or are at risk of developing the disease. Implementing prevention strategies for these women can be beneficial to the health of both the mother and her children.[11]

Osteoporosis

Osteoporosis affects approximately 44 million Americans aged 50 years and older.[12] Although men experience osteoporosis, 80% of Americans with the disease are women. In addition, women who are white or Asian have a higher prevalence of osteoporosis than do women who are black or Hispanic.[13] Osteoporotic fractures led to more than 500,000 hospitalizations, more than 800,000 emergency room encounters, and more than 2.6 million physician office visits in 1995 in the United States.[14] In addition, nearly 180,000 individuals were placed in nursing homes in 1995 as a result of osteoporotic fractures.[14] Studies show that the annual direct care expenditures for osteoporotic fractures range from $12.2 to $17.2 billion, and women account for 82% of this amount.[14]

Several strategies have been identified that can help women reach optimal peak bone mass and continue building new bone tissue with age to prevent osteoporosis. These strategies include adequate calcium and vitamin intake, adequate physical activity, maintaining a healthy body weight, smoking abstinence, alcohol control, avoiding long-term use of medications known to increase risk of osteoporosis, taking medications known to lower osteoporosis risk, and teaching fall prevention.[15] A proactive approach by healthcare professionals in assessing their patients' risks for osteoporosis can lead to early implementation of prevention strategies and a better outcome for many women. Healthcare professionals should work together to identify at-risk patients and provide appropriate therapy.

Pregnancy and Physical Activity

In the early 20th century, physical activity was discouraged during pregnancy because of theoretical concerns that exercise would injure the fetus and the mother during this time by (1) decreasing the oxygen available to the mother and fetus, (2) causing hypothermia-induced fetal distress or birth abnormalities, or (3) increasing uterine contractions.[16,17] As a result, women were advised not to engage in physical activity and to simply be sedentary during the pregnancy period.[16] Current studies, however, show that healthy women with uncomplicated pregnancies do not need to limit their exercise for fear of these adverse events.[17] Data show that women who engage in physical activity during pregnancy have about a 50% decreased risk for gestational diabetes compared with sedentary women.[16] Additionally, active women experience a 40% decrease in the incidence of preeclampsia compared with inactive women.[16] Other benefits to remaining physically active during the pregnancy include reduced weight gain, more rapid weight loss after pregnancy, improved mood, and improved sleep patterns.[18]

Regular exercise in pregnant women should only be done with a physician's knowledge and approval.[18] The overall risks and benefits to the mother and fetus should be considered by the patient and her physician before beginning or continuing a physical activity program.[18] In the absence of medical and obstetric complications, the American College of Sports Medicine recommends 30 minutes or more of moderate-intensity activity on most, if not all, days of the week in pregnant women.[17,18] Women who have participated in regular and consistent physical activity before the pregnancy should be able to maintain that program to some degree throughout the pregnancy.[18] Women who are just starting a program once they have become pregnant as a way to improve their health during pregnancy should begin very slowly and be careful not to overexert.[18] The safety of the mother and fetus should always be the primary concern, and therefore activities that place the mother at high risk of falling and of abdominal injury (e.g., kickboxing, horseback riding, ice hockey, soccer) should be avoided during pregnancy.[18] Additionally, exertion at altitudes of 6,000 feet or higher should be avoided, as should scuba diving during pregnancy because of the risk for decompression sickness in the fetus during this activity.[17,18] Pharmacists should advise their pregnant patients to consult with their physician regarding an appropriate exercise prescription while pregnant.

MINORITIES AND DISEASE PREVENTION

Similar to women, minority populations have traditionally been underrepresented in clinical research studies. More recently, however, data on minorities have become more frequently published to give researchers and healthcare professionals a clearer picture of the prevalence of disease in these populations. Knowing which diseases are more likely to occur in certain populations can allow healthcare professionals to target specific minorities for the prevention and treatment of those specific diseases. Much is still unknown as to why certain populations are more likely to incur certain diseases, but knowing disease prevalence information about certain minority populations can allow healthcare professionals to focus proven disease prevention strategies in those specific groups.

Several chronic diseases appear to disproportionately affect certain minority populations compared with other ethnic groups. The following list of disease prevalence statistics serves as an example of where healthcare professionals can focus attention on prevention strategies to decrease the prevalence of disease in certain populations:

- The incidence of hypertension in African Americans in New York City affects nearly one third of this population compared with only 22% of white Americans.[19,20]
- African Americans with hypertension have an 80% greater risk of dying of a **stroke** compared with the general population and have the highest stroke death rate of any ethnic population in general. The stroke death rate for African Americans is three to four times greater than for white Americans.[20–22]
- The incidence of coronary heart disease (CHD) is highest in white males (8.9%). CHD prevalence is next highest in black females (7.5%), followed by black males (7.4%), Mexican American males (5.6%), white females (5.4%), and finally Mexican American females (4.3%).[19]
- Obesity affects approximately 30% of all Americans regardless of race.[19] The incidence of obesity in African American females is 49% and for Mexican American females is 38.4%.[19] At the other end of the spectrum, Asian females have only a 7% incidence of obesity.[19]
- The prevalence of diabetes mellitus is approximately two times greater in American Indians and Alaskan Natives compared with the overall population (15.3% versus 7.3%, respectively). Other minority populations that rate above the general population are Hispanic blacks (11.7%) and Mexican Americans (9.6%). By comparison, non-Hispanic whites have a diabetes mellitus incidence of 4.8%.[19]
- Whites and Asian Americans have a greater prevalence for **osteoporosis** compared with African or Hispanic Americans.[13]

Disease prevention strategies can also be affected by income level. In 2003, approximately 30% of U.S. adults engaged in regular leisure time physical activity, while another 30% participated in some leisure time physical activity, and the remaining 40% of U.S. adults were inactive during their leisure time.[23] During this same year, about 50% of adults who were poor or near poor were inactive during leisure time compared with about 30% of adults who had an income that was twice that of poverty. Additionally, about 25% of adults who live in or near poverty engaged in regular amounts of leisure time physical activity compared with more than one third of adults living in families with higher incomes.[23] Therefore, adults living below or near poverty are less likely to participate in regular amounts of physical activity and are more likely to be inactive compared with adults who have greater amounts of income.[23] This means that individuals who have the least amount of income are at greater risk for certain diseases, such as cardiovascular disease, compared with higher-income individuals.

As discussed in Chapter 5 on health behavior change, it is important to understand the factors that influence participation in health prevention strategies. In the general population of the United States, the demographic factors known to positively affect physical activity participation include being male, younger, a non-smoker, leaner, more educated, and white, and having a self-reported view of overall good health.[24,25] Psychological factors that positively correlate with physical activity include higher **self-efficacy,** greater perceived benefits of physical activity, greater enjoyment, lower levels of depression, higher incidence of self-regulating behaviors, and fewer perceived barriers to physical activity.[24,25] Other positively correlated factors from social and environmental influences include increased support from family, friends, and healthcare providers, access to physical activity facilities, enjoyable climate and scenery, frequently seeing others participating in physical activity, neighborhoods conducive to walking, and perceived safety while participating in physical activity.[24,26–31]

A study conducted in 2003 was aimed at identifying factors that influenced participation in physical activity among African American men and women. Among this population, almost 40% are not meeting the Centers for Disease Control and Prevention and American College of Sports Medicine (CDC/ACSM) recommendations for physical activity, and almost 25% of African Americans are completely sedentary.[24] The goal of the study was to examine the demographic, psychological, social, and environmental factors associated with meeting the CDC/ACSM recommendations and to compare these factors in African American men and women.[24]

The sample cohort of men (n = 165) and women (n = 407) showed that a significant amount of men in the study were married compared with the women ($P < 0.001$) and that a significant difference existed between the men and women with respect to income ($P < 0.01$).[24] Additionally, a significantly greater amount of women were attempting to lose weight compared with the men ($P < 0.001$).[24] The results revealed that many positive correlates existed in both African American men and women and some negative correlates existed as well. African American men who were more likely to participate in physical activity were employed, had greater income, had a higher self-rating of health, rated physical activity efficacy higher, had greater physical activity enjoyment, and consumed more fruits and vegetables. The negative correlate with African American men was age. The positive correlates with African American women were employment, education, income, self-rating of health, physical activity self-efficacy, physical activity enjoyment, fruit and vegetable intake, reporting physical activity programs at their church, and attempting to lose weight. Negative correlates for African American women included age, number of chronic health conditions, and body mass index.[24]

Knowing which factors influence participation in physical activity and other disease prevention strategies can be of great help to healthcare professionals. The information above can help to identify African American individuals who might be more or less likely to participate in physical activity. It should be noted, however, that there is no substitute for personal consultation with patients to identify their specific barriers and needs when it comes to health behavior participation. Healthcare professionals can be involved at the individual, community, or societal level at getting more minorities involved in physical activity and other healthy behaviors.

Framingham Heart Study

A quick note should be made regarding the Framingham Heart Study as it is mentioned several times throughout this book. Several chapters and Appendix A use the Framingham Heart Study data to calculate an individual patient's risk for having a coronary event within the next 10 years. Knowing this risk level can help guide the intensity of treatment for patients. The Framingham Heart Study, however, has been criticized in the past for its underrepresentation of minority groups in their study and therefore the inability to use the Framingham data in certain populations. The National Institutes of Health, however, state that "Although the Framingham cohort is primarily white, the importance of the major CVD risk factors identified in this group have been shown in other studies to apply almost universally among racial and ethnic groups, even though the patterns of distribution may vary from group to group."[32] Therefore, Appendix A can and should be used as a means to identify the coronary risk for all patients.

THE PHARMACIST'S ROLE IN DISEASE PREVENTION IN WOMEN AND MINORITY POPULATIONS

As a prominent member of the healthcare workforce, pharmacists have an obligation to serve those individuals who may be underserved or underrepresented. Women and minorities in the past have been overlooked in research studies and publications, especially those involving disease prevention. Pharmacists, working closely with other healthcare professionals in a collaborative team approach, can identify and educate women and minority populations who may be at risk for certain diseases. Changes to the way disease prevention is approached in these populations can be done with individual patients themselves, or on a group and societal level. Educating minority groups at churches and community centers, as well as offering informational material in the pharmacy itself, can be an excellent place to start increasing awareness about certain diseases and the risks associated with them. Pharmacists can also get more involved at the national, state, and local government levels to help change regulations that make obtaining and participating in disease prevention strategies more widely available to all members of society. The literature may not have all the answers yet as to why certain populations are more at risk for certain diseases compared with others, but it is clear that participating in proven disease prevention strategies is a way to improve the health outcomes of all individuals.

REFERENCES

1. American Heart Association. Heart Disease and Stroke Statistics—2006 Update. Dallas: American Heart Association, 2006.
2. Mosca L, Appel LJ, Benjamin EJ, et al. Evidence-based guidelines for cardiovascular disease prevention in women. Circulation 2004;109:672–693.
3. U.S. Department of Health and Human Services. Physical activity and health: a report of the Surgeon General. Atlanta: U.S. Department of Health and Human Services, Centers for Disease Control and Prevention, National Center for Chronic Disease Prevention and Health Promotion, 1996.
4. Mokdad AH, Marks JS, Stroup DF, Gerberding JL. Actual causes of death in the United States, 2000. JAMA 2004;291:1238–1245.
5. American Cancer Society: Cancer facts and figures 2006. Atlanta: American Cancer Society. Available at: http://www.cancer.org/downloads/stt/CAFF06EsCsMc.pdf. Accessed March 30, 2006.
6. Ries LAG, Eisner MP, Kosary CL, et al., eds. SEER Cancer Statistics Review, 1975–2002. National Cancer Institute. Bethesda, MD. Available at: http://seer.cancer.gov/csr/1975_2002/, based on November 2004 SEER data submission, posted to the SEER web site 2005.

7. Davis L, Lindley C. Neoplastic disorders and their treatment: general principles. In: Koda-Kimble MA, ed. Applied Therapeutics: The Clinical Use of Drugs, 8th ed. Philadelphia: Lippincott Williams & Wilkins, 2005:88.1–88.35.

8. National Cancer Institute. Cigarette smoking and cancer: questions and answers. National Cancer Institute, U.S. National Institutes of Health, 2004. Available at: http://www.cancer.gov/cancertopics/factsheet/Tobacco/cancer. Accessed March 30, 2006.

9. American Cancer Society: Cancer facts and figures 2003. Atlanta: American Cancer Society, 2003.

10. Calle EE, Rodriguez C, Walker-Thurmond K, Thun MJ. Overweight, obesity, and mortality from cancer in a prospectively studied cohort of U.S. adults. N Engl J Med 2003;348:1625–1638.

11. Department of Health and Human Services. Diabetes and women's health across the life stages. U.S. Department of Health and Human Services, Centers for Disease Control and Prevention, October 2001.

12. National Osteoporosis Foundation: America's Bone Health: The State of Osteoporosis and Low Bone Mass. Washington, D.C.: National Osteoporosis Foundation, 2002.

13. Nichols DL, Essery EV. Osteoporosis and exercise. In: Kaminsky LA, et al., eds. ACSM's Resource Manual for Guidelines for Exercise Testing and Prescription, 5th ed. Baltimore: Lippincott Williams & Wilkins, 2006: 489–499.

14. U.S. Department of Health and Human Services. Bone Health and Osteoporosis: A Report of the Surgeon General. Rockville, MD: U.S. Department of Health and Human Services, Office of the Surgeon General, 2004.

15. National Institutes of Health. Osteoporosis Overview. National Institutes of Health, Osteoporosis and Related Bone Diseases, National Resource Center, June 2005. Available at: http://www.niams.nih.gov/bone/hi/overview.htm. Accessed March 9, 2006.

16. Dempsey JC, Butler CL, Williams MA. No need for a pregnant pause: physical activity may reduce the occurrence of gestational diabetes mellitus and preeclampsia. Exerc Sports Med Rev 2005;33:141–149.

17. Whaley MH, Brubaker PH, Otto RM, eds. ACSM's Guidelines for Exercise Testing and Prescription, 7th ed. Baltimore: Lippincott Williams & Wilkins, 2006:229–232.

18. Church T. General overview of preparticipation health screening and risk assessment. In: Kaminsky LA, et al., eds. ACSM's Resource Manual for Guidelines for Exercise Testing and Prescription, 5th ed. Baltimore: Lippincott Williams & Wilkins, 2006:115–121.

19. American Heart Association. Heart Disease and Stroke Statistics—2005 Update. Dallas: American Heart Association, 2005.

20. NYC Department of Health and Mental Hygiene. Management of hypertension in adults. City Health Information 2005;24:39–50.

21. Sacco RL, Boden-Albala B, Abel G, et al. Race-ethnic disparities in the impact of stroke risk factors: the Northern Manhattan Stroke Study. Stroke 2001;32:1725–1731.

22. Stansbury JP, Jia H, Williams LS, Vogel WB, Duncan PW. Ethnic disparities in stroke: epidemiology, acute care, and postacute outcomes. Stroke 2005;36:374–387.

23. U.S. Department of Health and Human Services. Health, United States, 2005 with chartbook on trends in the health of Americans. U.S. Department of Health and Human Services, Centers for Disease Control and Prevention, National Center for Health Statistics. DHHS Publication No. 2005-1232, November 2005.

24. Bopp M, Laken M, Butler K, Carter RE, McClorin L, Yancey A. Factors associated with physical activity among African-American men and women. Am J Prev Med 2006;30:340–346.

25. Trost SG, Owen N, Bibeau AE, Sallis FJ, Brown W. Correlates of adults' participation in physical activity: review and update. Med Sci Sports Exerc 2002;34:1996–2001.

26. Owen N, Leslie E, Salmon J, Fotheringham MJ. Environmental determinants of physical activity and sedentary behavior. Exerc Sport Sci Rev 2000;28:153–158.

27. Giles-Corti B, Donovan RJ. Relative influences of individual, social environmental, and physical environmental correlates of walking. Am J Public Health 2003;93:1583–1589.

28. Humpel N, Owen N, Leslie E. Environmental factors associated with adults' participation in physical activity: a review. Am J Prev Med 2002;22:188–199.

29. Ball K, Bauman A, Leslie E, Owen N. Perceived environmental aesthetics and convenience and company are associated with walking for exercise among Australian adults. Prev Med 2001;33:434–440.

30. Dannenberg AL, Jackson RJ, Frumkin H, et al. The impact of community design and land-use choices on public health: a scientific research agenda. Am J Public Health 2003;93:1500–1508.

31. Berrigan D, Troiano RP. The association between urban form and physical activity in U.S. adults. Am J Prev Med 2002;23(Suppl 1):74–79.

32. Department of Health and Human Services, National Institutes of Health, National Heart, Lung and Blood Institute. Framingham Heart Study. Available at: http://www.nhlbi.nih.gov/about/framingham/design.htm. Accessed May 1, 2006.

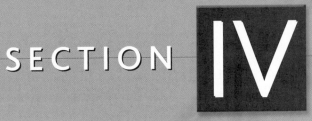

SECTION IV

APPENDICES

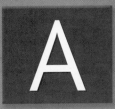

Framingham 10-Year Coronary Heart Disease Risk Assessment

Estimate of 10-Year Risk for Men

Age	Points
20–34	−9
35–39	−4
40–44	0
45–49	3
50–54	6
55–59	8
60–64	10
65–69	11
70–74	12
75–79	13

Total Cholesterol	Points				
	Age 20–39	Age 40–49	Age 50–59	Age 60–69	Age 70–79
<160	0	0	0	0	0
160–199	4	3	2	1	0
200–239	7	5	3	1	0
240–279	9	6	4	2	1
≥280	11	8	5	3	1

	Age 20–39	Age 40–49	Age 50–59	Age 60–69	Age 70–79
			Points		
Nonsmoker	0	0	0	0	0
Smoker	8	5	3	1	1

HDL (mg/dL)	Points
≥60	−1
50–59	0
40–49	1
<40	2

Systolic BP (mm Hg)	If Untreated	If Treated
<120	0	0
120–129	0	1
130–139	1	2
140–159	1	2
≥160	2	3

Point Total	10-Year Risk %
<0	<1
0	1
1	1
2	1
3	1
4	1
5	2
6	2
7	3
8	4
9	5
10	6
11	8
12	10
13	12
14	16
15	20
16	25
≥17	≥30

10-Year Risk = _____ %

Estimate of 10-Year Risk for Women

Age	Points
20–34	−7
35–39	−3
40–44	0
45–49	3
50–54	6
55–59	8
60–64	10
65–69	12
70–74	14
75–79	16

Total Cholesterol	Points				
	Age 20–39	Age 40–49	Age 50–59	Age 60–69	Age 70–79
<160	0	0	0	0	0
160–199	4	3	2	1	1
200–239	8	6	4	2	1
240–279	11	8	5	3	2
≥280	13	10	7	4	2

	Points				
	Age 20–39	Age 40–49	Age 50–59	Age 60–69	Age 70–79
Nonsmoker	0	0	0	0	0
Smoker	9	7	4	2	1

HDL (mg/dL)	Points
≥60	−1
50–59	0
40–49	1
<40	2

Systolic BP (mm Hg)	If Untreated	If Treated
<120	0	0
120–129	1	3
130–139	2	4
140–159	3	5
≥160	4	6

Point Total	10-Year Risk %
<9	<1
9	1
10	1
11	1
12	1
13	2
14	2
15	3
16	4
17	5
18	6
19	8
20	11
21	14
22	17
23	22
24	27
≥25	≥30

10-Year Risk = _____%

Source: National Institutes of Health, National Heart, Lung, and Blood Institute. Third report of the National Cholesterol Education Program (NCEP) Expert Panel on Detection, Evaluation, and Treatment of High Blood Cholesterol in Adults (Adult Treatment Panel III). NIH Publication No. 02-5215, September 2002.

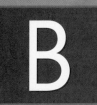

Body Mass Index Table

F ind height in the left-hand column and body weight in the columns to the right. The number at the top of that column will be the body mass index (BMI).

Body Mass Index (kg/m²)

	21	22	23	24	25	26	27	28	29	30	31
4′10″	100	105	110	115	119	124	129	134	138	143	148
4′11″	104	109	114	119	124	128	133	138	143	148	154
5′0″	107	112	118	123	128	133	138	143	148	153	158
5′1″	111	116	122	127	132	137	143	148	153	158	164
5′2″	115	120	126	131	136	142	147	153	158	164	170
5′3″	118	124	130	135	141	146	152	158	163	169	175
5′4″	122	128	134	140	145	151	157	163	169	174	181
5′5″	126	132	138	144	150	156	162	168	174	180	186
5′6″	130	136	142	148	155	161	167	173	179	186	192
5′7″	134	140	146	153	159	166	172	178	185	191	198
5′8″	138	144	151	158	164	171	177	184	190	197	204
5′9″	142	149	155	162	169	176	182	189	196	203	209
5′10″	146	153	160	167	174	181	188	195	202	207	216
5′11″	150	157	165	172	179	186	193	200	208	215	222
6′0″	154	162	169	177	184	191	199	206	213	221	229
6′1″	159	166	174	182	189	197	204	212	219	227	235
6′2″	163	171	179	186	194	202	210	218	225	233	242
6′3″	168	176	184	192	200	208	216	224	232	240	248
6′4″	172	180	189	197	205	213	221	230	238	246	255

Body Mass Index (BMI) Calculation:
BMI = [weight (kg)/height (m²)]

Body Mass Index (BMI) Categories:
Normal Weight: BMI = 18.5–24.9 kg/m²
Overweight: BMI = 25–29.9 kg/m²
Obese: BMI = 30 kg/m² or greater

Source: Clinical Guidelines on the Identification, Evaluation, and Treatment of Overweight and Obesity in Adults. Bethesda, MD: National Institutes of Health, U.S. Department of Health and Human Services, 1998. NIH Publication No. 98-4083.

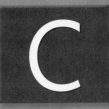

Case Study Answers

CHAPTER 6: HYPERTENSION

SOAP Notes

S: "I want to lower my blood pressure and become more healthy."

O: Vitals: Height: 5'8"   Weight: 240 lb   BMI: 36.5 kg/m²
HR: 76 beats/min   BP: 194/88 mm Hg
Current medications: HCTZ 25 mg daily, metoprolol 50 mg daily, simvastatin 20 mg daily
Chronic diseases: Hypertension, hyperlipidemia, obesity
Risk factors for heart disease: Hypertension, hyperlipidemia, obesity, sedentary lifestyle, age
Caloric intake to maintain current body weight: 3,775 kcal/day
Current physical activity program: None
Framingham risk score: 16% risk for CHD in the next 10 years
CHD risk category: Moderately high risk (based on a Framingham of 16% and having more than two risk factors)

A:
1. High blood pressure (not managed with HCTZ 25 mg and now added metoprolol 50 mg daily)
2. High blood cholesterol (managed with simvastatin 20 mg daily)
3. Obesity
4. Sedentary lifestyle

P:
1. Initiate a blood pressure management program
2. Modify lifestyle to follow DASH eating plan, exercise, and lose weight

Exercise Program

Goals:

Short Term (4 weeks)

1. Participate in 30 minutes of light to moderate physical activity on most days of the week
2. Keep blood pressure <140/90 mm Hg
3. Promote healthy lifestyle

Long Term (6 months)

1. Maintain a consistent blood pressure <120/80 mm Hg
2. Decrease cardiovascular disease risk
3. Be physically active for at least 30 minutes on most days of the week with a moderate level of activity
4. Lose 10% of body weight (achieve body weight of approximately 215 lb)

Exercise Prescription

Activity	Frequency	Duration	Intensity	Progression
Aerobic (walking, biking, swimming, or swim aerobics)	3–4 times/week	15–20 minutes (can divide into two sessions/day)	Light to moderate	Add 5 minutes to the duration each week up to 30 minutes, then increase frequency one additional day per week up to most days of the week, then increase to a moderate level of activity
Resistance training (all major muscle groups)	2–3 days/week		1 set of 10–12 repetitions	Increase to two sets after 2 weeks, then increase to three sets after 4 weeks. Add weight to maintain 12–15 repetitions as needed
Flexibility (all major muscle groups)	3 days/week		Maintain each stretch 20–30 seconds	
Warm-up and cool-down	Before and after each aerobic and resistance training session	5–10 minutes	Low	

Increase overall daily physical activity by doing yard work, household chores, taking stairs at work, taking a 10-minute brisk walk at lunchtime and after work

Reassessment and Follow-Up

Assess progress every other week for first 4 weeks, then every other month for first 6 months, then 2–3 times per year thereafter.

Dietary Intervention

Goals:

Short Term (1 week)

1. Assess current eating habits
2. Assess barriers for changing eating habits

Medium range (1–4 weeks)

1. Reduce sodium, saturated fat, cholesterol
2. Increase calcium, potassium, and magnesium
3. Reduce daily caloric intake by 250–350 kcal/day

Long Term (>4 weeks)

1. Maintain DASH eating plan
2. Lose weight at a rate of approximately 1 lb per week
3. Reassess patient goals and set new goals (further weight loss or weight maintenance)

Dietary Suggestions

1. Increase fruits and vegetable intake to 4–5 servings each per day
2. Decrease total caloric intake by 250–350 kcal/day
3. Decrease total fat by 10% and saturated fat by 10% by limiting fried foods and fast food
4. Reduce dietary cholesterol 150 mg/day by eating low-fat or fat-free dairy foods and lean cuts of meat
5. Increase complex carbohydrate intake by 7% with more fruits and vegetables and grains, but limit sweets
6. Increase fiber intake by 22 g/day with fruits, vegetables, nuts, and seeds
7. Decrease sodium intake by 600 mg/day by limiting processed foods

Reassessment and Follow-Up

Assess progress weekly for the first 4 weeks, then monthly for the first 6 months, then 2–3 times per year thereafter.

CHAPTER 7: DYSLIPIDEMIA

SOAP Notes

S: "I am here to fill this prescription to lower my cholesterol."
O: Vitals: Height: 5'10"   Weight: 210 lb   BMI: 30.1 kg/m^2
    HR: 85 beats/min   BP: 124/78 mm Hg

Labs: Total cholesterol: 265 mg/dL
Triglyceride: 176 mg/dL
LDL: 195 mg/dL
HDL: 35 mg/dL

Current medications: simvastatin 20 mg daily (new prescription)

Chronic diseases: hyperlipidemia (new diagnosis)

Risk factors for heart disease: Hyperlipidemia, family history (father had AMI at age 50 years), obesity, sedentary lifestyle

Caloric intake to maintain current body weight: 3,557 kcal/day

Framingham risk score: 4% risk for CHD in the next 10 years

CHD risk category: Moderate risk (based on a Framingham of less than 10% and having more than two risk factors)

A:

1. Hyperlipidemia
2. Obesity
3. Family history for heart disease
4. Sedentary lifestyle

P:

1. Start simvastatin 20 mg daily
2. Assess patient's readiness to change lifestyle habits
3. Initiate exercise program 2–4 times per week initially, then 5–6 times per week
4. Consume diet consistent with NCEP ATP III guidelines of low fat, low cholesterol
5. Decrease daily caloric intake to promote weight loss

Exercise Program
Goals:

Short Term (4 weeks)

1. Promote healthy lifestyle
2. Exercise 2–4 times per week

Long Term (6–12 months)

1. Decrease cardiovascular disease risk
2. Decrease serum cholesterol, LDL, and triglyceride and increase HDL
3. Achieve healthy body weight
4. Exercise most days of the week

Exercise Prescription

Activity	Frequency	Duration	Intensity	Progression
Aerobic (walking or biking)	2–3 times/week	10–20 minutes	Moderate	Add 5 minutes to duration each week up to 45 minutes, then increase frequency one additional day per week up to most days of the week

Activity	Frequency	Duration	Intensity	Progression
Resistance training (all major muscle groups)	3 days/week		1 set of 10–12 repetitions	Increase to two sets after 2 weeks then increase to three sets after 4 weeks. Add weight to maintain 10–12 repetitions as needed
Flexibility (all major muscle groups)	3 days/week		Maintain each stretch 20–30 seconds	
Warm-up and cool-down	Before and after each aerobic and resistance training session	5–10 min	Low	

Increase overall daily physical activities by taking the stairs instead of elevators, parking farther away in parking lots, walking the family pet, etc.

Reassessment and Follow-Up

Assess progress weekly for first 4 weeks, then monthly for first 6 months, then 2–3 times per year thereafter.

Dietary Intervention
Goals:

Short Term (4 weeks)

1. Assess current eating habits
2. Initiate NCEP ATP III suggested dietary intake
3. Reduce total caloric intake to promote weight loss

Long Term (>4 weeks)

1. Maintain NCEP ATP III suggested dietary intake
2. Decrease body weight
3. Maintain healthy body weight

Dietary Suggestions

1. Decrease total caloric intake by 300 kcal/day
2. Decrease daily total fat intake by 5% initially (first 2 weeks) then by another 5–10% during the next 2–4 weeks
3. Decrease saturated fat intake by half during the first 2 weeks
4. Substitute high-fat foods for those with whole grains, fruits, and vegetables

Reassessment and Follow-Up

Assess progress weekly for first 4 weeks, then monthly for first 6 months, then 2–3 times per year thereafter.

CHAPTER 8: CORONARY HEART DISEASE

SOAP Notes

S: The patient has filled out the required health history forms at the request of his wife but believes he is healthy and does not require a program such as yours.

O: Vitals: Height: 5′8″   Weight: 160 lb   BMI: 24 kg/m²
HR: 72 beats/min   BP: 118/76 mm Hg   Age: 46 years
Current medications: Occasional ibuprofen
Chronic diseases: Undiagnosed dyslipidemia
Risk factors for heart disease: Age, family history, current smoker, low HDL-cholesterol, elevated triglycerides
Caloric intake to maintain current body weight: 1,610 kcal/day
Current average caloric intake per day: 1,634 kcal/day
Current physical activity program: No specific program but attains an average of 8,650 steps per day with occupational activities
Framingham Risk Score: 6% for CHD in the next 10 years
CHD risk category: Moderate risk (based on a Framingham score of less than 10% and having more than two risk factors)

A:

1. Multiple risk factors for CHD
2. Current smoker
3. Undiagnosed dyslipidemia
4. Possibly disinterested in a lifestyle modification program
5. Adequate caloric intake

P:

1. Educate J.L. on the CHD risks of smoking, dyslipidemia, and family history
2. Initiate a smoking-cessation program
3. Modify lifestyle to increase physical activity
4. Inform J.L.'s physician of his undiagnosed dyslipidemia

Exercise Program
Goals:

Short Term (4 weeks)

1. Educate about the benefits of participating in physical activity to decrease the risk of CHD
2. Participate in 30 minutes of moderate-intensity physical activity on most days of the week

Long Term (6 months)

1. Reeducate about the benefits of physical activity
2. Adhere to 30 minutes of moderate-intensity physical activity on most days of the week
3. Decrease risk for CHD

Exercise Prescription

Activity	Frequency	Duration	Intensity	Progression
Aerobic (walking, biking, swimming, jogging, rowing)	3–4 times/week	20–30 minutes (can divide into two sessions/day)	Moderate	Add 5 minutes to the duration each week up to 30 minutes, then increase frequency one additional day per week up to most days of the week, then increase to a moderate level of activity
Resistance training (all major muscle groups)	2–3 days/week		1 set of 10–12 repetitions	Increase to two sets after 2 weeks, then increase to three sets after 4 weeks. Add weight to maintain 12–15 repetitions as needed
Flexibility (all major muscle groups)	3 days/week		Maintain each stretch 20–30 seconds	
Warm-up and cool-down	Before and after each aerobic and resistance training session	5–10 minutes	Low	

Maintain physical activity at work, participate in sporting activities such as basketball, racquetball, or tennis

Reassessment and Follow-Up

Assess progress every other week for first 4 weeks, then every other month for first 6 months, then 2–3 times per year thereafter.

Dietary Intervention
Goals:

Short Term (4 weeks)

1. Educate about the importance of a healthy eating plan
2. Increase fruit and vegetable intake
3. Increase dietary fiber intake
4. Decrease sodium intake
5. Maintain current caloric intake

Long Term (>4 weeks)

1. Reeducate about the importance of a healthy eating plan
2. Adhere to new dietary changes
3. Decrease risk for cardiovascular disease

Dietary Suggestions

1. Increase fruit and vegetable intake to 4–5 servings each per day
2. Gradually increase dietary fiber intake to 31 g per day
3. Decrease sodium intake by about 1,000–1,500 mg per day by limiting processed foods

Reassessment and Follow-Up

Assess progress weekly for the first 4 weeks, then monthly for the first 6 months, then 2–3 times per year thereafter.

Smoking-Cessation Program

Brief Smoking-Cessation Documentation

Patient information:

Name: J.L.   Date: October 1
Height: 5′8″   Weight: 160 lb   Age: 46 years
Comorbidities: Undiagnosed dyslipidemia
Medications: Occasional ibuprofen
Family history: Positive for CHD (father MI at age 54 years)
Smoking history: 1 ppd for 30 years

ASK	Current smoker, never has tried a quit attempt
ADVISE	Statement was made to J.L. that along with his numerous other risk factors for heart disease, he is at both a significant short-term and long-term risk for heart attack, stroke, and thromboembolism. Also, smoking can impact the health of his spouse. J.L. was informed that the pharmacist and pharmacy staff could assist him if he would like to quit.
ASSESS	J.L. states that his wife has also tried to get him to quit smoking for years. J.L. states that he is now willing to make a quit attempt and will participate in the brief intervention program that the pharmacy offers.
ASSIST	A quit date was set for 1 week from today (October 8).

J.L. was advised to tell his family, friends, and coworkers that he is quitting and to ask for their support.

J.L. was advised to remove all tobacco products from his home, car, and any other place he might have them. In addition, he was advised to have his house and car cleaned to remove smoky odors and establish a "clean or fresh start" to his quit attempt.

Counseling advice consisted of telling J.L.:

- Do not smoke even a single puff after the quit date.
- His trigger is break times at work and driving in the car, and he was advised to chew nicotine gum and perform activities that take his mind off of smoking.
- Avoid time pressures and stress at work and home by being well organized.
- Learn to anticipate and avoid temptation.

- Exercise by walking with a partner, such as his wife, on most days of the week to decrease weight gain and to feel good about himself.
- Encourage J.L. to talk about the quitting process, such as reasons for quitting and concerns and worries about quitting.

Pharmacotherapy recommendation:

- Nicotine gum 2 mg, up to 24 pieces per day as needed. This is available OTC and has been shown to delay weight gain. Counsel J.L. about side effects of mouth soreness and dyspepsia.

ARRANGE   A follow-up phone call was arranged for the day before the quit date (October 7) and 1 week after the quit date (October 15).

CHAPTER 9: STROKE

SOAP Notes

S: Patient feels that her resting blood pressure may be a little high and would like suggestions to help bring it into the appropriate range.

O: Vitals: Height: 4'10"   Weight: 125 lb   BMI: 19.2 kg/m^2
    HR: 58 beats/min   BP: 164/88 mm Hg   Age: 57 years
    Current medications: Amlodipine 5 mg daily
    Chronic diseases: Hypertension
    Risk factors for heart disease: Age, family history, current smoker, hypertension
    Caloric intake to maintain current body weight: 1,990 kcal/day
    Current average caloric intake per day: 2,000 kcal/day
    Current physical activity program: Walks on treadmill three times per week for 20 minutes
    Framingham risk score: Not applicable (no lipid panel)

A:

1. Treated but uncontrolled hypertension
2. Current smoker
3. Family history of CHD and stroke
4. Good nutritional habits
5. Good exercise habits but below recommended amounts

P:

1. Call patient's physician regarding blood pressure medication and control
2. Initiate a smoking-cessation program
3. Modify lifestyle to increase physical activity
4. Monitor blood pressure long term

Exercise Program

Goals:

Short Term (4 weeks)

1. Participate in 30 minutes of moderate intensity physical activity on most days of the week

Long Term (6 months)

1. Adhere to 30 minutes of moderate intensity physical activity on most days of the week
2. Decrease risk for stroke and CHD

Exercise Prescription

Activity	Frequency	Duration	Intensity	Progression
Aerobic (walking, biking, swimming, jogging, rowing)	5–7 times/week	30 minutes (can divide into two sessions/day)	Moderate	Add 5 minutes to the duration each week up to 30 minutes, then increase frequency one additional day per week up to most days of the week
Resistance training (all major muscle groups)	2–3 days/week		1 set of 10–12 repetitions	Increase to two sets after 2 weeks, then increase to three sets after 4 weeks. Add weight to maintain 12–15 repetitions as needed
Flexibility (all major muscle groups)	3 days/week		Maintain each stretch 20–30 seconds	
Warm-up and cool-down	Before and after each aerobic and resistance training session	5–10 minutes	Low	

Maintain physical activity at work by playing with children in games outside and inside

Reassessment and Follow-Up

Assess progress every other week for first 4 weeks, then every other month for first 6 months, then 2–3 times per year thereafter.

Dietary Intervention
Goals:

Short and Long Term

1. Maintain current eating habits
2. Maintain concentration on low-sodium, low-saturated fat eating plan
3. Maintain at least five servings of fruits and vegetables per day
4. Decrease risk for stroke and CHD

Dietary Suggestions

1. Decrease sodium intake by about 500 mg per day
2. Maintain at least five servings of fruits and vegetables per day

Reassessment and Follow-Up

Assess progress every other week for the first 4 weeks, then monthly for the first 6 months, then 2–3 times per year thereafter.

Smoking-Cessation Program

Brief Smoking Cessation Documentation

Patient information:
Name: A.P.   Date: April 10
Height: 4'10"   Weight: 125 lb   Age: 57 years
Comorbidities: Hypertension
Medications: Amlodipine 5 mg daily
Family history: Positive for stroke, CHD, and diabetes mellitus
Smoking history: 1.5 ppd for 33 years

ASK	Current smoker, has tried to quit 5 to 7 times in the past 15 years
ADVISE	Statement was made to A.P. that along with her numerous other risk factors for heart disease, she is at both a significant short-term and long-term risk for heart attack, stroke, and thromboembolism. A.P. was informed that the pharmacist and pharmacy staff could assist her if she would like to quit.
ASSESS	A.P. states that this is not a good time to try quitting as she has "significant family matters" that she is currently dealing with. She states that she may be interested sometime in the future.
ASSIST	A quit date was not set for A.P. at this time as she is not currently interested. Counseling advice for A.P. consisted of:

- Reminding her of the significant risk of CHD and stroke that smoking brings to her health.
- Reminding her that the pharmacy staff would be very happy and eager to help her make a quit attempt when she is again ready.
- Advising her that there are currently several pharmacologic products now available to help her increase her chances of quitting.

ARRANGE	Follow-up with A.P. regarding her interest in quitting at each visit she makes to the pharmacy for prescription refills and wellness visits.

CHAPTER 10: PERIPHERAL ARTERIAL DISEASE

SOAP Notes

S: The patient expressed interest in the disease prevention program and would like to enroll.

O: Vitals: Height: 5'7"   Weight: 135 lb   BMI: 21.2 kg/m^2
HR: 88 beats/min   BP: 138/88 mm Hg   Age: 32 years old

Current medications: NPH and regular insulin before breakfast and dinner
Chronic diseases: Type 1 diabetes mellitus
Risk factors for heart disease: Diabetes, current smoker, sedentary lifestyle
Caloric intake to maintain current body weight: 1,942 kcal/day
Current average caloric intake per day: 2,054 kcal/day
Current physical activity program: None
Framingham risk score: not applicable (no lipid panel)

A:

1. Multiple risk factors for PAD and cardiovascular disease
2. Type 1 diabetes mellitus with unknown hemoglobin A_{1c}
3. Current smoker of 1 ppd for 15 years
4. Sedentary lifestyle
5. Diet high in saturated fat, cholesterol, and sodium
6. Unknown blood lipids

P:

1. Educate B.N. on the atherosclerotic risks of diabetes, smoking, and sedentary lifestyle
2. Initiate a smoking cessation program
3. Modify lifestyle to increase physical activity
4. Modify current eating habits to decrease amounts of saturated fats, cholesterol, and sodium
5. Obtain hemoglobin A_{1c} and lipid panel

Exercise Program

Goals:

Short Term (4 weeks)

1. Educate about the benefits of participating in physical activity to decrease the risk of atherosclerosis
2. Participate in 30 minutes of moderate-intensity physical activity on 3 to 4 days of the week

Long Term (6 months)

1. Reeducate about the benefits of physical activity
2. Adhere to 30 minutes of moderate-intensity physical activity on most days of the week
3. Decrease risk for cardiovascular disease

Exercise Prescription

Activity	Frequency	Duration	Intensity	Progression
Aerobic (walking, biking, swimming, jogging, rowing)	3–4 times/week	20–30 minutes (can divide into two sessions/day)	Light to moderate	Add 5 minutes to the duration each week up to 30 minutes, then increase frequency one additional day per week up to most days of the week, then

Activity	Frequency	Duration	Intensity	Progression
				increase to a moderate level of activity
Resistance training (all major muscle groups)	2–3 days/week		1 set of 10–12 repetitions	Increase to two sets after 2 weeks, then increase to three sets after 4 weeks. Add weight to maintain 12–15 repetitions as needed
Flexibility (all major muscle groups)	3 days/week		Maintain each stretch 20–30 seconds	
Warm-up and cool-down	Before and after each aerobic and resistance training session	5–10 minutes	Low	

Increase overall daily physical activity by doing yard work and household chores, taking stairs at work, taking a 10-minute brisk walk at lunchtime and after work

Reassessment and Follow-Up

Assess progress every other week for first 4 weeks, then every other month for first 6 months, then 2–3 times per year thereafter.

Dietary Intervention
Goals:

Short Term (4 weeks)

1. Educate about the importance of a healthy eating plan
2. Decrease frequency of fast food consumption
3. Increase fruit and vegetable intake
4. Increase dietary fiber intake
5. Decrease saturated fat, cholesterol, and sodium intake
6. Maintain current calorie intake

Long Term (>4 weeks)

1. Reeducate about the importance of a healthy eating plan
2. Adhere to new dietary changes
3. Decrease risk for cardiovascular disease

Dietary Suggestions

1. Increase fruit and vegetable intake to 4–5 servings each per day
2. Decrease total fat by 10% and saturated fat by 5% by limiting fried foods and fast food

3. Reduce dietary cholesterol 125 mg/day by eating low-fat or fat-free dairy foods and lean cuts of meat
4. Increase complex carbohydrate intake by 10% with more fruits and vegetables and grains, but limit sweets
5. Gradually increase fiber intake by 13 g/day with fruits, vegetables, nuts, and seeds
6. Decrease sodium intake by 1,500–2,000 mg/day by limiting processed and fast foods

Reassessment and Follow-Up

Assess progress weekly for the first 4 weeks, then monthly for the first 6 months, then 2–3 times per year thereafter.

Smoking-Cessation Program

Brief Smoking Cessation Documentation

Patient information:
Name: B.N.   Date: January 15
Height: 5′7″   Weight: 135 lb   Age: 32 years
Comorbidities: Type 1 diabetes mellitus
Medications: NPH and regular insulin before breakfast and dinner
Family history: Distant family history (uncle) for CHD
Smoking history: 1 ppd for 15 years

ASK	Current smoker, never has tried a quit attempt
ADVISE	Statement was made to B.N. that along with her other risk factors for heart disease (diabetes and sedentary lifestyle), she is at risk for heart attack, stroke, thrombo-embolism, and peripheral arterial disease. B.N. was informed that the pharmacists and pharmacy staff could assist her if she would like to make a quit attempt.
ASSESS	B.N. states that she has thought about quitting for a few years but did not know how. B.N. states that she is willing to make a quit attempt and will participate in the brief intervention program that the pharmacy offers.
ASSIST	A quit date was set for 1 week from today (January 22)

B.N. was advised to tell her family, friends, and coworkers that she is quitting and to ask for their support.

B.N. was advised to remove all tobacco products from her home, car, and any other place she might have them. In addition, she was advised to have her house and car cleaned to remove smoky odors and establish a "clean or fresh start" to her quit attempt.

Counseling advice consisted of telling B.N.:

■ Do not smoke even a single puff after the quit date.
■ Her triggers are going to the bar after work with coworkers as well as after eating meals. Therefore, she is advised to tell coworkers about her quit attempt and to avoid smoky bars that may cause her to begin smoking again. Also, she is advised to try chewing gum after meals and to engage in an activity that will distract her from wanting to smoke (e.g., taking a walk).
■ Avoid time pressures and stress at work and home by being well organized.
■ Learn to anticipate and avoid temptation.
■ Increase overall physical activity level by setting aside time to exercise each day.
■ Encourage B.N. to talk about the quitting process such as reasons for quitting and concerns and worries about quitting.

Pharmacotherapy recommendation:

■ Nicotine gum 2 mg, up to 24 pieces per day as needed. This is available OTC and has been shown to delay weight gain. Counsel B.N. about side effects of mouth soreness and dyspepsia.

ARRANGE   A follow-up phone call was arranged for the day before the quit date (January 21) and 1 week after the quit date (January 29).

CHAPTER 11: HEART FAILURE

SOAP Notes

S: The patient states that she is interested in becoming healthier through exercise and weight loss.

O: Vitals: Height: 5′4″   Weight: 199 lb   BMI: 34 kg/m^2

HR: 82 beats/min   BP: 128/82 mm Hg   Age: 45 years

Current medications: Hydrochlorothiazide 12.5 mg/day, rosuvastatin 10 mg/day

Risk factors for heart disease: Hypertension, hyperlipidemia, obesity, sedentary lifestyle

Current eating plan: None specific

Caloric intake to maintain current body weight: 2,073.5 kcal/day

Current physical activity program: None

Framingham risk score: <1% for CHD in next 10 years

CHD risk category: Moderate risk (based on a Framingham of less than 10% and having more than two risk factors)

A:

1.   Hypertension (controlled with HCTZ 12.5 mg/day)
2.   Dyslipidemia (controlled with rosuvastatin 10 mg/day)
3.   Obesity
4.   Sedentary lifestyle

P:

1.   Modify lifestyle behaviors to incorporate physical activity and dietary changes

Exercise Program

Goals:

Short Term (4 weeks)

1.   Increase overall daily activities
2.   Participate in 30 minutes of moderate physical activity on most days of the week

Long Term (6 months)

1.   Participate in 30 to 45 minutes of accumulated physical activity 5 to 7 days/week
2.   Lose 10% body weight (achieve body weight of approximately 180 lb)
3.   Decrease risk for coronary heart disease and heart failure

Exercise Prescription

Activity	Frequency	Duration	Intensity	Progression
Aerobic (walking, bicycling, aerobic machines at local fitness club)	3–4 times/week	20 minutes (can divide into two sessions/day)	Moderate (walking inside or outside 3.5–4 mph)	Add 5 minutes to the duration each week up to 30 minutes, then increase frequency one additional day per week up to most days of the week
Resistance training (all major muscle groups)	2–3 days/week		1 set of 10–12 repetitions	Increase to two sets after 2 weeks, then increase to three sets after 4 weeks. Add weight to maintain 12–15 repetitions as needed
Flexibility (all major muscle groups)	3 days/week		Maintain each stretch 20–30 seconds	
Warm-up and cool-down	Before and after each aerobic and resistance training session	5–10 minutes	Low	

Increase overall daily physical activity by playing with children inside and outside of the home, doing yard work and household chores, taking stairs whenever possible, parking farther away from stores

Reassessment and Follow-Up

Assess progress every other week for first 4 weeks, then every other month for first 6 months, then 2–3 times per year thereafter.

Dietary Intervention
Goals:

Short Term (1 week)

1. Assess eating habits
2. Assess barriers for changing eating habits

Medium range (1 to 4 weeks)

1. Reduce total calories by 300 kcal/day
2. Reduce saturated fats, cholesterol, and sodium
3. Replace eating "fast food" with healthier choices of premade snacks, lunches, and dinners if "eating on the run" is necessary

Long Range (>4 weeks)

1. Lose weight at approximately 0.87 lb per week until weight loss goal is reached
2. Maintain reduction in calories/day by eating smaller portion sizes
3. Continue to avoid frequently eating "fast food"

Dietary Suggestions

1. Increase fruit and vegetable intake to 4–5 servings each per day
2. Decrease total caloric intake by 300 kcal/day
3. Decrease total fat by 10% and saturated fat by 10% by limiting fried foods and fast food
4. Reduce dietary cholesterol at least 150 mg/day by eating low-fat or fat-free dairy foods and lean cuts of meat
5. Increase complex carbohydrate intake by 10% with more fruits and vegetables and grains, but limit sweets
6. Gradually increase fiber intake by 20 g/day with fruits, vegetables, nuts, and seeds
7. Decrease sodium intake by 1,000 mg/day by limiting processed foods

Reassessment and Follow-Up

Assess progress weekly for the first 4 weeks, then monthly for the first 6 months, then 2–3 times per year thereafter.

Weight-Loss Program

Weight-Loss Program Worksheet

Name: _BJ_
Date of initial consultation: _April 15, 2006_
Gender: Male / **Female**
Age: _45_ yr
Height: _64_ inches
Height: _1.63_ m (calculate by multiplying height in inches by 0.0254)
Weight: _199_ lb
Weight: _90.5_ kg (calculate by dividing weight in pounds by 2.2)
PA = Physical activity coefficient (calculate using the following table)

	Sedentary	Low active	Active	Very active
Male	1.0	1.11	1.25	1.48
Female	**1.0**	1.12	1.27	1.45

STEP 1: Calculate Body Mass Index (BMI) and Classify
BMI = [weight (kg) / height (m^2)]
BMI = [_90.5_ kg / (_1.63_ m)^2]
BMI = _34.1_ kg/m^2

Classification of overweight and obesity according to BMI (circle)

<18.5 kg/m^2	Underweight
18.5–24.9 kg/m^2	Normal
25–29.9 kg/m^2	Overweight
30–34.9 kg/m^2	**Obesity Class I**
35–39.9 kg/m^2	Obesity Class II
≥40 kg/m^2	Obesity Class III or Extreme Obesity

STEP 2: Calculate the Estimated Energy Requirement (EER)

Males aged > 19 years:

EER = 662 − 9.53 × age (yr) + PA × [15.9 × weight (kg) + 540 × height (m)]

EER = 662 − 9.53 × _____ yr + _____ × [15.9 × _____ kg + 540 × _____ m]

EER = _____ kcal

Females aged > 19 years:

EER = 354 − 6.91 × age (yr) + PA × [9.36 × weight (kg) + 726 × height (m)]

EER = 354 − 6.91 × _45_ yr + _1.0_ × [9.36 × _90.5_ kg + 726 × _1.63_ m]

EER = _2,073.5_ kcal

STEP 3: Calculate current caloric intake and eating patterns

Day 1 total calories: _2,801_ kcal

Day 2 total calories: _2,597_ kcal

Day 3 total calories: _2,634_ kcal

Day 4 total calories: _____ kcal

Average total daily calories: _2,687_ kcal

Suggested caloric deficit in food consumption per day: _300_ kcal (multiply by 7 to get weekly caloric deficit) = _2,100_ kcal)

STEP 4: Design Exercise Prescription and Calculate Energy Expenditure

Examples of physical activity the patient prefers: _walking, indoors or outdoors_

_____

_____

Weight-loss goals:

1. _Lose 10% body weight in 6 months_ _____

_____

2. _Decrease risk for coronary heart disease_ _____

_____

3. _____

Exercise Prescription:

    Mode: _walking_

      –associated MET level: _5.0_

    Intensity: _50–70% MHR_ (% max heart rate or RPE)

    Duration: _30_ minutes

    Frequency: _4_ times per week

    Rate of Progression: _Focus should be on increasing duration (30–45 min) and frequency (5–7 times/week) over intensity (70+% MHR)_

_____

Energy expenditure:

(METs × 3.5 × body weight in kg) / 200 = kcal/min

(_5.0_ × 3.5 × _90.5_ kg) / 200 = _7.9_ kcal/min (calories expended per minute of activity)

Multiply answer by the duration = calories expended per exercise session (kcal/session)

_7.9_ kcal /min × _30_ minutes = _237_ kcal/session

Multiply answer by frequency = calories expended per week (kcal/week)

_237_ kcal/session × _4_ times per week = _948_ kcal/week

STEP 5: Design a Weight Loss Program

A. Current body weight: _199_ lb
B. Weight loss goal: _10%_
C. Weight loss goal in pounds: _20_ lb (Step A × Step B)
D. Goal body weight: _180_ lb (Step A – Step C)
E. Goal BMI classification: _Obesity Class I_ (Obtain from chart in STEP 1)
F. Weekly calories decreased from food consumption: _2,100_ kcal (Obtain from STEP 3)
G. Caloric expenditure per week from physical activity: _948_ kcal (Obtain from STEP 4)
H. Total weekly caloric deficit: _3,048_ kcal (Step F + Step G)
I. Amount of body weight lost per week: _0.87_ lb (Step H/3,500 kcal)
J. Approximate time to achieve the goal weight: _23_ weeks (Step C/Step I)

CHAPTER 12: DIABETES MELLITUS

SOAP Notes

S: Patient states that she is having difficulty keeping her blood glucose in proper range, especially on the weekends.

O: Vitals: Height: 5′6″ Weight: 130 lb BMI: 20.9 kg/m^2
HR: 78 beats/min BP: 116/72 mm Hg Age: 21 years
Fasting blood glucose: 105 mg/dL HbA_{1c}: 7.0%
Current medications: NPH and regular insulin before breakfast and dinner
Chronic diseases: Type 1 diabetes mellitus
Risk factors for diabetes complications: Cardiovascular disease risk factors = diabetes mellitus, family history, sedentary lifestyle
Caloric intake to maintain current body weight: 1,980 kcal/day
Current average caloric intake per day: 1,910 kcal/day
Alcohol consumption: 5 drinks per night on Thursday through Saturday
Current physical activity program: None
Framingham risk score: Not applicable (no lipid panel)

A:

1. Type 1 diabetes mellitus on insulin × 6 years
2. Sedentary lifestyle
3. Family history of CHD
4. No specific diet
5. High alcohol intake three days per week

P:

1. Counsel patient regarding alcohol intake and blood glucose changes
2. Suggest dietary changes to improve glucose control and decrease risks for CVD
3. Modify lifestyle to increase physical activity

Exercise Program

Goals:

Short Term (4 weeks)

1. Participate in 30 minutes of moderate-intensity physical activity on most days of the week

2. Monitor blood glucose before and after exercise sessions and adjust carbohydrate intake accordingly
3. Increase physical work capacity

Long Term (6 months)

1. Adhere to 30 minutes of moderate-intensity physical activity on most days of the week (maintain at least 150 minutes of moderate intensity activity per week)
2. Monitor blood glucose before and after exercise sessions and adjust carbohydrate intake accordingly
3. Decrease risk for CVD

Exercise Prescription

Activity	Frequency	Duration	Intensity	Progression
Aerobic (walking, biking, swimming, jogging, rowing)	5–7 times/week	30 minutes (can divide into two to three sessions/day)	Moderate	Add 5 minutes to the duration each week up to 30 minutes, then increase frequency one additional day per week up to most days of the week
Resistance training (all major muscle groups)	2–3 days/week		1 set of 15–20 repetitions	Increase to two sets after 2 weeks. Add weight to maintain 15–20 repetitions as needed
Flexibility (all major muscle groups)	3 days/week		Maintain each stretch 20–30 seconds	
Warm-up and cool-down	Before and after each aerobic and resistance training session	5–10 minutes	Low	

Increase daily lifestyle activity by walking to work, taking stairs rather than elevators, and taking daily walks with the dog

Reassessment and Follow-Up

Assess progress every other week for first 4 weeks, then every other month for first 6 months, then 2–3 times per year thereafter.

Dietary Intervention
Goals:

Short and Long Term

1. Decrease alcohol intake
2. Maintain a consistent intake of carbohydrates

3. Monitor blood glucose before and after exercise and adjust carbohydrate accordingly
4. Decrease risk for CVD

Dietary Suggestions

1. Limit alcohol intake to one drink per day
2. Increase carbohydrate intake to 55% of total calories and maintain a consistent intake throughout the day. Most carbohydrate intake should come from whole grains, fruits, vegetables, and low-fat dairy products
3. Increase monounsaturated fat intake to 13% of total calories
4. Maintain a combined carbohydrate and monounsaturated fat intake of 60 to 70% of total calories
5. Decrease saturated fat intake to less than 10% of total calories
6. Increase protein intake to 15 to 20% of total calories
7. Gradually increase fiber intake to 20–30 g/day

Assessment and Follow-Up

Assess progress every other week for the first 4 weeks, then monthly for the first 6 months, then 2–3 times per year thereafter.

CHAPTER 13: OBESITY

SOAP Notes

S: "What can I do to lose weight that I have gained since the birth of my children?"

O: Vitals: Height: 5′3″   Weight: 180 lb   BMI: 32 kg/m²
   HR: 90 beats/min   BP: 117/66 mm Hg   Age: 38 years
   Current Medications: None
   Chronic Diseases: Obesity
   Risk factors for heart disease: Obesity, sedentary lifestyle
   Caloric intake to maintain current body weight: 2,574 kcal/day
   Current physical activity program: None (but is active caring for her three children)
   Framingham risk score: Not applicable (no lipid panel)

A:

1. Obese
2. Sedentary lifestyle

P:

1. Assess patient's readiness to change lifestyle habits and barriers to change
2. Decrease daily caloric intake by 500 kcal/day
3. Initiate an exercise program 3–4 times per week initially, then 6+ times per week

Exercise Program
Goals:

Short Term (4 weeks)

1. Participate in safe activities
2. Promote healthy lifestyle
3. Participate in physical activity 3–4 times per week

Long Term (6 months)

1. Decrease cardiovascular disease risk
2. Be physically active on most days of the week (150 minutes of exercise/week progressing to >300 minutes/week)
3. Lose 10% of body weight (achieve body weight of approximately 160 lb)

Exercise Prescription

Activity	Frequency	Duration	Intensity	Progression
Aerobic (walking, biking, swimming, or swim aerobics)	3–4 times/week	15–20 minutes (can divide into two sessions/day)	Light to moderate	Add 5 minutes to the duration each week up to 60 minutes, then increase frequency one additional day per week up to most days of the week
Resistance training (all major muscle groups)	2–3 days/week		1 set of 10–12 repetitions	Increase to two sets after 2 weeks, then increase to three sets after 4 weeks. Add weight to maintain 12–15 repetitions as needed
Flexibility (all major muscle groups)	3 days/week		Maintain each stretch 20–30 seconds	
Warm-up and cool-down	Before and after each aerobic and resistance training session	5–10 minutes	Low	

Increase overall daily physical activity by actively playing with kids at home, taking kids for a walk or to the park. Set aside part of the day with kids to be a physical activity time when everyone becomes active playing games

Reassessment and Follow-Up

Assess progress weekly for first 4 weeks, then monthly for first 6 months, then 2–3 times per year thereafter.

Dietary Intervention
Goals:

Short Term (2 weeks)

1. Assess current eating habits
2. Assess readiness for change
3. Assess barriers for changing eating habits

    4. Stop gaining weight

    5. Reduce daily caloric intake by 500 kcal/day

Medium range (2 weeks–6 months)

    1. Lose weight at a rate of approximately 1 lb/week

Long Term (>6 months)

    1. Maintain weight loss

    2. Reassess patient goals and set new goals (further weight loss or weight maintenance)

Dietary Suggestions

    1. Decrease total calorie intake by 500 kcal/day

    2. Increase carbohydrate intake by 10%

    3. Decrease total fat intake by 15% with a decrease in saturated fat intake of 5–10%

    4. Increase fiber intake to 20 g/day by substituting high-fat foods with whole grains, fruits, and vegetables

    5. Increase calcium intake to 1,000–1,500 mg/day

Reassessment and Follow-Up

Assess progress weekly for the first 4 weeks, then monthly for the first 6 months, then 2–3 times per year thereafter.

Weight-Loss Program Worksheet

Name: _JM_
Date of initial consultation: _October 31, 2006_
Gender: Male / **Female**
Age: _38_ yr
Height: _63_ inches
Height: _1.60_ m (calculate by multiplying height in inches by 0.0254)
Weight: _180_ lb
Weight: _81.8_ kg (calculate by dividing weight in pounds by 2.2)
PA = Physical activity coefficient (calculate using the following table)

	Sedentary	Low active	Active	Very active
Male	1.0	1.11	1.25	1.48
Female	**1.0**	1.12	1.27	1.45

STEP 1: Calculate Body Mass Index (BMI) and Classify
BMI = [weight (kg) / height (m²)]
BMI = [_81.8_ kg / (_1.60_ m)²]
BMI = _32_ kg/m²

Classification of overweight and obesity according to BMI (circle)

<18.5 kg/m²	Underweight
18.5–24.9 kg/m²	Normal
25–29.9 kg/m²	Overweight
30–34.9 kg/m²	**Obesity Class I**
35–39.9 kg/m²	Obesity Class II
≥40 kg/m²	Obesity Class III or Extreme Obesity

STEP 2: Calculate the Estimated Energy Requirement (EER)

Males aged > 19 years:

EER = 662 − 9.53 × age (yr) + PA × [15.9 × weight (kg) + 540 × height (m)]

EER = 662 − 9.53 × _____ yr + _____ × [15.9 × _____ kg + 540 × _____ m]

EER = _____ kcal

Females aged > 19 years:

EER = 354 − 6.91 × age (yr) + PA × [9.36 × weight (kg) + 726 × height (m)]

EER = 354 − 6.91 × _38_ yr + _1.0_ × [9.36 × _81.8_ kg + 726 × _1.60_ m]

EER = _2,019_ kcal

STEP 3: Calculate current caloric intake and eating patterns

Day 1 total calories: _2,695_ kcal

Day 2 total calories: _2,870_ kcal

Day 3 total calories: _2,715_ kcal

Day 4 total calories: _2,819_ kcal

Average total daily calories: _2,775_ kcal

Suggested caloric deficit in food consumption per day: _500_ kcal (multiply by 7 to get weekly caloric deficit = _3,500_ kcal)

STEP 4: Design Exercise Prescription and Calculate Energy Expenditure

Examples of physical activity the patient prefers: _walking, swimming, water aerobics_

Weight loss goals:

1. _Stop gaining weight_

2. _Lose at least 10% body weight within 6 months_

3. _Maintain weight loss through regular participation in physical activity and following a proper nutrition plan_

Exercise Prescription:

> Mode: _walking_
> –associated MET level: _3.8_
> Intensity: _50–70%_ (% max heart rate or RPE)
> Duration: _20_ minutes
> Frequency: _3_ times per week
> Rate of Progression: _Add 5 minutes to duration each week up to 60 minutes, then increase frequency 1 additional day per week up to 5 to 6 days per week_

Energy expenditure:

(METs × 3.5 × body weight in kg) / 200 = kcal/min

(_3.8_ × 3.5 × _81.8_ kg)/200 = _5.4_ kcal/min (calories expended per minute of activity)

Multiply answer by the duration = calories expended per exercise session (kcal/session)

_5.4_ kcal/min × _20_ minutes = _108_ kcal/session

Multiply answer by frequency = calories expended per week (kcal/week)

_108_ kcal/session × _3_ times per week = _324_ kcal/week

STEP 5: Design a Weight-Loss Program

A. Current body weight: _180_ lb

B. Weight loss goal: _10_ %

C. Weight loss goal in pounds: _18_ lb (Step A × Step B)

D. Goal body weight: _162_ lb (Step A − Step C)

E. Goal BMI classification: _Overweight_ (Obtain from chart in STEP 1)
F. Weekly calories decreased from food consumption: _500_ kcal (Obtain from STEP 3)
G. Caloric expenditure per week from physical activity: _324_ kcal (Obtain from STEP 4)
H. Total weekly caloric deficit: _3,824_ kcal (Step F + Step G)
I. Amount of body weight lost per week: _1.09_ lb (Step H/3,500 kcal)
J. Approximate time to achieve the goal weight: _16.5_ weeks (Step C/Step I)

(Note: This is estimated using the initial physical activity recommendation and would change if the patient progressively increased physical activity duration and frequency as suggested.)

CHAPTER 14: METABOLIC SYNDROME

SOAP Notes

S: L.L. states that he has not seen a doctor in 15 years and his wife feels that he is out of shape and overweight, so she would like him to join the pharmacy's wellness program.
O: Vitals: Height: 6′0″   Weight: 273 lb
    BMI: 37.1 kg/m²   Waist circumference: 46 inches
    HR: 82 beats/min   BP: 138/90 mm Hg
    Smoker: Yes (1 pack per day × 25 years)
    Family history: Father had MI at age 43 years
    Fasting blood glucose: 108 mg/dL
    Total cholesterol: 240 mg/dL
    LDL cholesterol: 185 mg/dL
    HDL cholesterol: 25 mg/dL
    Triglycerides: 360 mg/dL
    Current medications: None
    Chronic diseases: None diagnosed
    Risk factors for cardiovascular disease: Smoker, obese, dyslipidemia, elevated blood pressure, elevated blood glucose, sedentary lifestyle, family history
    Caloric intake to maintain current body weight: 3,204 kcal/day
    Current average caloric intake per day: 3,426 kcal/day
    Alcohol consumption: 6–10 drinks/week
    Current physical activity program: None
    Baseline pedometer reading: 3,865 steps/day average
    Framingham risk score: 16% risk for CHD within the next 10 years
    CHD risk category: Moderately high risk (based on a Framingham score of 10–20% and having two or more risk factors)

A:

1. Obese
2. Current smoker (1 ppd × 25 yr)
3. Elevated blood cholesterol
4. Dyslipidemia
5. Elevated fasting glucose
6. Atherogenic diet
7. Sedentary lifestyle
8. Positive family history of CHD
9. No current physician and no physical examination for 15 years

P:

1. Counsel patient regarding risk factors for cardiovascular disease
2. Recommend smoking-cessation program
3. Recommend weight-loss program
4. Recommend lifestyle modifications of increased physical activity and nutritional changes
5. Recommend he obtain a physician for a physical examination with the recommendation of beginning aspirin 81 mg daily to decrease CVD risk

Exercise Program
Goals:

Short Term (4 weeks)

1. Participate in 30 minutes of accumulated moderate-intensity physical activity on most days of the week (walking for 10 minutes three times per day during truck stops)
2. Increase daily physical activity by increasing overall activity

Long Term (6 months)

1. Participate in 30–60 minutes of moderate intensity physical activity on most days of the week
2. Lose 10% body weight in 6 months
3. Decrease risk for CVD

Exercise Prescription

Activity	Frequency	Duration	Intensity	Progression
Aerobic (walking, biking)	5 times/week	30 minutes (can divide into two to three sessions/day)	Light to moderate	Add 5 minutes to the duration each week up to 30 minutes, then increase frequency one additional day per week up to most days of the week
Resistance training (all major muscle groups)	2 days/week		1 set of 15–20 repetitions	Increase to two sets after 2 weeks. Add weight to maintain 15–20 repetitions as needed
Flexibility (all major muscle groups)	3 days/week		Maintain each stretch 20–30 seconds	
Warm-up and cool-down	Before and after each aerobic and resistance training session	5–10 minutes	Low	

Increase daily lifestyle activity by taking stairs rather than elevators, walking dog when home, taking walks with spouse

Reassessment and Follow-Up

Assess progress every other week for first 4 weeks, then every other month for first 6 months, then 2–3 times per year thereafter.

Dietary Intervention
Goals:

Short Term (2 weeks)

1. Assess readiness for change
2. Overcome barriers to healthy eating
3. Stop gaining weight
4. Reduce daily caloric intake by 400 kcal/day

Medium range (2–6 months)

1. Lose weight at a rate of approximately 1 to 1.5 pounds/week
2. Develop and adhere to a healthy eating plan

Long Term (>6 months)

1. Maintain weight loss
2. Reassess goals and set new goals for weight loss and weight maintenance
3. Decrease risk for CVD

Dietary Suggestions

1. Decrease daily calorie intake by 400 kcal/day
2. Decrease total fat intake
3. Decrease saturated fat intake by at least half
4. Decrease dietary cholesterol intake
5. Increase fiber intake (gradually) by 10–15 g/day
6. Increase intake of whole grains, fruits, vegetables, and low-fat dairy products
7. Decrease intake of simple, refined sugars
8. Decrease intake of sodium

Reassessment and Follow-Up

Assess progress every other week for the first 4 weeks, then monthly for the first 6 months, then 2–3 times per year thereafter.

Weight-Loss Program

Weight-Loss Program Worksheet

Name: _LL_
Date of initial consultation: _August 31, 2006_
Gender: **Male** /Female
Age: _44_ yr
Height: _72_ inches
Height: _1.83_ meters (calculate by multiplying height in inches by 0.0254)
Weight: _273_ lb

Weight: _124.1_ kg (calculate by dividing weight in pounds by 2.2)
PA = Physical activity coefficient (calculate using the following table)

	Sedentary	Low active	Active	Very active
Male	**1.0**	1.11	1.25	1.48
Female	1.0	1.12	1.27	1.45

STEP 1: Calculate Body Mass Index (BMI) and Classify
BMI = [weight (kg) / height (m^2)]
BMI = [_124.1_ kg / (_1.83_ m)^2]
BMI = _37.1_ kg/m^2

Classification of overweight and obesity according to BMI (circle)
<18.5 kg/m^2 Underweight
18.5–24.9 kg/m^2 Normal
25–29.9 kg/m^2 Overweight
30–34.9 kg/m^2 Obesity Class I
35–39.9 kg/m^2   **Obesity Class II**
≥40 kg/m^2 Obesity Class III or Extreme Obesity

STEP 2: Calculate the Estimated Energy Requirements (EER)
Males aged > 19 years:
EER = 662 − 9.53 × age (yr) + PA × [15.9 × weight (kg) + 540 × height (m)]
EER = 662 − 9.53 × _44_ yr + _1.0_ × [15.9 × _124.1_ kg + 540 × _1.83_ m
EER = _3,204_ kcal

Females aged > 19 years:
EER = 354 − 6.91 × age (yr) + PA × [9.36 × weight (kg) + 726 × height (m)]
EER = 354 − 6.91 × _____ yr + _____ × [9.36 × _____ kg + 726 × _____ m
EER = _____ kcal

STEP 3: Calculate current caloric intake and eating patterns
Day 1 total calories: _3,810_ kcal
Day 2 total calories: _3,015_ kcal
Day 3 total calories: _3,560_ kcal
Day 4 total calories: _3,320_ kcal
Average total daily calories: _3,426_ kcal
Suggested caloric deficit in food consumption per day: _400_ kcal
Suggested caloric deficit in food consumption per week: _2,800_ kcal (multiply by 7 to get weekly caloric deficit)

STEP 4: Design Exercise Prescription and Calculate Energy Expenditure
Examples of physical activity the patient prefers: _walking when on the road at work, bicycling when at home_
Weight loss goals:

1. _Lose 10% body weight within 6 months_

2. _Manage blood pressure, blood glucose, and blood lipids_

3. _Decrease risk for coronary heart disease_

Exercise Prescription:
  Mode: _walking_
    –associated MET level: _3.8_
  Intensity: _50–60% MHR_ (% max heart rate or RPE)
  Duration: _30_ minutes (accumulated: 10 min 3×/day)
  Frequency: _5_ times per week
  Rate of Progression: _Focus should be on increasing duration (30–60 min) and frequency (5–7 times/week) over intensity_

Energy expenditure:
(METs × 3.5 × body weight in kg) / 200 = kcal/min
(_3.8_ × 3.5 × _124.1_ kg)/200 = _8.3_ kcal/min (calories expended per minute of activity)
Multiply answer by the duration = calories expended per exercise session (kcal/session)
_8.3_ kcal/min × _30_ minutes = _249_ kcal/session
Multiply answer by frequency = calories expended per week (kcal/week)
_249_ kcal/session × _5_ times per week = _1,245_ kcal/week

STEP 5: Design a Weight Loss Program
A. Current body weight: _273_ lb
B. Weight loss goal: _10_%
C. Weight loss goal in pounds: _27_ lb (Step A × Step B)
D. Goal body weight: _246_ lb (Step A – Step C)
E. Goal BMI classification: _Obesity Class II_ (Obtain from chart in STEP 1)
F. Weekly calories decreased from food consumption: _2,800_ kcal (Obtain from STEP 3)
G. Caloric expenditure per week from physical activity: _1,245_ kcal (Obtain from STEP 4)
H. Total weekly caloric deficit: _4,045_ kcal (Step F + Step G)
I. Amount of body weight lost per week: _1.16_ lb (Step H/3,500 kcal)
J. Approximate time to achieve the goal weight: _23_ weeks (Step C / Step I): _5.8_ months (Step J/4)

(Note: This is estimated using the initial physical activity recommendation and would change if the patient progressively increased physical activity duration and frequency as suggested.)

Smoking-Cessation Program

Brief Smoking-Cessation Documentation

Patient information:
Name: L.L. Date: August 31
Height: 6′0″ Weight: 273 lb Age: 44 years
Comorbidities: None diagnosed
Medications: None
Family history: Positive for CHD
Smoking history: 1 ppd for 25 years

ASK   Current smoker, never has tried a quit attempt

ADVISE   Statement was made to L.L. that along with his numerous other risk factors for heart disease, he is at both a significant short-term and long-term risk for heart attack, stroke, and thromboembolism. Also, smoking can impact the health of his children and spouse. L.L. was informed that the pharmacist and pharmacy staff could assist him if he would like to quit.

ASSESS   L.L. states that his wife is also a smoker and should also quit. L.L. states that he is now willing to make a quit attempt along with his wife and will participate in the brief intervention program that the pharmacy offers.

ASSIST   A quit date was set for 1 week from today (September 7)

L.L. was advised to tell his family, friends, and coworkers that he is quitting and to ask for their support.

L.L. was advised to remove all tobacco products from his home, car, work truck, and any other place he might have them. In addition, he was advised to have his house and work truck cleaned to remove smoky odors and establish a "clean or fresh start" to his quit attempt.

Counseling advice consisted of telling L.L.:

- Do not smoke even a single puff after the quit date.
- His triggers are truck stops and he was advised to take a walk for several weeks instead of sitting in the restaurant.
- Avoid time pressures and stress at work and home by being well organized
- Learn to anticipate and avoid temptation.
- Exercise by walking with a partner on most days of the week to decrease weight gain and to feel good about himself.
- Encourage L.L. to talk about the quitting process such as reasons for quitting and concerns and worries about quitting.

Pharmacotherapy recommendation:

- Nicotine gum 2 mg, up to 24 pieces per day as needed. This is available OTC and has been shown to delay weight gain. Counsel L.L. about side effects of mouth soreness and dyspepsia.

ARRANGE   A follow-up phone call was arranged for the day before the quit date (September 6) and one week after the quit date (September 14)

CHAPTER 15: CANCER

SOAP Notes

S: G.D. states that he has a family history of cancer and would like to do what he can to try to prevent cancer in himself.

O: Vitals: Height: 6′4″   Weight: 195 lb
BMI: 23.8 kg/m^2 Age: 25 years old
HR: 60 beats/min   BP: 110/70 mm Hg
Smoker: No
Family history: Yes—breast cancer in mother and grandmother, colon cancer in grandfather
Current medications: Ibuprofen 400 mg prn for sore shoulder
Chronic diseases: None
Risk factors for cardiovascular disease: None
Caloric intake to maintain current body weight: 3,487 kcal/day
Current average caloric intake per day: 3,500 kcal/day
Alcohol consumption: None
Current physical activity program: Active playing basketball and water skiing 2–3 times per week
Framingham risk score: Not applicable (no lipid panel)

A:

1. Family history of breast cancer in mother and grandmother, colon cancer in grandfather
2. Physically active but no regular exercise program

P:

1. Counsel patient regarding risk factors (lifestyle, environmental, occupational, genetic, medications) for cancer
2. Counsel patient regarding lifestyle modifications that have been shown to decrease cancer risks
3. Recommend a regular exercise program that can decrease cancer risk and improve overall health and continuation of participation in various sports
4. Recommend dietary changes that coincide with cancer-reducing strategies as well as those recommended for overall health

Exercise Program

Goals:

Short Term (4 weeks)
1. Participate in 30 minutes of accumulated moderate to vigorous physical activity 3–5 days per week
2. Increase daily physical activity by participating in activities of daily living
3. Continue participating in various sports 2–3 times per week

Long Term (6 months)

1. Participate in 30–45 minutes or more of moderate to vigorous intensity physical activity 5 days or more per week
2. Decrease overall risk for cancer and other diseases
3. Continue participating in various sports 2–3 times per week

Exercise Prescription

Activity	Frequency	Duration	Intensity	Progression
Aerobic (jogging, biking, swimming, stair climbing, basketball, racquetball, tennis, volleyball, water skiing)	3–5 times per week initially, up to 5+ times per week	20 minutes initially, 30–45 minutes or more ideally (can divide into several sessions/day)	Moderate to vigorous	Add 5 minutes to the duration each week up to 30–45 minutes or more
Resistance training (all major muscle groups)	2–3 days/week		3 sets of 8–12 repetitions	Begin with two sets and increase to three sets after 1–2 weeks. Add weight to maintain 8–12 repetitions as needed

Activity	Frequency	Duration	Intensity	Progression
Flexibility (all major muscle groups)	At least 3 days per week, but ideally before and after exercise sessions	Maintain each stretch 15–30 seconds, 2–4 sets per stretch		
Warm-up and cool-down	Before and after each aerobic and resistance training session	5–10 minutes	Low	

Increase daily lifestyle activity by taking stairs rather than elevators, parking farther away from entrances of buildings

Reassessment and Follow-Up

Assess progress every other week for first 4 weeks, then every other month for first 6 months, then 2–3 times per year thereafter.

Dietary Intervention
Goals:

Short Term (4 weeks)

1. Assess readiness for change
2. Overcome barriers to healthy eating
3. Develop and adhere to a healthy eating plan that is consistent with cancer-reducing strategies

Long Term (>6 months)

1. Maintain an optimal caloric intake and a healthy eating plan
2. Decrease risk for cancer

Dietary Suggestions

1. Increase intake of fruits and vegetables to about 9 servings/day
2. Increase fiber intake by eating more fruits and vegetables and whole-grain foods
3. Decrease intake of saturated fats by about 2% of total calories/day
4. Decrease cholesterol intake by about 30 mg/day
5. Decrease sodium intake by about 300 mg/day

Reassessment and Follow-Up

Assess progress every other week for the first 4 weeks, then every other month for the first 6 months, then 2–3 times per year thereafter.

CHAPTER 16: OSTEOPOROSIS

SOAP Notes

S: L.K. states that her grandmother has osteoporosis and would like to know what she can do to decrease her risk for the disease.

O: Vitals: Height: 5′1″   Weight: 105 lb
BMI: 19.9 kg/m²   Age: 27 years old
HR: 75 beats/min   BP: 110/68 mmHg
Smoker: Yes (1 pack per day × 10 years)
Family history: grandmother has osteoporosis
Current medications: None
Chronic diseases: None diagnosed
Risk factors for cardiovascular disease: sedentary lifestyle, smoking
Caloric intake to maintain current body weight: 1,739 kcal/day
Current average caloric intake per day: 1,750 kcal/day
Alcohol consumption: 2–3 drinks per week
Current physical activity program: none
Framingham risk score: Not available (no lipid panel)

A:

1.   Sedentary
2.   Current smoker (1 ppd × 10 yr)
3.   Low calcium intake
4.   Grandmother has osteoporosis

P:

1.   Counsel patient regarding risk factors for osteoporosis
2.   Recommend smoking-cessation program
3.   Recommend lifestyle modifications to increase weight-bearing physical activity and nutritional changes to add more calcium

Exercise Program

Goals:

Short Term (4 weeks)
1.   Participate in 30 minutes of moderate-intensity weight-bearing physical activity 3 days/week
2.   Participate in resistance training activities 2 days/week
3.   Increase daily physical activity by increasing overall activity

Long Term (6 months)

1.   Participate in 30–60 minutes of moderate to high intensity weight-bearing physical activity 3–5 days/week
2.   Participate in resistance training activities 2–3 days/week
3.   Maintain bone mass

Exercise Prescription

Activity	Frequency	Duration	Intensity	Progression
Aerobic (jogging or walking with intermittent jogging, stair climbing, jump roping, tennis, basketball, volleyball)	3–5 times/week	30 minutes (can divide into two to three sessions/day)	Moderate	Gradually add more load to the bones by jogging more often and playing activities that require jumping
Resistance training (all major muscle groups)	2 days/week		1 set of 8–12 repetitions	Increase to two sets after 2 weeks. Add weight to maintain 8–12 repetitions as needed
Flexibility (all major muscle groups)	3–5 days/week		Maintain each stretch 20–30 seconds	
Warm-up and cool-down	Before and after each aerobic and resistance training session	5–10 minutes	Low	

Increase daily lifestyle activity by taking stairs rather than elevators, walking dog when home, taking walks with family and friends, taking stairs rather than elevator

Reassessment and Follow-Up

Assess progress every other week for first 4 weeks, then every other month for first 6 months, then 2–3 times per year thereafter.

Dietary Intervention
Goals:

Short Term (2 weeks) to Long Term (>6 months)

1. Double the amount of calcium in food intake
2. Maintain or slightly increase caloric intake
3. Maintain other aspects of nutritional consumption

Dietary Suggestions

1. Increase calcium intake by 500–700 mg/day (e.g., low-fat dairy products such as milk and yogurt)
2. Increase intake of low-fat dairy products and fresh fruits and vegetable that are high in calcium
3. Possibly take supplements if calcium intake is not achieved with food intake
4. Exercise outside to obtain adequate vitamin D intake from sunlight
5. Increase fiber content by 5 g/day with whole grains and fresh fruits and vegetables

Reassessment and Follow-Up

Assess progress every other week for the first 4 weeks, then monthly for the first 6 months, then 2–3 times per year thereafter.

Smoking-Cessation Program

Brief Smoking-Cessation Documentation

Patient information:
Name: L.K.   Date: March 9
Height: 5'1"   Weight: 105 lb   Age: 27 years
Comorbidities: None diagnosed
Medications: None
Family history: None for CHD, positive for osteoporosis
Smoking history: 1 ppd for 10 years

ASK	Current smoker, never has tried a quit attempt
ADVISE	Statement was made to L.K. that smoking places her at higher risk for osteoporosis and heart disease. Also, smoking can impact the health of her friends and family through secondhand smoke. L.K. was informed that the pharmacist and pharmacy staff could assist her if she would like to quit.
ASSESS	L.K. states that her grandmother smoked and that this may have contributed to her getting osteoporosis. L.K. states that she is now willing to make a quit attempt and will participate in the brief intervention program that the pharmacy offers.
ASSIST	A quit date was set for 1 week from today (March 16)

ASSIST L.K. was advised to tell her family, friends, and coworkers that she is quitting and to ask for their support.

L.K. was advised to remove all tobacco products from her home, car, work, and any other place she might have them. In addition, she was advised to have her house and car cleaned to remove smoky odors and establish a "clean or fresh start" to her quit attempt.

Counseling advice consisted of telling L.K.:

■ Do not smoke even a single puff after the quit date.
■ Her triggers are being around others who smoke and going to the bars. Advise her to avoid going to the bars and to be with those who do not smoke for several weeks.
■ Avoid time pressures and stress at work and home by being well organized.
■ Learn to anticipate and avoid temptation.
■ Exercise by walking with a partner on most days of the week to decrease weight gain and to feel good about herself.
■ Encourage L.K. to talk about the quitting process such as reasons for quitting and concerns and worries about quitting.

Pharmacotherapy recommendation:

■ Nicotine gum 2 mg, up to 24 pieces per day as needed. This is available OTC and has been shown to delay weight gain. Counsel L.K. about side effects of mouth soreness and dyspepsia.

ARRANGE   A follow-up phone call was arranged for the day before the quit date (March 15) and one week after the quit date (March 23).

CHAPTER 17: OSTEOARTHRITIS

SOAP Notes

S: E.P. states that she has osteoarthritis and does not like to take medications. She would like to participate in the pharmacy's osteoarthritis disease-management program.

O: Vitals: Height: 5'6"   Weight: 190 lb
   BMI: 30.5 kg/m²   Age: 73 years old
   HR: 76 beats/min   BP: 116/78 mm Hg
   Smoker: No
   Family history: None
   Current medications: Hydrochlorothiazide 50 mg daily, acetaminophen 1,000 mg every 6–8 hours
   Chronic diseases: Osteoarthritis, hypertension
   Risk factors for cardiovascular disease: Obesity, hypertension, sedentary lifestyle
   Caloric intake to maintain current body weight: 1,874 kcal/day
   Current average caloric intake per day: 2,150 kcal/day
   Alcohol consumption: None
   Current physical activity program: None
   Framingham risk score: Not available (no lipid panel)

A:

1. Osteoarthritis
2. Hypertension
3. Obesity
4. Sedentary lifestyle

P:

1. Counsel patient regarding proper management (pharmacologic and non-pharmacologic) of osteoarthritis
2. Counsel patient regarding risk factors for osteoarthritis
3. Counsel patient regarding risk factors for cardiovascular disease
4. Recommend weight-loss program
5. Recommend increased physical activity to help manage osteoarthritis symptoms and aid in weight loss
6. Recommend dietary changes to aid in weight loss and assist in the management of her hypertension

Exercise Program

Goals:

Short Term (4 weeks)

1. Participate in 20–30 minutes of accumulated light to moderate physical activity 3 days/week
2. Increase daily physical activity by participating in activities of daily living

Long Term (6 months)

1. Participate in 30–60 minutes of light to moderate intensity physical activity 3–5 days/week
2. Lose 10% body weight in 6 months

3. Improve symptoms of osteoarthritis
4. Improve functional status
5. Maintain quality of life
6. Decrease risk for CVD

Exercise Prescription

Activity	Frequency	Duration	Intensity	Progression
Aerobic (walking, biking, swimming, water aerobics)	3 times/week, initially and 3–5 times/week ideally	10 minutes initially, 30–60 minutes ideally (can divide into several sessions/day or one session with resting breaks if needed)	Light to moderate	Add 5 minutes to the duration each week up to 30–60 minutes, emphasizing duration over intensity
Resistance training (all major muscle groups)	2–3 days/week		2 sets of 10–12 repetitions	Begin with one set and increase to two sets after 2 weeks. Add weight to maintain 10–12 repetitions as needed
Flexibility (all major muscle groups)	Initially 2–3 days/week, ideally 5–7 days per week	Maintain each stretch 15–30 seconds, 2–4 sets per stretch		
Warm-up and cool-down	Before and after each aerobic and resistance training session	5–10 minutes	Low	

Increase daily lifestyle activity by taking stairs rather than elevators, walking dog when home, taking walks with spouse

Reassessment and Follow-Up

Assess progress every other week for first 4 weeks, then every other month for first 6 months, then 2–3 times per year thereafter.

Dietary Intervention
Goals:

Short Term (2 weeks)

1. Assess readiness for change
2. Overcome barriers to healthy eating
3. Reduce daily caloric intake by 350 kcal/day

Medium range (2–6 months)

1. Lose weight at a rate of approximately 1–1.5 pounds/week
2. Develop and adhere to a healthy eating plan

Long Term (>6 months)

1. Maintain weight loss
2. Reassess goals and set new goals for weight loss or weight maintenance
3. Decrease risk for CVD

Dietary Suggestions

1. Decrease daily calorie intake by 350 kcal/day
2. Decrease total fat intake by 6%
3. Decrease saturated fat intake by 4%
4. Decrease dietary cholesterol intake 100 mg/day
5. Increase fiber intake (gradually) by 11 g/day
6. Increase intake of whole grains, fruits, vegetables, and low-fat dairy products
7. Decrease sodium intake by 500 mg/day
8. Increase calcium intake by 240 mg/day

Reassessment and Follow-Up

Assess progress every other week for the first 4 weeks, then monthly for the first 6 months, then 2–3 times per year thereafter.

Weight-Loss Program

Weight-Loss Program Worksheet

Name: *EP*
Date of initial consultation: *March 22, 2006*
Gender: Male / **Female**
Age: *73* yr
Height: *66* inches
Height: *1.68* m (calculate by multiplying height in inches by 0.0254)
Weight: *190* lb
Weight: *86* kg (calculate by dividing weight in pounds by 2.2)
PA = Physical activity coefficient (calculate using the following table)

	Sedentary	Low active	Active	Very active
Male	1.0	1.11	1.25	1.48
Female	**1.0**	1.12	1.27	1.45

STEP 1: Calculate Body Mass Index (BMI) and Classify
BMI = [weight (kg) / height (m^2)]
BMI = [*86* kg / (*1.68* m)^2]
BMI = *30.5* kg/m^2

Classification of overweight and obesity according to BMI (circle)
<18.5 kg/m^2 Underweight
18.5–24.9 kg/m^2 Normal

25–29.9 kg/m²	Overweight
30–34.9 kg/m²	**Obesity Class I**
35–39.9 kg/m²	Obesity Class II
≥40 kg/m²	Obesity Class III or Extreme Obesity

STEP 2: Calculate the Estimated Energy Requirement (EER)

Males aged > 19 years:

EER = $662 - 9.53 \times$ age (yr) + PA $\times [15.9 \times$ weight (kg) + $540 \times$ height (m)]

EER = $662 - 9.53 \times$ ___ yr + ___ $\times [15.9 \times$ ___ kg + $540 \times$ ___ m

EER = ___ kcal

Females aged > 19 years:

EER = $354 - 6.91 \times$ age (yr) + PA $\times [9.36 \times$ weight (kg) + $726 \times$ height (m)]

EER = $354 - 6.91 \times$ *73* yr + *1.0* $\times [9.36 \times$ *86* kg + $726 \times$ *1.68* m

EER = *1,874* kcal

STEP 3: Calculate current caloric intake and eating patterns

Day 1 total calories: *2,050* kcal

Day 2 total calories: *2,250* kcal

Day 3 total calories: *2,130* kcal

Day 4 total calories: *2,170* kcal

Average total daily calories: *2,150* kcal

Suggested caloric deficit in food consumption per day: *350* kcal

Suggested caloric deficit in food consumption per week: *2,450* kcal (multiply by 7 to get weekly caloric deficit)

STEP 4: Design Exercise Prescription and Calculate Energy Expenditure

Examples of physical activity the patient prefers: *walking, bicycling, swimming, water aerobics (water aerobics will be used for the exercise prescription calculation)*

Weight loss goals:

1. *Lose 10% body weight within 6 months*

2. *Manage osteoarthritis symptoms and blood pressure*

3. *Decrease risk for coronary cardiovascular disease*

Exercise Prescription:

    Mode: *water aerobics*

      –associated MET level: *4.0*

    Intensity: *50–60% MHR* (% max heart rate or RPE)

    Duration: *30* minutes

    Frequency: *3* times per week

    Rate of Progression: *Focus should be on increasing duration (30–60 min) and frequency (5–7 times/week) over intensity*

Energy expenditure:

(METs $\times 3.5 \times$ body weight in kg) / 200 = kcal/min

($4.0 \times 3.5 \times 86$ kg) / 200 = *6.0* kcal/min (calories expended per minute of activity)

Multiply answer by the duration = calories expended per exercise session (kcal/session)
_6.0_ kcal/min × _30_ minutes = _180_ kcal/session
Multiply answer by frequency = calories expended per week (kcal/week)
_180_ kcal/session × _3_ times per week = _540_ kcal/week

STEP 5: Design a Weight Loss Program
A. Current body weight: _190_ lb
B. Weight loss goal: _10_%
C. Weight loss goal in pounds: _19_ lb (Step A × Step B)
D. Goal body weight: _171_ lb (Step A–Step C)
E. Goal BMI classification: _Overweight_ (Obtain from chart in STEP 1)
F. Weekly calories decreased from food consumption: _2,450_ kcal (Obtain from STEP 3)
G. Caloric expenditure per week from physical activity: _540_ kcal (Obtain from STEP 4)
H. Total weekly caloric deficit: _2,990_ kcal (Step F + Step G)
I. Amount of body weight lost per week: _0.85_ lb (Step H / 3,500 kcal)
J. Approximate time to achieve the goal weight: _22.4_ weeks (Step C/Step I): _5.6_ months (Step J/4)

CHAPTER 18: CHRONIC LUNG DISEASE

SOAP Notes

S: R.O. states, "During track practice I have trouble breathing. Is it because I am out of shape?"

O: Vitals: Height: 5′3″   Weight: 100 lb
BMI: 17.8 kg/m²   Age: 14 years
HR: 74 beats/min   BP: 110/60 mm Hg
Smoker: No
Family history: Mother has asthma
Current medications: None
Chronic diseases: Seasonal allergies
Risk factors for cardiovascular disease: None
Caloric intake to maintain current body weight: NA
Current average caloric intake per day: NA
Alcohol consumption: None
Current physical activity program: Member of the high school track team

A:

1. Exercise induces asthma-like symptoms during and after track practice
2. Seasonal allergies especially during the spring season

P:

1. Recommend R.O. visit her pediatrician about the possibility of asthma or exercise-induced asthma
2. Provide R.O. and her mother counseling and written information about EIA
3. Suggest to R.O. that her pediatrician provide her track coach with a note and information regarding her diagnosis
4. Instruct R.O. of ways in which she can self-manage her asthma symptoms by using peak flowmeter, proper medication, and the Borg RPE scale to assess her exercise intensity

Exercise Program

Goals:

1. Obtain evaluation from pediatrician regarding symptoms
2. Understand how to self-manage symptoms through the use of a peak flow-meter, proper medication, and the Borg RPE scale
3. Participate on the track team and be symptom free
4. Participate in any physical activity and be symptom free

Exercise Prescription

Activity	Frequency	Duration	Intensity	Progression
Jogging, running, cycling, swimming	3–7 times/week	30–45 minutes/session	Light to moderate, Borg RPE 11–14	Maintain current level
Resistance training (all major muscle groups)	2–3 days/week	2 sets of 10–12 repetitions	To fatigue	Maintain current level
Flexibility (all major muscle groups)	Initially 3–7 days/week	Maintain each stretch 20–60 seconds, 2–4 sets per stretch		
Warm-up and cool-down	Before and after each aerobic and resistance training session	5–10 minutes	Low, Borg RPE <10	
Maintain daily lifestyle activity by taking stairs rather than elevators, walking dog when home				

Reassessment and Follow-Up

Follow-up in 1 week to ensure pediatrician visit has occurred or is scheduled. Follow-up weekly for first months to ensure symptoms are under control and then periodically thereafter.

Glossary

A

acute coronary syndrome: A nonspecific term used to describe a number of emergent chest pain situations such as a myocardial infarction (MI) or heart attack, stable or unstable angina pectoris, and coronary artery vasospasm.

adenosine triphosphate (ATP): An energy-rich compound that releases free energy to power all forms of biologic work when the terminal phosphate bond is broken.

angina pectoris: A situation describing a decreased amount of blood perfusing the heart.

asthma: A chronic inflammatory disorder caused by a complex interaction between inflammatory cells and mediators that results in airway inflammation and hyperreactivity of the bronchial smooth muscles, which cause variable degrees of airway obstruction.

atherosclerosis: The process by which lipids are deposited on the inner layer of the arteries, and the fibrosis and thickening of the arterial wall.

atherosclerotic disease: See atherosclerosis.

B

basal metabolic rate (BMR): The energy that is required to complete cellular processes in the body necessary to sustain normal physiologic activities.

body composition: The relative amount of muscle, fat, bone, and other vital parts of the body.

body mass index (BMI): A method used to define obesity that uses a ratio of a person's height and weight.

Borg rating of perceived exertion (RPE): A way to monitor physical activity intensity based on how the patient feels.

C

caloric deficit: Also called negative caloric balance; when a person's net daily calories at the end of the day are fewer than those required to maintain current body weight, resulting in weight loss.

calorie: A measure of energy; a small calorie is the energy it takes to raise the temperature of 1 g of water 1°Celsius; a large Calorie is also referred to as a kilocalorie (kcal) or 1,000 small calories.

cancer: Also referred to as a neoplasm, tumor, or malignancy; a group of more than 100 diseases that are characterized by an uncontrolled growth and spread of abnormal cells.

cardiac output: The volume of blood ejected from the heart during a particular unit of time (i.e., per minute).

cardiorespiratory endurance: The ability of the body's circulatory and respiratory systems to supply fuel and oxygen during sustained physical activity.

cardiovascular disease (CVD): A broad term used to describe illnesses associated with the heart or vasculature system.

cholesterol: An important component of maintaining normal physiologic functioning that significantly increases the risk for cardiovascular disease when excess amounts are in the bloodstream.

chronic bronchitis: A disorder of excessive mucus secretion into the bronchial tree that is accompanied by a chronic cough.

chronic lung disease: A long-term pulmonary disorder such as asthma, chronic obstructive pulmonary disease (COPD), chronic bronchitis, emphysema, chronic rhinitis, cystic fibrosis, and drug-induced pulmonary diseases.

chronic obstructive pulmonary disease (COPD): A group of pulmonary diseases including emphysema, chronic bronchitis, and in some cases asthma that cause airflow blockage and breathing-related problems.

chylomicrons: Triglyceride-rich lipoproteins formed in the intestine and found in the blood after a dietary intake high in fat.

claudication: A primary symptom of peripheral arterial disease that is characterized by walking-induced pain in one or both legs (as a result of insufficient blood flow to the muscles) that does not subside until rest.

coronary heart disease (CHD): Also called ischemic heart disease; a complex disease process that ultimately results in an imbalance in the amount of oxygen that is able to supply the heart compared with the demand that it requires to function properly.

D

degenerative joint disease: See osteoarthritis.

diabetes mellitus: A syndrome that results from an absolute or relative lack of insulin to the cells of the body.

diastolic blood pressure: The force of blood against the walls of the arteries during diastole, or when blood is filling the ventricles of the heart.

dyslipidemia: A combination of increased blood lipid levels and lipoprotein concentrations that can be caused by environmental, genetic, and pathologic risk factors.

E

emphysema: A pulmonary disorder in which there is abnormal enlargement of the airspaces in the lungs with permanent damage to the bronchial walls.

endothelial dysfunction: Damage to the endothelium as a result of smoking and diseases such as diabetes, obesity, hypertension, and others that can play a critical role in the early stages of atherosclerosis.

endothelium: A monolayer of cells that line the interior lumen of arteries.

energy: The ability to perform work; is revealed only when change takes place.

essential body fat: A minimum amount of fat needed for the body to function normally. It is essential in the brain, heart, cell membranes, nerve tissue, and bone marrow.

essential hypertension: A patient diagnosed with high blood pressure for which there is no identifiable cause. Also, the most common type of hypertension.

estimated energy requirements (EER): The estimated number of calories needed to consume each day to meet the body's metabolic needs and to maintain current body weight.

exercise: Physical activity that is planned or structured and involves repetitive bodily movements done to improve or maintain one or more of the components of physical fitness.

exercise-induced asthma (EIA): Transient airway obstruction caused by participating in physical activity that usually occurs in cold or dry environments.

exercise-induced bronchospasm (EIB): See exercise-induced asthma.

exercise physiology: A subspecialty within the science of physiology that specifically looks at how organs, tissues, and cells in the body function as they relate to physical movement.

F

fat-free mass: Also called lean body mass; the portion of body composition that primarily consists of muscle tissue and internal organs.

fatty acids: Aliphatic acids that may be saturated or unsaturated and contain only carbon, oxygen, and hydrogen.

flexibility: The range of motion around the joint.

H

health literacy: The ability to read, understand, and use health information.

heart failure (HF): The inability of the heart to adequately deliver oxygen to the body.

hemorrhagic stroke: A stroke caused by bleeding in the brain.

high-density lipoprotein (HDL): Performs reverse cholesterol transport by taking excess cholesterol from tissues, such as coronary arteries, to be metabolized.

hypertension: Also called high blood pressure; an individual who has one of the three following criteria: (1) a systolic blood pressure of 140 mm Hg or higher, or a diastolic blood pressure of 90 mm Hg or higher; (2) taking antihypertensive medication; or (3) being told at least twice by a physician or other health professional that he or she has hypertension.

I

intermediate-density lipoprotein (IDL): A subfraction of LDL and is included in the LDL measurement in clinical practice.

ischemia: A term used to describe a situation in which little or no blood flow is getting to the heart muscle, brain, or other organs and tissues.

ischemic heart disease: Also called coronary heart disease; a complex disease process that ultimately results in an imbalance in the amount of oxygen that is able to supply the heart compared with the demand that it requires to function properly.

ischemic stroke: A stroke caused by lack of oxygen to the brain.

K

kcal (kilocalorie): 1,000 calories (used interchangeably with calorie); see calorie.

L

low-density lipoprotein (LDL): The major cholesterol transport lipoprotein; is mostly derived from LDL catabolism and cellular synthesis.

M

maximal aerobic power: See maximal oxygen uptake.

maximal oxygen consumption or uptake ($\dot{V}o_2$ max): The physiologic plateau of oxygen consumption.

metabolic equivalent (MET): A method to characterize physical activity at different levels of effort based on the amount of oxygen used by the body during that activity.

metabolic syndrome: A "constellation" of metabolic risk factors in one individual that includes atherogenic dyslipidemia (elevated triglycerides and apolipoprotein B, small LDL particles, and low HDL cholesterol concentrations), elevated blood pressure, elevated plasma glucose, a prothrombotic state, and a proinflammatory state.

monounsaturated fatty acid (MUFA): Fatty acids that contain a single double bond.

muscular endurance: The ability of the muscle to continue to perform without fatigue.

muscular strength: The ability of the muscle to exert force during an activity.

myocardial infarction (MI): A medical emergency in which little or no blood is circulating through the heart and often accompanied by chest pain and electrocardiogram (ECG) changes.

N

negative caloric balance: See caloric deficit.

net daily calories: The number of calories consumed in a day minus the number of calories expended through physical activity and metabolic activity.

O

obesity: Excess body fat that often leads to additional and significant health problems.

osteoarthritis: A degeneration of the articular cartilage as well as the underlying subchondral bone of a joint that can occur in any joint, but most commonly occurs in the knees, hips, hands, and spine.

osteoblasts: Cells that are responsible for building new bone to replace the bone that has been removed by the osteoclasts.

osteoclasts: Cells that are responsible for the degradation (also called resorption) of old bone.

osteoporosis: Means "porous bone;" characterized by low bone mass and a structural deterioration of bone tissue resulting in bone fragility and an increased risk of fractures of the hip, spine, and wrist.

oxygen consumption: The process by which the body takes in oxygen and uses it to move muscles during activity, especially aerobic activity.

P

peripheral arterial disease (PAD): Atherosclerosis of the lower extremity arteries diagnosed by the presence of lower-extremity pain with exertion, often called claudication, or absent or markedly diminished pulses on physical examination.

pharmacodynamics: The study of biochemical and physiologic effects of drugs and their mechanism of action.

pharmacokinetics: A discipline within pharmacology that studies a drug's absorption, distribution, metabolism, and excretion to predict how the drug will perform once it is administered.

physical activity: Any bodily movement produced by skeletal muscles that results in the expenditure of energy.

physical fitness: Components of exercise that include cardiorespiratory endurance (aerobic fitness), muscular strength, muscular endurance, flexibility, and body composition.

physical inactivity: A lack of any regular pattern of physical activity beyond that required for daily functioning.

polyunsaturated fatty acid (PUFA): Fatty acids that have two or more double bonds, which make the compound open to hydrogenation.

positive caloric balance: The net daily calorie intake is greater than what is required, resulting in weight gain.

prehypertension: An individual who has a systolic pressure of 120 to 139 mm Hg, or a diastolic pressure of 80 to 89 mm Hg in addition to not taking antihypertensive medication and having not been told by a physician or other health professional that he or she has hypertension.

primordial prevention: The concept of preventing chronic diseases through the prevention of the risk factors that cause diseases.

S

saturated fatty acid: Fatty acids that have all the chemical bonds filled; have been shown to be highly atherogenic.

self-efficacy: A fundamental concept in behavior change that states that for patients to make change they must believe in themselves and have confidence that they can execute the desired behavior.

storage fat: Excess body fat that is not required for the body to function normally.

stroke: A sudden onset of focal neurologic deficit that lasts for 24 hours or longer; thought to be caused by the vascular system.

systolic blood pressure: The force of blood against the walls of the arteries during systole, or when blood is ejected from the ventricles of the heart.

T

total body fat: A portion of the body composition that consists of both essential fat and storage fat.

***trans* fatty acid:** Unsaturated fatty acid in which hydrogen is on the opposite side of the double bond.

transient ischemic attack (TIA): The same definition as a stroke, but lasts for less than 24 hours and usually less than 30 minutes.

triglycerides: Glycerol (triacylglycerol) that has been esterified from three fatty acids; the main constituent of stored energy in adipose tissue that can contribute to the development of atherosclerosis and pancreatitis.

type 1 diabetes mellitus: An absolute lack of insulin or the inability of the pancreas to make and secrete insulin.

type 2 diabetes mellitus: A relative lack of insulin; accounts for 90 to 95% of all diabetics.

U

unsaturated fatty acid: Fatty acids that contain double or triple bonds available for hydrogenation.

V

very low-density lipoprotein (VLDL): Synthesized in the liver; primary transport mechanism for endogenous triglyceride.

V̇o₂ max: See maximal oxygen uptake.

Index

Page numbers in *italics* denote figures; those followed by a t denote tables.

A

Abdominal aortic aneurysm, 136

Abdominal obesity
metabolic syndrome and, 231
stroke risk and, 162

ABI (*See* Ankle-brachial index)

ACE inhibitors, 53t, 126t, 143, 150, 150t, 158t, 176t

Acetaminophen, 270

ACSM (*See* American College of Sports Medicine)

Activities of daily living (ADL), 298–299

Acute coronary syndrome (ACS), 134, 145, 359

ADA (*See* American Diabetes Association; American Dietetic Association)

Adenosine triphosphate (ATP), 32, 139, 359

ADL (*See* Activities of daily living)

Adolescents (*See also* Children)
exercise recommendations for, 245
metabolic syndrome among, 228

Adult-onset diabetes mellitus, 197 (*See also* Type 2 diabetes mellitus)

Adult Treatment Panel III (ATP III), 134, 136–137, 138
on coronary heart disease, 152
on metabolic syndrome, 227–228, 228, 230
nutritional guidelines, 232, 233
on peripheral artery disease, 178
on stroke, 164

Aerobic exercise, 32, *34,* 35–36, 65
for cancer survivors, 246
coronary heart disease and, 139–140, 153
diabetes and, 208
metabolic syndrome and, 234–235
osteoarthritis and, 268
stroke and, 165, 167

Aerobic metabolism, 32

African Americans
childhood obesity among, 288

coronary heart disease among, 305
diabetes among, 198
hypertension among, 305
metabolic syndrome among, 229
obesity among, 305
physical activity by, 306
smoking rates among, 86

Age/aging (*See also* Older adults)
impact of, 296–297
metabolic syndrome and, 228
smoking and, 86

AHA (*See* American Heart Association)

Alaska Natives, diabetes mellitus among, 198, 305

Alcohol consumption
beneficial health effects of, 25–26
calories in, 7
cancer and, 243
chronic disease and, 6
diabetes and, 205–206
disease prevention and, 24–26
heart failure and, 188

Alcohol consumption (*cont.*)
  hypertension and, 122, 123t
  osteoporosis and, 253, 254
  recommended amounts of,
    18
Aldosterone receptor blockers,
    126t, 188t
Allergens, 275
α₁-Antitrypsin replacement
    therapy, 276t
α-blockers, 126t
α-glucosidase inhibitors, 202t
Amenorrhea, 258
American Cancer Society, 245
American College of Cardiology
  exercise recommendations
    for post-myocardial
    infarction, 149
  Guidelines for the Manage-
    ment of Patients with
    Peripheral Arterial
    Disease, 175–176,
    177, 179
  heart failure guidelines,
    187, 188
American College of Sports
    Medicine (ACSM), 16,
    29
  aerobic exercise recommen-
    dations, 35
    for older adults, 298
  exercise recommendations,
    41, 43, 46, 153, 180, 306
    for asthma patients, 279
    for cancer survivors, 247
    for diabetes patients, 208
    for hypertension patients,
      128
    to lower cancer risk, 245
    for obese/overweight
      patients, 66, 224
    for osteoarthritis patients,
      268
    for osteoporosis patients,
      259, 260t
    for peripheral arterial dis-
      ease patients, 177
    for pregnant women, 304
  resistance training recom-
    mendations, 36
American Diabetes Asso-
    ciation (ADA), 203
American Dietetic Association
    (ADA), 16

American Heart Association
    (AHA), 11, 29, 106, 138
  diet and stroke risk recom-
    mendations, 163
  dietary recommendations
    for children and ado-
    lescents, 292–293
  exercise recommendations,
    41, 179, 180
    for peripheral arterial dis-
      ease patients, 177
    for post-myocardial
      infarction patients,
      149
  on fatty acid intake, 233
  Go Red for Women cam-
    paign, 301
  Guidelines for the Manage-
    ment of Patients with
    Peripheral Arterial
    Disease, 175–176, 177,
    179
  heart failure guidelines,
    187, 188
  on metabolic syndrome, 228
  on prevention of cardio-
    vascular disease in
    women, 302
  promotion of physical activ-
    ity and, 153
  Scientific Statement for
    healthcare profession-
    als, 155
American Indians, diabetes
    mellitus among, 198,
    305
American Pharmacists
    Association, 140, 260
Amiodarone, 54t
Amlodipine, 168
Angina pectoris, 145, 146, 359
Angiotensin-converting enzyme
    (ACE) inhibitors, 53t,
    126t, 148, 150, 150t,
    176t, 188t
Angiotensin II antagonists, 126t
Angiotensin II receptor block-
    ers (ARB), 148, 188t
Ankle-brachial index (ABI), 174
Anticholinergics, 276t
Anticoagulants, 163t
Antihypertensive drugs, 124,
    126t
Antimicrobial agents, 276t
Antioxidants, 14, 302

Antiplatelets, 150t, 163t, 176t,
    231t
Aortoiliac atherosclerosis, 174
ARB (*See* Angiotensin II recep-
    tor blockers)
Arthritis (*See also* Osteoarthritis)
  physical activity and, 30
Arthritis Foundation, 268, 269
Asheville Project, on asthma,
    113, 281–282
Asian Americans
  osteoporosis among, 252,
    304, 305
  smoking rates among, 86
Aspirin therapy, 54t, 150, 231t,
    302
Asthma, 273, 359
  Asheville Project, 113,
    281–282
  case study, 282
  exercise-induced, 277
  medications for, 276t, 277
  nutritional recommenda-
    tions for people with,
    278–279, 279t
  pathophysiology of, 274, 275t
  pharmacist-managed care
    of, 113
  physical activity and,
    279–280, 281t
  prevalence of, 274
  prevention of, 275–278, 276t
  secondhand smoke and, 90
  smoking and, 277
  treatment of, 275–278, 276t
Atenolol, 53t
Atherogenic diet, 231
Atherosclerosis, 86–87, 134,
    135, 146, 173, 359
  heart failure and, 187
  prehypertension and, 130
  stroke and, 160, 162
Atherosclerotic disease, 359
Atherosclerotic process, 293
Atherothrombosis, 146
ATP (*See* Adenosine
    triphosphate)
ATP III (*See* Adult Treatment
    Panel III)
Autonomic neuropathy, 212t

B
Banded gastroplasty, 221
Basal metabolic rate (BMR), 7,
    296–297, 359

B-complex vitamins, 14, 15t
Behavioral counseling, smoking cessation and, 92–93
Behavioral Risk Factor Surveillance System (BRFSS), 104
Behavior change, 103–113
    program adherence and barriers to, 106–108, 107t
        healthcare system and provider related, 107t, 108
        patient-related, 106–108
        pharmacy practice and, 112–113
    strategies, 108–112
        motivational counseling, 111–112
        patient-related, 109t
        program-related, 110–111t
    theories and models, 104–106
        5 A's behavioral intervention protocol, 105–106
        health belief model, 105
        social cognitive theory, 106
        transtheoretical model of change, 105
Behavior therapy, 68
    for coronary heart disease, 151, 152t
    for obesity, 220, 220t
Benzodiazepines, 94
Benzphetamine, 68t
β₂ agonists, 276t
β-blockers, 94, 126t, 150, 150t, 176t, 188t
    exercise interaction, 50, 52, 53t, 276
    target heart rate and, 41
β-carotene, 14
Bicycling, 42t
Biguanides, 202t
Bile acid sequestrants, 137t
Biotin, 14
Bisphosphonates, 254t
Blacks (See African Americans)

Blood pressure (See also Diastolic blood pressure; Systolic blood pressure)
    classification of, 121t
    sibutramine effects on, 68
    stroke risk and, 161
BMI (See Body mass index)
BMR (See Basal metabolic rate)
Body composition, 30, 59–60, 359
    defined, 60
Body fat, 60
    essential, 60, 360
    storage, 60, 363
    subcutaneous, 60
    total, 60, 362
Body mass index (BMI), 59–60, 59t, 359
    calculating, 70, 72, 80
    in childhood obesity, 288
    desired, in women, 302
    metabolic syndrome and, 231
    obesity and, 216
    sedentary patients with normal BMI vs. active patients with obese BMI, 66–67
    stroke risk and, 162
    table, 315
    weight loss and, 61
Body weight
    hypertension and, 126
    osteoporosis and, 254
Bone health, overtraining and, 258
Bone loss, 297
Bone mass, resistance training and, 36
Bone remodeling, 252
Borg rating of perceived exertion (RPE), 40, 40–41, 279–280, 359
Breast cancer, 240, 303
    alcohol consumption and, 25
    exercise and, 153, 180
    obesity and, 57, 217t, 243
    physical activity and, 243
BRFSS (See Behavioral Risk Factor Surveillance System)
Bronchitis, chronic, 273, 274, 275, 360

Bronchodilators, 54t
Bupropion, 176t
Bupropion SR, 94, 96t, 99
Butter, margarine vs., 12–13

C
Caffeine, 94, 95
Calcitonin, 254t
Calcium, 15t
    diabetes and, 205
    heart failure and, 191t
    hypertension and, 124, 126, 127t
    older adults and, 297
    for osteoporosis, 254t, 255–257, 256t, 304
    recommended daily amount of, 20t
Calcium-channel blockers, 53t, 126t
Caloric balance, 62–63
Caloric balance equation, 62–63
Caloric deficit, 63, 221, 267, 359
Caloric intake
    aging and, 297
    calculating, 71, 73–78, 78, 81
    estimation of, 9t
    of fats, 138
    recommended
        adult, 9t
        children, 293
Calories, 7, 359
    counting, 22–23
    food labeling and, 21, 21–22, 23
    net daily, 63, 361
Cancer, 239–248, 359 (See also individual cancers)
    body mass index and, 67
    economic costs of, 240
    health risks of, 240
    lifestyle behaviors and, 6
    nutrition and, 5, 243–245, 245t
        obesity, 57, 217t, 243
        program adherence, 244–245, 244t
    overview, 239
    pathophysiology of, 240, 241t
    pharmacy practice application, 247–248
    physical activity and, 245–247, 246t
    prevalence of, 240

Cancer (*cont.*)
  prevention of, 240–243, 242t
    physical activity and, 243
    tobacco use, 86, 87t,
      88–89, 242–243
  treatment of, 240–243
  women and, 303
Carbohydrates, 6, 9–10
  diabetes mellitus and, 204,
    205t, 210
  dietary recommendations
    for coronary heart disease
      patients, 153t
    for heart failure patients,
      191t
    for hypertension patients,
      127t
    for osteoporosis patients,
      256t
    for peripheral arterial dis-
      ease patients, 179t
    for stroke patients, 165t
  energy derived from, 7
  recommended amounts of,
    18, 20t
Cardiac output, 50, 121, 186,
    359
  aging and, 296
Cardiac rehabilitation, 150
  exercise and, 154
Cardiogenic emboli, 160
Cardiorespiratory endurance,
    30, 359–360
Cardiovascular disease (CVD),
    145, 360
  diabetes and, 203
  diet and, 16
  economic costs of, 134
  hypertension and, 121
  lifestyle behaviors and, 6
  metabolic syndrome and, 227
  peripheral arterial disease
    and, 174
  physical activity and, 29, 65,
    164
  prehypertension and, 129
  risk of, in older adults, 299
  smoking and, 85, 86–88, 87t
  women and, 301–302, 303
Cardiovascular function, in
    older adults, 298
Carvedilol, 53t
Case studies
  cancer, 247–248, 346–348

chronic lung disease, 282,
    356–357
coronary heart disease,
    155–156, 322–325
diabetes mellitus, 212–213,
    335–337
dyslipidemia, 142, 319–322
heart failure, 193–194,
    331–335
hypertension, 130–131,
    317–319
metabolic syndrome, 236,
    341–346
obesity, 225, 337–341
osteoarthritis, 270,
    351–356
osteoporosis, 261, 349–351
peripheral arterial disease,
    181, 327–331
smoking cessation, 100–101,
    324–325, 327, 330–331,
    345–346, 351
stroke, 168–169, 325–327
weight control, 72–82,
    333–335, 339–341,
    343–345, 354–356
CDE (*See* Certified diabetes
    educator)
Centers for Disease Control
    and Prevention (CDC)
  on childhood obesity, 288
  on chronic disease, 1
  exercise recommendations,
    35, 41, 43, 46, 153, 180,
    279, 306
Central α_2 agonists, 126t
Cerebral infarction, 160
Cerebrovascular disease,
    hypertension and, 120
Certified diabetes educator
    (CDE), 211
CHD (*See* Coronary heart
    disease)
Childhood obesity, 218–219,
    287, 288–289
  causes of, 288–289
  nutrition and, 292–293
  physical activity and,
    291–292
  prevention of, 289–291
    community organization
      involvement, 290
    family involvement, 291

federal, state, and local
    government involve-
    ment, 289
  healthcare provider
    involvement, 290
  industry and media
    involvement, 289–290
  pharmacist's role in,
    293–294
  school system involve-
    ment, 290–291
Children, 287–294
  dietary recommendations
    for, 293
    calcium, 256
  disease prevention in, 287
  exercise recommendations
    for, 245
  metabolic syndrome
    among, 228
Chlorpromazine, 94
Chocolate, disease prevention
    and dark, 24
Cholesterol, 360 (*See also*
    High-density lipopro-
    tein (HDL) cholesterol;
    Low-density lipoprotein
    (LDL) cholesterol)
  blood levels of, 134
    coronary heart disease
      and, 149
    in dyslipidemia, 134
    heart failure and, 187
    managing, 136
    metabolic syndrome and,
      233
    stroke risk and, 162
    in women, 302
  dietary, 13
    average daily intake, 138
    childhood intake of, 293
    diabetes and, 204–205,
      205t
    food labeling and, 22
    foods high in, 12t
    hypertension and, 124
    nutrition and, 6
    recommendations
      for dyslipidemia
        patients, 139t
      for heart failure patients,
        191t
      for hypertension
        patients, 127t

for osteoporosis patients, 256t

recommended amounts of, 18, 20t

stroke prevention and, 162, 165t

Chronic bronchitis, 273, 274, 275, 360

Chronic diseases, 117

nutrition and, 5–6

obesity and, 57

Chronic kidney disease (CKD), coronary heart disease and, 147–148

Chronic lung disease, 242–243, 273–282, 360

economic costs of, 274

health risks of, 274

nutrition and, 278–279, 279t

overview, 273–274

pathophysiology of, 274–275, 275t

asthma, 274

COPD, 274–275

pharmacy practice application, 280–282

case study, 282

physical activity and, 279–280, 281t

prevalence of, 274

prevention of, 275–278

treatment of, 275–278, 276t, 278t

Chronic obstructive pulmonary disease (COPD), 273, 274, 360

nutritional recommendations for people with, 279t

obesity and, 57

pathophysiology of, 274–275, 275t

physical activity and, 278, 280, 281t

prevention of, 275–278, 276t

smoking and, 277

treatment of, 275–278, 276t

medications for, 276t

Chronic rhinitis, 273

Chylomicrons, 135, 360

CKD (*See* Chronic kidney disease)

Claudication, 174, 360

Clinical Guidelines on the Identification, Evaluation, and Treatment of Overweight and Obesity in Adults, 216, 218

Clonidine, 95, 97t

Clozapine, 94

Colon cancer, 240

obesity and, 57, 217t, 243

physical activity and, 30, 153, 180, 243

in women, 303

Community interventions, to increase physical activity, 151

Community organization role in preventing childhood obesity, 290, 294

Commuting, stroke risk and, 165–166

Complex carbohydrates, 9, 10, 11t

Congenital cardiovascular defects, 145

Congestive heart failure (*See* Heart failure)

Consumer nutrition, 19–22

Cool-down, 35

COPD (*See* Chronic obstructive pulmonary disease)

Coronary artery disease

heart failure and, 187, 193

obesity and, 217t

physical activity and lowered risk of, 30

Coronary artery vasospasm, 145

Coronary heart disease (CHD), 145–156, 360

aging and, 296

alcohol consumption and, 25

body mass index and, 67

as cause of death, 134

chronic kidney disease and, 147–148

dietary cholesterol and, 13

dietary fiber and, 10

economic costs of, 146

environmental risk factors, 147t

ethnicity and, 305

exercise prescription and, 45

Framingham Heart Study, 311–314

health behaviors contributing to, 104

health risks, 146

hypertension and, 120

lipoproteins and, 136

metabolic syndrome and, 228

nutrition and, 152, 153t

overview, 145–146

pathophysiology of, 146–148, 147t

peripheral arterial disease and, 174

pharmacy practice application, 154–156

case study, 155–156

physical activity and, 30, 139, 153–154, 154t

prevalence of, 146

prevention of, 148–152

primary coronary heart disease, 148–149

secondary coronary heart disease, 149–150

risk factors for, 188

smoking cessation and, 90

stress and, 229

trans fatty acids and, 12, 138

treatment of

behavior therapy, 151–152, 152t

drug therapy, 150, 150t

in women, 301, 302

Corticosteroids, 276t

CP (creatine phosphate), 32

CVD (*See* Cardiovascular disease)

Cystic fibrosis, 273

D

Daily activities, *34*

Dance, 42t

DASH (Dietary Approaches to Stop Hypertension) eating plan, 17, 122, 123t, 124, 127t, 190–191, 255

Degenerative joint disease, 263, 360 (*See also* Osteoarthritis)

Delayed onset muscle soreness (DOMS), 141

Depression

exercise and, 153, 180

Depression (*cont.*)
  non-adherence and, 112–113
  obesity and, 217t
Diabetes mellitus, 112,
    197–213, 360 (*See also*
    Type 1 diabetes melli-
    tus; Type 2 diabetes
    mellitus)
  body fat and, 60
  chronic kidney disease and,
    147, 148
  dietary therapy and, 63
  dyslipidemia and, 136
  economic costs of, 198
  ethnicity and, 305
  gestational, 198, 303, 304
  health risks of, 198
  heart failure and, 188
  lifestyle behaviors and, 6
  lower extremity disease and,
    176–177
  nutrition and, 5, 203–206,
    205t, 221
    alcohol and, 205–206
    carbohydrates and, 204
    dietary fats and, 204–205
    protein and, 204
    vitamins and minerals,
      205
  obesity and, 217t
  overview, 197
  pathophysiology of,
    198–199, 200t
  peripheral arterial disease
    and, 174, 175
  pharmacist-managed care
    of, 113
  pharmacy practice applica-
    tion, 211–213
    case study, 212–213
  physical activity and, 30,
    206–211, 207t
    safety considerations,
      210–211, 211t, 212t
  prevalence of, 198
  prevention of, 200–203
  stroke and, 162
  treatment of, 200–203, 202t
  women and, 302, 303
Diabetes Prevention Program,
    201–202
Diabetic neuropathy, 208
Diastolic blood pressure, 120,
    360

heart failure and, 187
physical activity and, 128
sibutramine and, 68, 221
stroke risk and, 161
Diet (*See also* Nutrition)
  dietary suggestions (case
    studies)
    cancer, 348
    coronary heart disease, 324
    diabetes mellitus, 337
    dyslipidemia, 321
    hypertension, 319
    metabolic syndrome, 343
    obesity, 339
    osteoarthritis, 354
    osteoporosis, 350
    peripheral arterial disease,
      329–330, 333
    stroke, 327
  dietary therapy, 63–65
  poor, as cause of death, 85
  very low-calorie, 63, 64, 222
Dietary Approaches to Stop
    Hypertension (DASH)
    eating plan, 17, 122,
    123t, 124, 127t,
    190–191, 255
Dietary fiber, 9, 10, 11t
  diabetes and, 205t
  hypertension and, 124, 126
  recommendations
    for coronary heart disease
      patients, 153t
    for dyslipidemia patients,
      139t
    for heart failure patients,
      191t
    for hypertension patients,
      127t
    for osteoporosis patients,
      256t
    for peripheral arterial dis-
      ease patients, 179t
  recommended daily amount
    of, 20t
Dietary Guidelines for
    Americans 2005, 9,
    16–18, 19, 23, 138, 164,
    178, 190, 232, 244, 255,
    279, 297
Diethylpropion, 68t
Digoxin, 53t, 188t
  pharmacokinetic and exer-
    cise interaction, 189

Disaccharides, 10
Disease prevention
  alcohol and, 24–26
  in children, 287
  dark chocolate and, 24
  income level and, 305–306
  key minerals and, 15t
  key vitamins and, 15t
  lifestyle modification and, 1–3
  in minorities, 305–307
  in older adults, 295–296
  physical activity and, 30–31
  in women, 301–305
Diseases
  chronic, 5–6, 57, 117
  obesity-related, 217t
  resulting from hypertension,
    123t
  smoking-related, 86–89, 87t
Diuretics, 126t, 188t
DOMS (*See* Delayed onset
    muscle soreness)
Drug-exercise interaction,
    50–52, 53–54t
Drug-induced hypertension,
    122t
Drugs
  antihypertensive, 124, 126t
  asthma, 276t, 277
  COPD, 276t, 277
  coronary heart disease, 150,
    150t
  diabetes, 201, 202t
  dyslipidemia, 137t
  heart failure, 188t
  metabolic syndrome, 231t
  obesity, 68, 220–221, 221t
  optimal medication therapy,
    280–281
  osteoarthritis, 265t
  osteoporosis, 254t
  osteoporosis and, 254
  peripheral arterial disease,
    176, 176t
  smoking and, 94–95
  smoking cessation, 94–95,
    96–97t, 99–100
  stroke or TIA, 163t
Dyslipidemia, 133–142, 360
  coronary heart disease and,
    149
  defined, 134
  depression and, 112
  diabetes and, 203

diet and, 16
  dietary therapy, 63
economic costs of, 134
health risks of, 134
heart failure risk and, 193
metabolic syndrome and, 227
nutrition and, 138, 139t, 221
overview, 133
overweight and, 148
pathophysiology of,
  134–136, 135t
peripheral arterial disease
  and, 174
pharmacy practice and,
  140–142, 155
  case study, 142
physical activity and, 139–140,
  140t
prevention of, 136–137
stroke and, 162
treatment of, 136–137

E
Economic costs
  of cancer, 240
  of chronic diseases, 1–2, 30
  of chronic lung disease, 274
  of coronary heart disease, 146
  of diabetes mellitus, 198
  of dyslipidemia, 134
  of heart failure, 186
  of hypertension, 120
  of metabolic syndrome, 228
  of obesity, 30, 57, 59, 216
  of osteoarthritis, 264
  of osteoporosis, 252
  of stroke, 160
Education, smoking preva-
  lence and, 86
EER (See Estimated energy
  requirements)
Eggs, as source of cholesterol,
  13, 138
EIA (See Exercise-induced
  asthma)
EIB (See Exercise-induced
  bronchospasm)
Emphysema, 273, 274, 275,
  360
Endothelial dysfunction, 24,
  174, 360
  smoking and, 87–88
Endothelium, 87–88, 360
End-stage renal disease, 147

Energy, 6, 360
  defined, 32
  estimated energy require-
    ments, 7–8, 8t, 70, 72,
    77, 80, 360
  food as, 6–16
  stored, 135
Energy expenditure
  calculating, 71, 73t, 78–79
  caloric intake and, 288
  goals, 44
Environmental risk factors
  for asthma and COPD,
    275t
  for cancer, 241t
  for coronary heart disease,
    147t
  for diabetes mellitus, 200t
  for dyslipidemia, 135t
  for heart failure, 187
  for metabolic syndrome,
    229t
  for obesity, 217t
  for osteoarthritis, 265t
  for osteoporosis, 253t
  for peripheral arterial dis-
    ease, 175t
  for stroke, 161t
Epidemic, defined, 288
Epinephrine, 88
Essential body fat, 60, 360
Essential hypertension, 120,
  122t, 360
Estimated energy requirements
  (EER), 7–8, 360
  calculating, 70, 72, 77, 80
  estimating, 8t
Estrogens, for osteoporosis,
  254t
Ethnicity
  childhood obesity and, 288
  diabetes mellitus and, 198
  obesity and, 216
  osteoporosis and, 252, 304
  smoking and, 86
Etiology, of hypertension,
  120–121, 122t
Exercise, 360 (See also Aerobic
  exercise; Physical activity; Resistance training)
  accumulating time through-
    out day, 292
  aging and, 296
  asthma and, 277

bone health and overtraining in women, 258
for cancer survivors, 246–247
claudication and, 174
coronary heart disease and,
  134, 149
defined, 30
diabetes mellitus and, 197
digoxin pharmacokinetics
  and, 189
footwear and, 208
heart failure and, 186
metabolic syndrome and,
  231
muscle pain and, 141
nutrition and, 6
osteoarthritis and, 265
peripheral arterial disease
  and, 176–177
stretching, 34, 37, 167
stroke risk and, 165–166
weight-bearing, 258–259, 260t
Exercise-induced asthma
  (EIA), 277, 280, 360
Exercise-induced broncho-
  spasm (EIB), 277, 360
Exercise physiology, 32–33, 360
  energy, 32
  oxygen consumption, 32–33
Exercise prescriptions
  legal issues with, 45–46
  principles, 37–44
    duration, 41–43
    energy expenditure goals,
      44
    frequency, 43
    intensity, 38
    metabolic equivalent
      level, 41, 42t
    patient goals, 37–38
    rate of perceived exer-
      tion, 40, 40–41
    rate of progression, 43–44
    talk test, 39
    target heart rate, 39–40
    type of physical activity, 38
  sample, 78–79, 81
    cancer, 347–348
    chronic lung disease, 357
    coronary heart disease, 323
    diabetes mellitus, 336
    dyslipidemia, 320–321
    heart failure, 332
    hypertension, 318

Exercise prescriptions, sample (*cont.*)
  metabolic syndrome, 342
  obesity, 338
  osteoarthritis, 353
  osteoporosis, 350
  peripheral arterial disease, 328–329
  stroke, 326
Exertion, rate of perceived, *40*, 40–41
Expert Panel on Detection, Evaluation, and Treatment of High Blood Cholesterol in Adults (*See* Adult Treatment Panel III)
Extratreatment social support, 99
  smoking cessation and, 93, 93t, 99

F
Falls
  decreasing risk for, 298
  prevention of, 254
Family role in preventing childhood obesity, 291
Fat-free mass, 60, 360
Fats, 6, 10–13
  diabetes and dietary, 204–205, 205t
  energy derived from, 7
  food labeling and, 22
  monounsaturated (*See* Monounsaturated fats)
  polyunsaturated (*See* Polyunsaturated fats)
  recommendations for hypertension patients, 127t
  recommendations for osteoporosis patients, 256t
  recommended amounts of, 18, 20t
  saturated (*See* Saturated fats)
Fatty acids, 10–11, 135, 360
  monounsaturated, 11, 12t, 361
  polyunsaturated, 11, 12t, 362
  saturated, 11, 12t, 233, 362
  trans, 11–12, 138, 152, 205, 233, 362

  unsaturated, 11, 12t, 138, 152, 153t, 233, 362
FDA (*See* Food and Drug Administration)
Federal government, role in childhood obesity, 289
Female-type obesity, 60
Fexofenadine, 46
Fiber (*See* Dietary fiber)
Fibric acid derivatives, 137t
Fibric acids, myopathy and, 141
Financial barriers to program adherence, 107
5 A's behavioral intervention protocol, 105–106
Flavonoids, 24
Flecainide, 94
Flexibility, 360
  aging and, 298
  defined, 30
  exercises
    for obese patients, 224
    for osteoarthritis patients, 268
    for stroke survivors, 167
Fluid needs, of older adults, 297
Fluvoxamine, 94, 95
Folate, 14, 15t, 205
Folic acid, 17
Food allergens, asthma and, 278
Food and Drug Administration (FDA), 68, 94, 204, 220
Food diary, 73, *74–77*
Food labeling/labels, 19–22, *21, 23,* 257
Food(s)
  as energy, 6–16
  food groups to encourage, 17–18
  high in protein, 14t
  high in saturated/unsaturated fatty acids and cholesterol, 12t
Footwear, exercise and, 208
Framingham Heart Study, 136, 174, 230, 307
  Point Score Table, 302, 311–314
Fructose, 10
Fruits
  lowering cancer risk and eating, 243

  lowering stroke risk and eating, 163, 165t
  recommended amounts of, 17–18, 20t

G
Galactose, 10
Gastric bypass, 221
Gender (*See also* Men; Women)
  metabolic syndrome and, 228
  osteoporosis and, 252, 253
Genetics
  cancer risk and, 240
  hypertension and, 120
Gestational diabetes, 198, 303, 304
Glucose, 10
Glycemic control, exercise and, 209, 210
Government role in preventing childhood obesity, 289, 294
Grains, whole, 10, 18, 20t

H
Haloperidol, 94
HDL (*See under* High-density lipoprotein)
Health behavior change (*See* Behavior change)
Health belief model, 105
Healthcare provider role in preventing childhood obesity, 290
Healthcare system, U.S.
  barriers to program adherence and, 107t, 108
  chronic disease costs and, 1–2
  effect of disease prevention on, 2t
Health literacy, 108, 360
Health risks
  of cancer, 240
  of chronic lung disease, 274
  of coronary heart disease, 146
  of diabetes mellitus, 198
  of dyslipidemia, 134
  of heart failure, 186
  of hypertension, 120
  of metabolic syndrome, 228
  of obesity, 216
  of osteoarthritis, 263–264

of osteoporosis, 252
of peripheral arterial disease, 174
of stroke, 160
Healthy People 2010, 86
Heart attack (*See* Myocardial infarction)
Heart disease
  atherosclerotic process and, 293
  nutrition and, 5
  pre-diabetes and, 198
  type 2 diabetes and, 199
Heart failure (HF), 145, 177, 185–194, 360
  economic costs of, 186
  health risks of, 186
  Heart Failure Guidelines, 188
  hypertension and, 120
  nutrition and, 190–191, 191t
  obesity and, 217t
  overview, 185
  pathophysiology of, 186–187, 187t
  pharmacy practice application, 193–194
    case study, 193–194
  physical activity and, 191–192, 192t
  prevalence of, 185–186
  prevention of, 187–190
  sibutramine and, 68
  treatment of, 187–190, 188t, 190t
Hemorrhagic stroke, 159, 160–161, 360
Heparin, 94
HF (*See* Heart failure)
High blood pressure (*See* Hypertension)
High-density lipoprotein (HDL), 88, 135, 136, 361
High-density lipoprotein (HDL) cholesterol, 24
  (*See also* Cholesterol)
  alcohol consumption and, 25
  body fat and, 60
  exercise and levels of, 292
  increasing, 136, 139
  metabolic syndrome and, 227
  type 2 diabetes and, 199
Hispanics
  childhood obesity among, 288

diabetes mellitus among, 305
  smoking rates among, 86
HIV/AIDS, depression and, 112
HMG-CoA (3-hydroxy-3-methylglutaryl co-enzyme A), 162
HMG-CoA reductase inhibitors (statins), 137t, 141, 162, 176t
Hormone therapy, 302
Household physical activities, 33, 42t
Human insulin inhalation powder (Exubera), 95
Hydrochlorothiazide, 130, 193, 270
Hyperglycemia, 198
  defined, 210
  signs and symptoms, 211t
Hyperlipidemia, 134
  heart failure and, 187
  lifestyle behaviors and, 6
  obesity and, 57
  physical activity and, 30
  stroke and, 162
Hypertension, 119–131, 145, 361
  in African Americans, 305
  alcohol consumption and, 25
  body fat and, 60
  body mass index and, 67
  chronic kidney disease and, 147
  controlling, 89
  coronary heart disease and, 149
  defined, 120
  depression and, 112
  diabetes and, 198, 199, 203
  diet and, 16
    dietary therapy, 63
  disease outcomes from, 123t
  economic costs of, 120
  essential, 120, 122t, 360
  etiology of, 120–121, 122t
  exercise and, 48–49, 153, 292
  health risks associated with, 120
  heart failure and, 187–188, 193
  lifestyle behaviors and, 6
  nutrition and, 221
  obesity and, 57, 217t
  overview, 119

overweight and, 148
  pathophysiology of, 120–121, 122t
  peripheral arterial disease and, 174
  pharmacy practice application, 129–131
    case study, 130–131
  physical activity and, 30
  prehypertension, 129–130
  prevalence of, 120
  prevention and treatment of, 121–129, 123t
    antihypertensive agents, 126t
    nutrition and, 124–127, 127t
    physical activity and, 128–129, 129t
    program adherence recommendations, 125t
  secondary, 120, 122t
  sodium intake and, 18
  stroke and, 161–162
  in women, 302
Hypoglycemia
  defined, 210
  signs and symptoms, 211t
Hypoplastic aortoiliac syndrome, 175

I
IDL (*See* Intermediate-density lipoprotein)
Illicit drug use, heart failure and, 188
Income
  disease prevention and, 305–306
  smoking prevalence and, 86
Industry involvement in childhood obesity, 289–290
Injury
  avoiding activity-induced, 47t
  obesity and risk of orthopedic, 66
Institute of Medicine (IOM), 108, 287, 288, 289, 290
Insulin, 202t, 210
  effects of physical activity on levels of, 54–55, 54t
  exercise and injecting, 210–211
  interaction with smoking, 94, 95

Intermediate-density lipoprotein (IDL), 135, 361
Intratreatment social support, 99
IOM (*See* Institute of Medicine)
Iron, 15t, 17
Ischemia, 146, 159, 361
Ischemic heart disease, 112, 361 (*See also* Coronary heart disease)
Ischemic stroke, 145, 159, 179, 361
  environmental factors increasing risk of, 161t

J
JNC 7 (Seventh Report of the Joint National Committee of Prevention, Detection, Evaluation, and Treatment of High Blood Pressure), 120, 124, 152, 164, 178

K
kcal (kilocalorie), 7, 361
Kidney disease, chronic, 147–148
Knee osteoarthritis, 265, 268

L
Lactose, 10
LDL (*See under* Low-density lipoprotein)
Lean body mass, 360
Lecithin, 135
LED (*See* Lower extremity disease)
Legal issues with prescribing exercise, 45–46
Leisure time
  physical activity, *34,* 42t, 305–306
  stroke risk and, 165–166
Leukotriene receptor antagonists, 276t
Life expectancy, 295
Lifestyle modifications
  cancer risk and, 241, 242t
  coronary heart disease and, 151, 152t
  disease prevention through, 1–3
  heart failure and, 188, 190

systolic blood pressure reductions and, 123t
  type 2 diabetes mellitus and, 200–201
Lifestyle therapies, therapeutic lifestyle changes, 134
Lipase inhibitors, 68t, 221t
Lipitor, 100
Lipoproteins, 135 (*See also* High-density lipoprotein; Low-density lipoprotein)
Local government, role in preventing childhood obesity, 289
Log books, 109t
Loop diuretics, 126t
Low-density lipoprotein (LDL), 88, 135, 136, 361
Low-density lipoprotein (LDL) cholesterol, 11 (*See also* Cholesterol)
  body fat and, 60
  diabetes and, 205
  metabolic syndrome and, 227
  reducing levels of, 134, 135, 136, 138, 139, 152, 164, 179, 233
Lower-extremity arterial disease, 173 (*See also* Peripheral arterial disease)
Lower-extremity disease (LED), 176–177
Lung cancer, 240, 242, 243
  smoking and, 88–89
  in women, 303
Lung disease, chronic (*See* Chronic lung disease)

M
Macronutrients, 7
Magnesium
  disease prevention and, 15t
  hypertension and, 124, 126, 127t
  recommendations
    daily amounts, 20t
    for heart failure patients, 191t
    for osteoporosis patients, 256t, 257
Male-type obesity, 60

Malignancy (*See* Cancer)
Maltose, 10
Margarine, butter *vs.,* 12–13
Maximal aerobic power, 32, 296, 298, 361
Maximal oxygen consumption or uptake (VO$_2$ max), 32, 296, 298, 361
Maximum heart rate (MHR), 39
Meat, recommended daily amount of, 20t
Media role in prevention of childhood obesity, 289–290
Medical nutrition therapy (MNT), 203
Medication adherence, 103–104
  depression and, 112–113
Medication-induced myopathy, 141
Medication non-adherence, 103
Men
  estimate of 10-year risk of coronary heart disease, 311–314
  metabolic syndrome and, 228
  osteoporosis and, 252, 253
  smoking among, 86
Menopause, bone loss during, 252
Mental stress, metabolic syndrome and, 229–230
Metabolic equivalent (MET) levels, 41, 42t, 44, 79, 292, 361
Metabolic syndrome, 227–236, 361
  defined, 227
  dyslipidemia and, 136
  economic costs of, 228
  health risks of, 228
  heart failure and, 188
  lifestyle behaviors and, 6
  mental stress and, 229–230
  nutrition and, 232–233, 234t
  overview, 227
  pathophysiology of, 228–230, 229t
  pharmacy practice application, 235–236

physical activity and, 139,
  233–235, 235t, 292
prevalence of, 227–228
prevention of, 230–232
treatment of, 230–232, 231t,
  232t
Metabolism, 7
Metastatic bone disease, exercise and, 247
Methylxanthines, 276t
Metoprolol, 48, 130
  target heart rate and, 41
Mexican Americans
  coronary heart disease
    among, 305
  diabetes mellitus among,
    198, 305
  metabolic syndrome and, 228
  obesity among, 305
Mexiletine, 94
MHR (*See* Maximum heart rate)
MI (*See* Myocardial infarction)
Milk
  food labels, *23*
  recommended daily amount
    of, 18, 20t
Minerals, 6, 14–15
  diabetes and, 205
  disease prevention and, 15t
Minorities (*See also* African
    Americans; Hispanics)
  disease prevention in,
    305–307
    Framingham Heart Study,
      307
    pharmacist's role in, 307
MNT (*See* Medical nutrition
    therapy)
Mobility, peripheral arterial
    disease/lower extremity
    disease and, 177
Monosaccharides, 10
Monounsaturated fats, 138, 139t
  diabetes and, 204, 205t
  in diet, 233
  for patients with coronary
    heart disease, 152, 153t
  for patients with peripheral
    arterial disease, 179t
  to treat and prevent stroke,
    165t
Monounsaturated fatty acid
    (MUFA), 11, 361
  foods high in, 12t
Morbidity, smoking and, 148

Mortality
  from cancer, 239
  from cardiovascular disease,
    146
  from coronary heart dis-
    ease, 134, 146
  from diabetes mellitus, 197
  smoking and, 148
Motivational counseling,
    111–112
Motivational intervention, 98t
Motivational readiness for
    change, stages for, 105
MUFA (*See* Monounsaturated
    fatty acid)
Muscle pain, with exercise *vs.*
    medication-induced
    myopathy, 141
Muscular endurance, 30, 361
Muscular strength, 30, 153,
    264, 298, 361
Myocardial infarction (MI),
    145, 146–147, 361
  coronary heart disease and,
    149
  heart failure and, 193
  peripheral arterial disease
    and, 174
  physical activity and, 234
  stroke and, 159
  tobacco use and, 87, 242
Myopathy, medication-
    induced, 141
MyPyramid Food Guidance
    System, 18–19, *19*
MyPyramid Tracker, 23, 73

N
National Cancer Institute, 244
National Cholesterol Educa-
    tion Program (NCEP),
    134, 141, 152, 155, 164,
    178, 228
National Heart, Lung, and
    Blood Institute, 228
National Institutes of Health,
    244, 307
  Consensus Development
    Panel on Physical
    Activity and Cardio-
    vascular Health, 41
Native Americans
  childhood obesity among,
    288
  smoking rates among, 86

NCEP (*See* National
    Cholesterol Education
    Program)
Negative caloric balance, 216,
    361
Negligent risk, 45
Neoplasm (*See* Cancer)
Nephropathy, 212t
Net daily calories, 63, 361
Neuromuscular exercise,
    167
Neuropathy
  autonomic, 212t
  diabetic, 208
  peripheral, 176, 212t
Niacin, 14, 137t
Nicotine, 90
Nicotine gum, 94, 96t, 99
Nicotine inhaler, 94, 96t
Nicotine lozenge, 94, 96t
Nicotine nasal spray, 94, 96t
Nicotine patch, 94, 96t
Nicotine replacement, 176t
Nitrates, 54t
Non-insulin-dependent
    diabetes mellitus
    (NIDDM), 197 (*See also*
    Type 2 diabetes melli-
    tus)
Non-sulfonylurea insulin sec-
    retagogues, 202t
Noradrenergic agents, 68t, 221t
Norepinephrine, 88
Nortriptyline, 95, 97t
NSAIDs (nonsteroidal anti-
    inflammatory drugs),
    265t
Nutrients
  adequate, within calorie
    needs, 17
  percent daily value, 22
Nutrition (*See also* Diet)
  aging and, 297
  alcohol and disease preven-
    tion and, 18, 24–26
  applications, 18–24
    counting calories, 22–23
    food labeling and con-
      sumer nutrition, *19,*
      19–22, *21, 23*
    USDA Food Guide, 18–19
  cancer and, 241, 243–245,
    245t
  obesity and, 243

Nutrition, cancer and (*cont.*)
  program adherence and, 244–245, 244t
  carbohydrates (*See* Carbohydrates)
  childhood obesity and, 292–293
  chronic diseases and, 5–6
  chronic lung disease and, 278–279, 279t
  consumer, 19–22
  coronary heart disease and, 152, 153t
  diabetes mellitus and, 201, 203–206, 205t
  Dietary Guidelines for Americans, 16–18
  dyslipidemia and, 138, 139t
  fats (*See* Fats)
  food as energy, 6–16
  for healthy living, 6
  heart failure and, 190–191, 191
  hypertension and, 124–127, 127t
  metabolic syndrome and, 232–233, 234t
  minerals, 6, 14–15, 15t
  obesity and, 221–222, 222t, 292–293
  osteoarthritis and, 266–267, 267t
  osteoporosis and, 255–257, 256t
    calcium and, 255–257
    other nutrients, 257
    vitamin D and, 257
  peripheral arterial disease and, 178–179, 179t
  protein (*See* Protein)
  stroke and, 163–164, 165t
  vitamins (*See* Vitamins)
  water, 16
  for women, 302
Nutritional analysis, 82
Nutrition Facts, 21, *21, 23*

O
Obesity, 215–225, 361 (*See also* Overweight)
  abdominal, 162, 231
  in African Americans, 305
  cancer and, 241, 243
  childhood, 218–219, 287, 288–289
  classification of, 59t
  coronary heart disease and, 148–149
  defined, 59, 216
  diabetes and, 199, 203
  diet and, 16, 267t
  disease outcomes, 217t
  economic costs of, 30, 57, 59, 216
  exercise and, 153, 179, 296
  health risks of, 216
  heart failure and, 188
  hypertension and, 120
  impact of, 57–59
  incidence of, 57
  lifespan of individuals with, 217–218
  lifestyle behaviors and, 6
  metabolic syndrome and, 228, 231
  nutrition and, 5, 221–222, 222t
  osteoarthritis and, 265
  overview, 215
  pathophysiology of, 216–218, 217t
  pharmacy practice application, 224–225
  physical activity and, 30, 222–224, 224t
  prevalence of, 215–216
  prevention of, 218–221
  stroke and, 162
  treatment for, 218–221
    behavior therapy, 220, 220t
    pharmacotherapy, 220–221, 221t
    surgery, 221
    weight-loss and weight-maintenance strategies, 219–220
  trends among U.S. adults, *58*
  in women, 302
Obesity Guidelines, 69
Occupational physical activity, stroke risk and, 165–166
Olanzapine, 94, 95
Older adults, 295–299
  impact of aging, 296–297
  nutrition and, 297
  overview, 295–296
  pharmacist's role, 299
  physical activity and, 298–299
    cardiovascular function, 298
    resistance training, 298–299
Omega-3-fatty acid, 243
Opioids, 94
Optimal medication therapy, 280–281
Oral contraceptives, 94, 95
Orlistat, 68, 68t, 220
Ortho Tri-Cyclen, 100
Osteoarthritis, 263–270, 361
  economic costs of, 264
  health risks of, 263–264
  nutrition and, 266–267, 267t
  obesity and, 57, 217t
  overview, 263
  pathophysiology of, 264, 265t
  pharmacy practice application, 270
  physical activity and, 38, 268–269, 269t
    People with Arthritis Can Exercise program, 268–269
  prevalence of, 263–264
  prevention of, 264–266
  treatment of, 264–266, 265t, 266t
Osteoblasts, 252, 361
Osteoclasts, 252, 361
Osteoporosis, 251–261, 361
  defined, 251
  diet and, 16
  economic costs of, 252
  health risks of, 252
  nutrition and, 5, 6, 255–257, 256t
    calcium and, 255–257
    other nutrients, 257
    vitamin D and, 257
  overview, 251
  pathophysiology of, 252–253, 253t
  pharmacy practice application, 259–261
  physical activity and, 30, 153, 180, 257–259, 260t
  prevalence of, 252
  prevention of, 253–255
  treatment of, 253–255, 254t, 255t
  in women, 304

Overtraining, bone health and, 258
Overuse phenomenon, 266
Overweight (*See also* Obesity)
    classification of, 59t
    coronary heart disease and, 148–149
    defined, 216
    diet and, 16
        with osteoarthritis, 267t
    impact of, 57–59
    metabolic syndrome and, 228
Oxygen consumption, 32–33, 361

P
PACE (*See* People with Arthritis Can Exercise)
PAD (*See* Peripheral arterial disease)
PAHs (*See* Polycyclic aromatic hydrocarbons)
Pancreatitis, 135
Pantothenic acid, 14
Parathyroid hormone, 254t
Parents, childhood obesity and, 291
Pathophysiology
    of cancer, 240, 241t
    of chronic lung disease, 274–275, 275t
    of coronary heart disease, 146–148, 147t
    of diabetes mellitus, 198–200, 200t
    of dyslipidemia, 134–136, 135t
    of heart failure, 186–187, 187t
    of hypertension, 120–121, 122t
    of metabolic syndrome, 228–230, 229t
    of obesity, 216–218, 217t
    of osteoarthritis, 264, 265t
    of osteoporosis, 252–253, 253t
    of peripheral arterial disease, 174–175, 175t
    of stroke, 160–161, 161t
Patient goals, for physical activity, 37–38
Patient-related barriers to program adherence, 106–108

Patient-related behavior change strategies, 109t
Pedometers, 35–36
Pentazocine, 94
People with Arthritis Can Exercise (PACE), 268–269
Perimenopause, bone loss during, 252
Peripheral arterial disease (PAD), 136, 145, 173–181, 361
    health risks of, 174
    nutrition and, 178–179, 179t
    overview, 173–174
    pathophysiology of, 174–175, 175t
    pharmacy practice application, 181
    physical activity and, 179–181, 180t
    prevalence of, 174
    prevention of, 175
    treatment of, 175–178, 176t, 178t
Peripheral neuropathy (PN), 176, 212t
Peripheral vascular disease (PVD), 145, 173 (*See also* Peripheral arterial disease)
Pharmacists
    role in childhood obesity, 293–294
    role in community interventions to increase physical activity, 151
    role in disease prevention in minorities, 307
        of peripheral arterial disease, 180, 181
        in women, 307
    role in providing lifestyle modification information, 2–33
    role in treating peripheral arterial disease, 178
    role with older adults, 299
    Rx for Change and, 89–90
Pharmacodynamics, 362
    physical activity and, 50–52, 53–54t
Pharmacokinetics, 362
    digoxin, 189

physical activity and, 52–55, 53–54t
Pharmacy practice applications
    cancer, 247–248
        case study, 247–248, 346–348
    chronic lung disease, 280–282
        case study, 282, 356–357
    coronary heart disease, 154–156
        case study, 155–156, 322–325
    diabetes mellitus, 211–213
        case study, 212–213, 335–337
    dyslipidemia, 140–142
        case study, 142, 319–322
    heart failure, 193–194
        case study, 193–194, 331–335
    hypertension, 129–131
        case study, 130–131, 317–319
    metabolic syndrome, 235–236
        case study, 235–236, 341–346
    obesity/overweight, 224–225
        case study, 225, 337–341
    osteoarthritis, 270
        case study, 270, 352–356
    osteoporosis, 259–261
        case study, 261, 349–351
    peripheral arterial disease, 181
        case study, 181, 327–331
    program adherence and, 112–113
    smoking cessation in, 100–101
        case studies, 100–101, 324–325, 327, 330–331, 345–346, 351
    stroke, 168–169
        case study, 168–169, 325–327
    weight control in, 69–82
        case study, 72–82
        weight-loss program worksheet, 70–72, 333–335, 339–341, 343–345, 354–356

Phendimetrazine, 68t
Phentermine, 68t
Phospholipids, in dyslipidemia, 134, 135
Phosphorus, for osteoporosis,
257
Physical activity, 29–55, 362
(*See also* Exercise)
activity-induced injuries,
avoiding, 47t
adults participating in recommended amounts
of, *31*
by African Americans, 306
aging and, 298–299
cardiovascular function,
298
resistance training,
298–299
angina pectoris and, 146
asthma and, 277
barriers to, overcoming,
49–50, 51–52t
basic exercise physiology,
32–33
cancer and, 241, 243,
245–247, 246t
childhood obesity and, 289,
291–292
chronic lung disease and,
279–280, 281t
community interventions to
increase, 151
components of, 33–37
aerobic conditioning,
35–36
resistance training,
36–37
warm-up and cool-down,
33–35
COPD and, 278
coronary heart disease and,
149, 153–154, 154t
defined, 29
diabetes mellitus and, 200,
206–211, 207t
safety considerations,
210–211, 211t, 212t
type 1, 209
type 2, 210
disease prevention and,
30–31
dyslipidemia and, 139–140,
140t

estimated energy require-
ments and, 7–8
health benefits of, 30–31, 31t
heart failure and, 191–192,
192t
hypertension and, 122, 123t,
128, 129t
income level and, 305–306
metabolic syndrome and,
231, 233–235, 235t
obesity and, 222–224, 224t
osteoarthritis and, 264,
268–269, 269t
People with Arthritis Can
Exercise program,
268–269
osteoporosis and, 253,
257–259
paradigm, *34*
peripheral arterial disease
and, 176–177, 179–181,
180t
pharmacodynamics and,
50–52, 53–54t
pharmacokinetics and,
52–55, 53–54t
pregnancy and, 304–305
prescribing, 45–49
legal issues, 45–46
sample prescriptions,
46–49
principles of exercise prescription, 37–44
duration, 41–43
energy expenditure goals,
44
frequency, 43
intensity, 38
metabolic equivalent
level, 41, 42t
patient goals, 37–38
rate of perceived exer-
tion, *40*, 40–41
rate of progression, 43–44
talk test, 39
target heart rate, 39–40
type of physical activity, 38
stretching, 37
stroke and, 162, 164–167,
167t
theophylline and, 276–277
as weight control strategy,
65–68, 219
in women, 302

Physical education, childhood
obesity and, 292
Physical fitness, 30, 128, 268,
362
Physical inactivity, 362
aging and, 296–297
cancer and, 241, 303
as cause of death, 85
coronary heart disease and,
149–150
defined, 29–30
metabolic syndrome and, 228
peripheral arterial disease
and, 179
stroke risk and, 162
Plant stanols, 13, 137t, 138, 233
Plant sterols, 13, 137t, 138, 233
PN (*See* Peripheral neuropathy)
Polycyclic aromatic hydrocarbons (PAHs), 94
Polysaccharides, 10
Polyunsaturated fats, 138, 139t
diabetes and, 205t
in diet, 233
recommendations
for chronic heart disease
patients, 152, 153t
for peripheral arterial disease patients, 179t
for stroke patients, 165t
Polyunsaturated fatty acid
(PUFA), 11, 362
foods high in, 12t
Positive caloric balance, 63, 362
Postmenopause, bone loss
during, 252
Potassium, 15t
heart failure and, 191t
hypertension and, 124, 126,
127t
osteoporosis and, 256t
recommended amounts of,
18, 20t
Potassium-sparing diuretics,
126t
Practical counseling, 92–93,
93t, 99
Pre-diabetes, 198
Preeclampsia, 304
Pregnancy, physical activity
and, 304–305
Prehypertension, 120, 121t,
129–130, 362
PREMIER trial, 126

Prevalence
  of asthma, 274
  of cancer, 240
  of childhood obesity, 288
  of chronic lung disease, 274
  of coronary heart disease,
    146
  of diabetes mellitus, 198
  of heart failure, 185–186
  of hypertension, 120
  of metabolic syndrome,
    227–228
  of obesity, 215–216
  of osteoarthritis, 263–264
  of osteoporosis, 252
  of peripheral arterial disease,
    174
  of stroke, 160
Prevention
  of cancer, 240–243
  of childhood obesity,
    289–291
  of chronic kidney disease,
    148
  of chronic lung disease,
    275–278
  of coronary heart disease,
    148–150
    primary, 148–149
    secondary, 149–150
  of diabetes mellitus,
    200–203
  of dyslipidemia, 136–137
  of heart failure, 187–190
  of hypertension, 121–129
  of metabolic syndrome,
    230–232
  of obesity, 218–221
  of osteoarthritis, 264–266
  of osteoporosis, 253–255
  of peripheral arterial disease,
    175
  of stroke, 161–163
Primordial prevention, 293, 362
Program adherence
  barriers to
    healthcare system and
      provider-related,
      107t, 108
    patient-related, 106–108,
      107t
  depression and, 113
  pharmacy practice and,
    112–113

recommendations
  for asthma and COPD
    patients, 278t
  for cancer patients,
    244–245, 244t
  for coronary heart disease
    patients, 152t
  for diabetes mellitus
    patients, 203t
  for dyslipidemia patients,
    137t
  for heart failure patients,
    190, 190t
  for hypertension patients,
    125t
  for metabolic syndrome
    patients, 232, 232t
  for osteoarthritis patients,
    266t
  for osteoporosis patients,
    255t
  for peripheral arterial
    disease patients,
    178t
  for stroke patients, 163,
    164t
  for weight-loss program,
    220t
Program-related behavior
  change strategies,
  110–111t
Progression of physical activity, 43–44
Project ImPACT: Lipidemia,
  155
Project ImPACT:
  Osteoporosis, 260
Propoxyphene, 94
Propranolol, 53t, 94
Prostate cancer, 57, 240, 243
Protein, 6, 13–14
  diabetes and, 204, 205t
  energy derived from, 7
  foods high in, 14t
  recommendations
    for coronary heart disease
      patients, 153t
    daily amounts, 20t
    for dyslipidemia patients,
      139t
    for heart failure patients,
      191t
    for osteoporosis patients,
      256t

for peripheral arterial disease patients, 179t
for stroke patients, 165t
Provider-related barriers to
  program adherence,
  107t, 108
PUFA (See Polyunsaturated
  fatty acid)
PVD (See Peripheral vascular
  disease)

R
Race (See also African
  Americans; Whites)
  childhood obesity and, 288
  Framingham Heart Study
    and, 307
  metabolic syndrome and, 228
  obesity and, 216, 218
  osteoporosis and, 252, 304
Rate of perceived exertion, 40,
  40–41
Recreational physical activities, 33, 34, 42t
Red wine, cancer and, 243
Reproductive diseases, smoking and, 87t
Resistance training, 34, 36–37
  for cancer survivors, 246
  coronary heart disease risk
    and, 139, 140
  for diabetic patients, 208
  for metabolic syndrome
    patients, 234, 235
  for obese patients, 224
  in older adults, 298–299
  for osteoporosis patients,
    259
  very low-calorie diets and, 64
  weight-control program
    and, 66
Respiratory disease, smoking
  and, 87t
Retinopathy, 212t
Rheumatic fever/heart disease, 145
Riboflavin, 14
Risk, negligent, 45
Rosuvastatin, 193
RPE (See Borg rating of perceived exertion)
Rx for Change: Clinician-
  Assisted Tobacco
  Cessation, 89–90

S
Safety
　exercise and diabetic
　　patient, 210–211, 211t,
　　212t
　physical activity in obese
　　patients and, 223
Saturated fats, 138, 139t
　in atherogenic diet, 231
　childhood intake of, 293
　coronary heart disease and,
　　149
　recommendations
　　for diabetes patients, 205t
　　for peripheral arterial dis-
　　　ease patients, 179t
　stroke prevention and, 165t
Saturated fatty acids, 11, 362
　cholesterol increases and
　　intake of, 233
　foods high in, 12t
School system, role in prevent-
　　ing childhood obesity,
　　290–291, 294
Secondary hypertension, 120,
　　122t
Secondhand smoke, 90
Sedentary activities, 34
Sedentary patients with nor-
　　mal BMI, 66–67
Selective estrogen receptor
　　modulator, 254t
Selective intestinal cholesterol
　　absorption inhibitors,
　　137t
Self-efficacy, 104, 106, 109t,
　　298, 306, 362
Self-management education,
　　diabetes, 202
Serotonergic agents, 68t, 221t
Seventh Report of the Joint
　　National Committee of
　　Prevention, Detection,
　　Evaluation, and
　　Treatment of High
　　Blood Pressure (JNC 7),
　　120, 124, 152, 164, 178
Sibutramine, 68, 68t, 220, 221
Simple carbohydrates, 9–10,
　　11t
Simvastatin, 130
Smoking (*See also* Tobacco use)
　asthma and, 277

cancer and, 241, 242–243,
　　303
as cause of death, 85, 148
as cause of disease, 86–89,
　　87t, 148
chronic lung disease and,
　　275
COPD and, 277
costs of, 86
drug interactions with, 94–95
heart failure and, 188
osteoporosis and, 254
peripheral arterial disease
　　and, 174–175
prevalence of, 85, 86
secondhand smoke, 90
stroke and, 162
Smoking cessation, 89–100,
　　89–101
　algorithm for, 91
　benefits of, 90
　chronic disease and, 6
　chronic lung disease and,
　　278
　diabetes mellitus and, 200,
　　201
　hypertension and, 123
　identification and assess-
　　ment of tobacco use
　　through brief interven-
　　tion, 91
　　through intensive inter-
　　　vention, 99–100
　pharmacotherapy for, 94–95,
　　96–97t, 99–100
　in pharmacy practice,
　　100–101
　　case studies, 100–101,
　　　324–325, 327,
　　　330–331, 345–346,
　　　351
　preventing relapse, 97–99
　Rx for Change, 89–90
　smokers unwilling to make
　　quit attempt, 95, 97
　smokers willing to make
　　quit attempt, 91–95
Smoking-related diseases,
　　86–89, 87t, 148
　cancer, 87t, 88–89
　cardiovascular disease,
　　86–88, 87t
Social cognitive theory, 106

Social support, 99
　program adherence and,
　　110t
　smoking cessation and, 93,
　　93t, 99
Sodium, 15t
　food labeling and, 22
　intake of
　　childhood, 293
　　heart failure and, 190, 191t
　　hypertension and, 120,
　　　122, 126
　　osteoporosis and, 256t
　　recommended, 18, 20t
Special populations, 285
Starches, 10, 11t
State government, role in
　　childhood obesity, 289
Statins, 137t, 162, 176t
　myopathy and, 141
Steps, daily
　number of, 33
　pedometers and, 35–36
Storage fat, 60, 362
Strength-building activity,
　　stroke and, 167
Stress, metabolic syndrome
　　and mental, 229–230
Stretching exercises, 34, 37
　stroke and, 167
Stroke, 145, 159–169, 362
　in African Americans, 305
　alcohol consumption and,
　　25
　atherosclerotic process and,
　　293
　defined, 160
　economic costs of, 160
　health risks of, 160
　hemorrhagic, 159, 160–161,
　　360
　incidence of, 159
　ischemic, 145, 159, 161t,
　　179, 361
　lifestyle behaviors and, 6
　nutrition and, 5, 163–164,
　　164t
　obesity and, 57, 217t
　overview, 159
　overweight and, 148
　pathophysiology of, 160–161,
　　161t
　peripheral arterial disease
　　and, 174

pharmacy practice application, 168–169
case study, 168–169
physical activity and, 30, 164–167, 167t
pre-diabetes and, 198
prehypertension and, 129
prevalence of, 160
prevention of, 161–163, 165t, 167t
smoking and, 87, 242
treatment of, 162–163, 163t
type 2 diabetes and, 199
Subcutaneous fat, 60
Sucrose, 10, 204
Sugars, 9–10, 11t
Sulfites, 279
Sulfonylureas, 202t
Surgery, weight-loss, 221
Sympathomimetic agents, 54t
Systolic blood pressure, 120, 362
heart failure and, 191
lifestyle changes and reduction in, 123t
physical activity and, 128
sibutramine and, 68, 221
stroke risk and, 161

T
Tacrine, 94, 95
Talk test, 39
Target heart rate, 39–40
Target organ damage, 121
Task Force on Community Preventive Services, 151
TEE (See Total energy expenditure)
Theophylline, 54t, 94, 95
physical activity and, 276–277
Therapeutic lifestyle changes (TLC), 134, 136–137, 232
Thiamin, 14
Thiazide diuretics, 126t
Thiazolidinediones, 202t
Thrombus, 160
TIA (See Transient ischemic attack)
TLC (See Therapeutic lifestyle changes)

Tobacco cessation (See Smoking cessation)
Tobacco-dependence counseling, 89
Tobacco use (See also Smoking)
algorithm for treating, 91
cancer and, 242–243
identification and assessment through brief intervention, 91–99, 92t, 93t
through intensive intervention, 99–100
Total body fat, 60, 362
Total energy expenditure (TEE), 44
calculating, 73t, 78–79
Total peripheral resistance (TPR), 128
Trans fats
intake in childhood, 293
intake in women, 302
Trans fatty acids, 11–12, 362
diabetes and, 205
lowering, 138, 152, 233
Transient ischemic attack (TIA), 160, 362
prevention of, 162
Transtheoretical model of change, 105
"Treating Tobacco Use and Dependence," 89
Treatment
of cancer, 240–243
of chronic lung disease, 275–278, 276t
of coronary heart disease, 150–152
behavior therapy, 151, 152t
drug therapy, 150, 150t
of diabetes mellitus, 200–203
of dyslipidemia, 136–137
of heart failure, 187–190, 188t
of hypertension, 121–129
of metabolic syndrome, 230–232
of obesity, 218–221
behavior therapy, 220, 220t
pharmacotherapy, 220–221, 221t
surgery, 221

weight-loss and weight-maintenance strategies, 219–220
of osteoarthritis, 264–266, 265t, 266t
of osteoporosis, 253–255, 254t, 255t
of peripheral arterial disease, 175–178
of stroke, 162–163, 163t
Triglycerides, 65, 362
in dyslipidemia, 134, 135
lowering levels of, 136
metabolic syndrome and elevated, 227
physical activity and levels of, 292
Trisaccharides, 10
Tumor (See Cancer)
Type 1 diabetes mellitus, 181, 197, 199, 362
alcohol intake and, 205–206
nutrition and, 206
pathophysiology of, 199
physical activity and, 209
Type 2 diabetes mellitus, 197, 199, 362
alcohol intake and, 206
body mass index and, 67
carbohydrates and, 204
diet and, 16
exercise and, 153
lifestyle modifications and, 200–201
metabolic syndrome and, 227, 230
nutrition and, 206
obesity and, 57
overweight and, 148
pathophysiology of, 199
physical activity and, 30, 179, 210
protein intake and, 204
in women, 303

U
Unsaturated fatty acids, 11, 362
foods high in, 12t
intake of, 138, 152, 153t, 233

U.S. Department of
Agriculture (USDA)
caloric intake table, 9, 9t
Dietary Guidelines for
Americans, 9, 16–18,
19, 23, 138, 164, 178,
190, 232, 244, 255, 279,
297
dietary tracking system, 73
Food Guide, 17, 18–19
MyPyramid Tracker, 23
U.S. Department of Health,
Education, and
Welfare, 85
U.S. Department of Health
and Human Services, 9,
16, 23, 86, 89, 138, 151,
198, 232
U.S. Surgeon General
exercise recommendations,
41, 43, 46, 180
Report on Bone Health and
Osteoporosis, 255–256
Report on Physical
Activities, 139, 234
report on smoking, 85
USDA (*See* U.S. Department of
Agriculture)

V
Varenicline (Chantix), 97t
Vascular diseases, depression
and, 112
Vasodilators, 126t
Vegetables
cancer risk and eating, 243
recommended amounts of,
17–18, 20t
stroke risk and eating, 163,
165t
Verapamil, 53t
Verenicline, 94
Very low-calorie diets (VLCD),
63, 222
resistance training and, 64
Very low-density lipoprotein
(VLDL), 88, 135, 136,
139, 362
Visceral fat, 60
Vitamins, 6, 14
A, 14, 15t

B₆, 14
B₁₂, 14, 15t, 17, 297
B-complex, 14, 15t
C (ascorbic acid), 14, 15t
D, 14, 15t, 17
older adults and, 297
osteoporosis and, 254t,
257
diabetes and, 205
E, 14, 15t
K, 14
VLCD (*See* Very low-calorie
diets)
VLDL (*See* Very low-density
lipoprotein)
VO₂ max (*See* Maximal oxygen
consumption or
uptake)

W
Walking
for cancer survivors, 246
metabolic equivalent levels
and, 42t
for osteoarthritis patients,
268
for peripheral arterial disease patients, 177
to treat and prevent stroke,
176
Warfarin, 54t
Warm-up, 33, 35
Water, as nutrient, 6, 16
Weight-bearing exercise, for
osteoporosis, 258–259,
260t
Weight control, 57–82
body composition and,
59–60
cessation of weight gain, 61
coronary heart disease and,
134
dyslipidemia and, 137
obesity, impact of, 57–59, *58*
osteoarthritis and, 265
overweight, impact of,
57–59
in pharmacy practice,
69–82, *70–72*
case study, 72–82, *80–82*
physical activity and, 223

strategies for, 62–69
behavior therapy, 68
combination therapy, 69
dietary therapy, 63–65
pharmacotherapy, 68
physical activity, 65–68
weight loss, 61–62
goals, 69
program
case study, 72–82
designing, 79, *82*
worksheet, *70–72,
80–82*, 333–335,
339–341, 343–345,
354–356
strategies for, 219–220
weight maintenance, 62, 65,
69
strategies for, 219–220
Whites
coronary heart disease
among, 305
diabetes among, 198
metabolic syndrome
among, 228
osteoporosis among, 252,
304, 305
smoking rates among, 86
WHO (*See* World Health
Organization)
Women
disease prevention in,
301–305
cancer, 303
cardiovascular disease,
301–302
diabetes mellitus, 303
osteoporosis, 252, 253,
304
pharmacist's role in, 307
pregnancy and physical
activity, 304–305
estimate of 10-year risk of
coronary heart disease,
313–314
metabolic syndrome and, 228
smoking among, 86
World Health Organization
(WHO), 103, 112